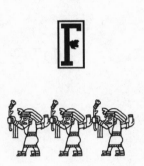

JOIE DAVIDOW

ILLUSTRATIONS BY
MIRO SALAZAR

A FIRESIDE BOOK
PUBLISHED BY SIMON & SCHUSTER

INFUSIONS

OF

HEALING

A Treasury of
Mexican-American
Herbal Remedies

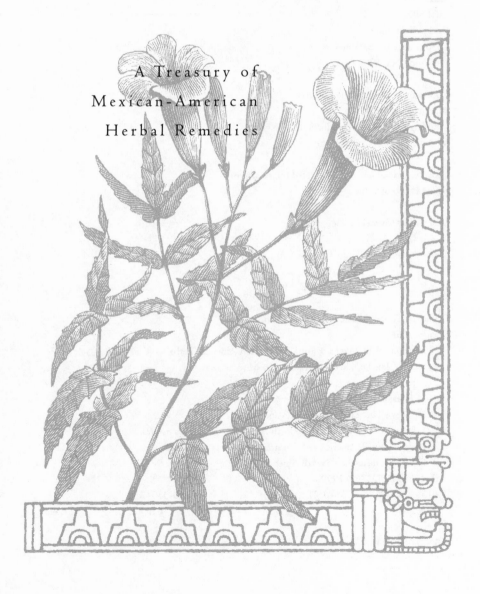

FIRESIDE
Rockefeller Center
1230 Avenue of the Americas
New York, NY 10020

FIRESIDE and colophon are registered trademarks of
Simon & Schuster, Inc.

Designed by Gabriel Levine

Manufactured in the United States of America

10   9   8   7   6   5   4   3   2   1

Library of Congress Cataloging-in-Publication Data
Davidow, Joie.
   Infusions of healing : a treasury of Mexican-American herbal
remedies / Joie Davidow ; illustrations by Miro Salazar.
      p.   cm.
   "A Fireside book."
   Includes bibliographical references and index.
      I. Herbs—Therapeutic use—North America.   2. Materia medica,
Vegetable—North America.   3. Mexican Americans—Medicine.
4. Traditional medicine—North America.   I. Title.
   RM666.H33D376   1999
   615'.321'0896872073—dc2I   99-34047
                                                      CIP

ISBN 0-684-85416-3

NOTE TO READERS

This publication contains the opinions and ideas of its author. It is intended to provide helpful and informative material on the subjects addressed in the publication. It is sold with the understanding that the author and publisher are not engaged in rendering medical, health, or any other kind of personal professional services in the book. The reader should be aware that any plant or substance can cause an allergic reaction in some people and should consult his or her medical, health, or other competent professional before adopting any of the suggestions in this book or drawing inferences from it.

The author and publisher specifically disclaim all responsibility for any liability, loss, or risk, personal or otherwise, which is incurred as a consequence, directly or indirectly, of the use and application of any of the contents of this book.

For my mother

CONTENTS

Part II
Plantas Que Curan: Healing Plants and Their Uses

Part III
Preparations for Herbs

INTRODUCTION

More than twenty years ago, I moved to Los Angeles from New York and settled into a Mexican-American neighborhood. The soothing cups of *manzanilla* and *yerba buena* tea offered at a neighbor's kitchen table, the rows of mysterious cellophane-packaged herbs hanging from the walls of the local *mercado*—these were my introduction to Mexican-American herbal healing.

As a writer and editor covering Los Angeles, first at the *L.A. Weekly*, then at *L.A. Style* magazine, I was constantly confronted with the Mexican-American culture that infuses the spirit of the city. At *L.A. Style* we produced a special "Latin L.A." issue, which inspired us to found a national Latino culture magazine called *Sí*. And from the ashes of the short-lived *Sí* magazine grew the seed of this book.

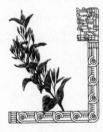
A journalist never knows where her work will take her. We are merely scribes, record keepers. And so it happened that I, an ordinary gringa, was entrusted with the task of assembling, for an English-speaking audience, part of the vast knowledge of herbal healing that has been passed down through the centuries: from the

Toltecs and the Maya to the Mexica, from the Mexica to the Franciscans, the Dominicans, and the Jesuits, from the friars to the settlers, from father to son, mother to daughter, *aubela a nieta, comadre a comadre.*

My research began not far from my own home, in the East L.A. living room of Ofelia Esparza, who led me through her childhood, recalling her mother's remedies, teaching me the now-familiar names: *malva, romero, epazote, popotillo.*

That afternoon I began an eighteen-month odyssey that has taken me throughout the southwestern United States and into Mexico. I have met with *curanderas* from the urban sprawl of East L.A. to the farmlands of southern New Mexico, walked the trails of botanical gardens from Pasadena to Cuernavaca, wandered the Mojave and Sonora deserts, and toured backyard gardens, examining and photographing medicinal plants. I have spent countless hours in the dusty stacks of the Benson Latin American Collection at the University of Texas, Austin, and in the cool inner sanctum of the L.A. Public Library's rare books department, delving into sixteenth-century Spanish accounts of indigenous Mexican herbal remedies.

I have tried to make this book a true treasury, to present this wealth of knowledge properly wrapped in the context of the culture that has nurtured it for so long. So in addition to including the lists of herbs and remedies, I have told the story of Aztec medicine, which is where it all began, and the stories of contemporary *curanderas* and *yerberas,* the healers, herbalists, and neighborhood grandmothers who are the caretakers of this knowledge today.

Of the more than 2,500 medicinal plants currently in use in Mexico, I cataloged only one-tenth, choosing the plants that are used most commonly and are most readily available in the United States. People may use an herb to treat an ailment simply because nothing else is available to them. Just because a field study reports that somebody somewhere used an herb for something, doesn't mean it works. So I tried to find further evidence of a plant's efficacy before I included it. I looked for some phytochemical action that would explain *why* a plant might remedy the ailment. For instance, if I heard that a certain herb was used to make a gargle for sore throat, I would look for some chemical constituent that might explain its anti-inflammatory properties. I listed only the remedies I found in several sources, and only if I found workable instructions on how to use them.

Many wonderful *comadres* helped me in my travels. Ginger Varney, Eileen Rosaly, and Chris Hardy were fellow sleuths, helping me search for knowledgeable healers in East L.A.

Denise Chávez took time away from writing her own book to show me around her hometown of Las Cruces, New Mexico, and introduced me to the herbalist Bonnie Ochoa. Jack Thompson in Las Vegas, New Mexico, Jan LaBrasca Skogin in Tucson, and Judy Fishman in Superior, Arizona, led me to local herbalists, *bótanicas*, and botanical gardens.

The *curandera* Mary Jane Garza generously allowed me to sit in on the group sessions she conducts with HIV patients in San Antonio, Texas, and put me in touch with her fellow healer, Elena Avila. And in Austin, Texas, Harry Pope invited me to share his home, and his friendship.

My research assistant, Melissa Blanco, cheerfully spent hours at the library and the copy machine, pulling in favors to help me gain access to important texts.

I am grateful to Becky Cabaza, my editor at Fireside/Simon & Schuster, for immediately wanting to publish the book, and for her unwavering enthusiasm and support. I would never have begun this project without the urging of my agent, Lisa Erbach Vance. And I would never have finished it without the constant encouragement of my *comadre* Esmeralda Santiago, who was always there to lift me up when my confidence failed me.

Finally, I thank my mother, Florence S. Davidow, who didn't live to see the book she told me I should write. She taught me to honor myself for the person I am, to spend my days doing work I believe in, and never to fear the consequences of following my chosen path. I hope I will continue to remember her lessons now that she is no longer here to remind me to keep going, even when the path seems to end.

PART I

FIVE CENTURIES
OF HEALING

¿Qué mágicas infusiones
de indios herbolarios
de mi patria, entre mis letras
el hechizo derramaron?

What are these magical infusions
of the Indian herbalists of my homeland,
that spill enchantment
over my pages?
—Sor Juana Inés de la Cruz (1648–1695)

Traditional Mexican-American medicine is *un rico menudo,* a rich stew, with a long list of ingredients: sixteenth-century Arab and European herbal medicines, ideas that date back to Hippocrates, twentieth-century patent medicines, plant medicines from Africa, herbal wisdom from North American native tribes. But the key ingredient is as old as Mesoamerica—the living legacy of the Aztecs, remnants of a vast treasury of herbal knowledge that has nearly vanished.

WAR OF THE WORLDS

When Hernando Cortés and his 553 men landed at Vera Cruz in 1519, they came face-to-face with a culture so vastly different from the one they had left in Europe, it was as though they had traveled by spaceship to a distant galaxy. The people of the Aztec empire viewed reality from a perspective that was almost incomprehensible to the Spanish. And the Aztecs were equally confounded by the Spaniards, whom they regarded as half gods, half monsters.

It could be argued that the more advanced culture lost the war, that the Spanish did not bring civilization to the New World but effectively demolished it. The Aztecs reigned for little more than a century, but during those decades, through constant warfare that expanded the boundaries of the empire from the Gulf Coast to the Pacific and trade routes that extended south through Honduras and Nicaragua, they acquired much of the collective knowledge of all the Mesoamerican peoples, inheriting the cultures of the Toltec, the Zapotec, the Mixtec, the Huaxtec, the Maya.

They were extraordinary astronomers who had developed a yearly calendar accurate within eleven minutes, and charted the movements of the stars, using only their own eyes to scan the skies. They were advanced mathematicians, spectacular craftsmen, accomplished architects and engineers. The Aztecs were artists—musicians, painters, sculptors, dancers. All members of the elite classes were poets. They valued skill with words as highly as skill with weapons and considered both to be necessary attributes. Vast libraries housed exquisitely painted fanlike volumes of fig-bark paper in which they recorded their philosophy, history, religion, literature, law, and scientific findings.

The conquistadors, marching into the Aztec capital of Tenochtitlán, were so overwhelmed by its splendor that they asked one another if they were dreaming. Crossing a wide causeway they entered a city of vast plazas, fountains, sculpture, and architecture of heroic proportions brightly decorated with colorful murals and glyphs. Floating gardens swayed in the lagoon. Flowering vines cascaded over the terraces of the townhouses. In one of his historic long letters to the king of Spain, Cortés expressed fear that no one would believe his description of a city so full of wonder that even the conquistadors themselves could hardly grasp what they were seeing. It has been called the Venice of the Americas because, like Venice, it was a magnificent city built on a series of canals. But it was more beautiful than Venice in one very important aspect: It was clean. So clean that a Spanish chronicler remarked that walking its streets he was "in no more danger of soiling his feet than he was of soiling his hands." A thousand workers washed and swept the streets and plazas each day. Clean water was brought into the city through aqueducts. Human waste was picked up from the houses daily, and public toilet facilities were placed at intervals along the great causeways that led into the city.

The Aztecs were meticulously clean in their person as well. They were offended by body odor, bathed daily, and used herbal deodorants and breath fresheners. Middle-class houses had private bathrooms, and there were public bathhouses throughout the city. Motecuhzoma II had more than a hundred bathrooms in his vast palace. He reportedly bathed and changed his clothes several times a day, never wearing a garment more than once.

The great capitals of Europe at that time, and for centuries afterward, were full of filth and misery. The rat-infested alleys were strewn with garbage and human waste. Chamber pots were emptied onto the streets, and clean running water was not even conceived of. The old adage that a man takes three baths in his lifetime, one at birth, one on his wedding day, and the last when he is a corpse about to be buried, was not far from the truth. The Spanish conquistadors were impressed that the Mexicans always greeted them by fumigating them with incense, which they took as a great honor. But we can only imagine what these men, unwashed and sweating in their heavy clothing and armor, must have smelled like to their fastidious hosts.

The Aztecs and the Spanish viewed one another with horror and awe, and each saw the face of a barbarian.

THE GLORY OF THE ANCIENT GARDENS

If their civilization had not been destroyed during the conquest, the Aztecs, like the Chinese, might have made a great contribution to the world through

21

their vast and ancient knowledge of herbal medicine. Within its borders, Mexico has arguably the greatest variety of plant life on earth. Its geography includes rugged mountain ranges and lush valleys, tropical jungles on the Caribbean coast and arid deserts that stretch to the Pacific in the north. The Aztecs had survived centuries of wandering from one terrain to another before founding their capital at Tenochtitlán. They had, of necessity, become expert botanists during their travels, forced to use whatever they could find growing around them for both food and medicine.

As the empire prospered, they became magnificent horticulturalists. In 1467 the great Motecuhzoma's grandfather, Motecuhzoma I, established an immense botanical garden at Huaxtepec, which his grandson later revived. It may well have been the first botanical garden on earth, and the most extensive collection of plants the world had ever seen. Trees, shrubs, herbs, and flowers were imported from all over the empire, along with gardeners trained in tending them. There were nearly two thousand varieties of plants in the garden—fruit trees, orchids from the tropics, stands of *ahuehuete* cypress—all artfully arranged to provide pleasure to the senses and planted for fragrance and color, light and shade. Pools, waterfalls, fountains, an aviary full of colorful exotic birds, and a zoo graced the grounds.

Although the garden at Huaxtepec was the largest in the empire, Motecuhzoma II also maintained a luxuriant garden at his palace in Tenochtitlán, another just outside the capital in the hills of Chapultepec, and yet another at the suburban palace in Ixtapalapa. In the allied state of Texcoco, the great "poet king," Nezahualcóyotl, maintained a glorious garden of his own. The Texcocan king was devoted to the study of plants and commissioned artists to paint examples of the various species for his library.

In all these gardens, medicinal plants were cultivated and studied. Aztec doctors used the gardens as laboratories, conducting experiments subsidized by the nobility and by the imperial government. The medicinal plants grown in the gardens were intended for the medical needs of the nobility, but commoners were invited to be treated at the gardens free of charge, in exchange for reporting the results to the medical researchers who practiced there.

Basic knowledge of herbal medicine was common. Nearly every family grew its own herbs and vegetables in a garden called *xochichinancalli*, literally "flower place enclosed by reeds." Even in the cities, families maintained roof gardens where they grew plants for food, medicine, and ornament.

Decades after the fall of the Aztec empire, Bernal Díaz del Castillo, who had been a soldier in the company of Cortés, remembered the gardens at Ixtapalapa in his memoir, *The True Story of the Conquest of New Spain.* "I could not get enough of it, of the variety of the trees and the aroma that each one had, of the terraces full of roses and other flowers, and the many fruits of the land . . . and I say again that as I stood there admiring it all, I did not believe that in the world there was any land such as this one. . . . Now all this is fallen, lost. None of it remains," he wrote sadly.

In the final assault on Tenochtitlán most of this glorious city was destroyed. What was left of the Aztec civilization was soon attacked by the Church. In 1528 the first archbishop of Mexico, Don Juan de Zumárraga, in his zealous determination to wipe out all traces of pagan religious practices, ordered the destruction of every book, every codex, every scrap of a hieroglyph. The great libraries of Texcoco, with their wealth of information about the medicinal plants, were piled onto an enormous bonfire. Spanish soldiers were instructed to seek out every book they could find to add to the pyre. It was a fervent reflection of what was going on in Spain at the time. Twenty years earlier, hot on the heels of the expulsion of the Moors, the Grand Inquisitor, Cardinal Ximenes, had ordered the same fate for every Arabic manuscript in Granada.

But in New Spain the Church must have been even more compelled to vanquish the demon, who they thought must be everywhere. The Spanish clergy saw a hellish, godless land where the people worshiped hideous idols to whom they offered bloody human sacrifice. The Church soon realized that every trace of Aztec culture would have to be demolished, because Aztec religion pervaded all of it.

THE FIFTH SUN

The Aztec practice of medicine, like every other aspect of Aztec life, was inseparable from their concept of the cosmos and their religious beliefs. Their very word for doctor, *tepati,* was derived from *teo,* sacred, and *patli,* medicine.

Religious mythology varied from region to region, but at the basis of Mesoamerican belief systems was the notion that the earth had been destroyed and recreated four times. The Aztecs believed that the first world was destroyed by ocelots, the second by hurricanes, the third by fiery rain, the fourth by floods. During the time of each of these four worlds, one of the sun gods reigned, each corresponding to one of the four elements: earth, wind, fire, and water. According to this system, we are now living in the fifth incarnation of the world, which is destined to be destroyed by earthquakes.

It was the Aztecs' mission to postpone this inevitable fifth cataclysm through their efforts on earth. All the previous worlds had been destroyed by warring gods. It was the job of the Aztecs to make sure that the current sun god, Tonatiuh, was kept well fed and in place so that the fifth world could continue.

There are many variations of the Aztec creation story, but it most commonly goes something like this: The gods built the current world in darkness. When their work was complete, the gods still felt lonely. They missed men and women, all of whom had perished in the destruction of the fourth world and whose remains were now in the lower region of Mictlán, which was presided over by the god and goddess Mictecacíhuatl and Mictlantecuhtli. So the plumed serpent god, Quetzalcóatl, journeyed down to the underworld to retrieve the bones of humanity. Mictecacíhuatl and Mictlantecuhtli agreed to release the bones, but then they tricked Quetzalcóatl by frightening him on his way back to the heavens. Quetzalcóatl dropped his bag of bones, and they all shattered. The poor god wept bitter tears. When he arrived at the celestial level of Tamoanchan, the place of birth, he didn't know what to say to his fellow gods. It was decided that the bones should be ground into powder. Then the gods pierced their male organs with maguey thorns so that they bled, and they sprinkled the powdered bones with their own blood. From this they made a paste, which they fashioned into human forms. Because they had been pasted together with shattered bones, these new men and women were weak, subject to death and disease. This fifth incarnation of humanity was a combination of the earthly, the old bones, and the divine, the blood of the gods. The gods had sacrificed their blood to recreate humanity, and now mankind would be forever in their debt, obliged to make blood sacrifices of their own in retribution. But man's debt to the gods was even greater. Humanity also owed the gods for the sun and the moon.

The earth had been recreated and repeopled, but all was still in darkness. So the gods gathered in the sacred city of Teotihuacán, where they built a big bonfire. In order to create a new sun to light the world, one of the gods would have to sacrifice himself by jumping into the fire. For four days the gods sat by this divine hearth, the *teotexcalli*. Nanahuatzin, a poor little pimply-faced god, volunteered to sacrifice himself. But the wealthy god, Tecuciztécatl, claimed precedence. Four times the wealthy god stepped up to the flames, but each time he lost his courage and stepped back again. At last it was the little pimply-faced god's turn. He stepped up to the fire and without hesitating leapt in. Great flames rose up, igniting the heavens in an explosion of red. The gods looked up to see the god Nanahuatzin emerge in the east. The new sun had risen.

Now Tecuciztécatl, the wealthy god, was ashamed and hurled himself into the bonfire. But by this time the fire was dying down, so the wealthy god burned slowly, emerging as the sun's pale reflection, the moon. The other gods looking on were so disgusted by the wealthy god's cowardly behavior, they threw a rabbit at him. When the Aztecs looked up at the moon, they saw on its surface the face of a rabbit where we see the face of a man.

Now the sun was in the sky, but it stood still. The gods asked it, "Why aren't you moving?" To which the sun replied, "Because I demand your kingdom and your blood." Hearing this, the gods fell down at once, sacrificing themselves to become the stars. But this still wasn't enough to keep the sun moving through the sky. It was now the job of mankind to make sure that the sun had enough energy to rise and set by feeding it with blood sacrifices.

According to the Judeo-Christian belief, humanity entrusts the world to an almighty God. We depend on God and are grateful for the earthly treasure that has been given to us. But the Aztecs' relationship with their gods was interdependent. The continued existence of the sun and moon, wind and rain, depended on mankind's ability to feed and appease the gods. At any time the gods could destroy the world just as they had done four times before. The Aztecs believed that they had been chosen to keep the gods well fed and happy. It was their mission to postpone the inevitable fifth cataclysm. Theirs was the struggle of good over evil, of light over darkness.

The Aztecs, like the Spanish, used their religious convictions to justify their imperialistic wars. The Aztecs went to war on the premise that it was their sacred duty to take captives for sacrifice to the gods. The Spanish went to war with the holy mission of proselytizing the Catholic faith, on the premise that it was their sacred duty to save the heathens. In very different ways they each made holy offerings of the souls of the people they vanquished.

KINGDOMS OF THE COSMOS

Western thought divides the natural from the supernatural, the miraculous from the ordinary, but to the Aztec mind it was all one and the same. The visible and the invisible, the spiritual and the material were all equally real.

Just as Christianity preaches that God is everywhere, the Aztecs believed that a multiplicity of gods was everywhere. Everything in the world had a divine origin, and the spirit of the gods was in every earthly thing. There were thirteen major deities and more than two hundred minor deities. Each god could have various names and manifestations. As the Aztecs conquered new territories, they absorbed the gods of the other Mesoamerican tribes so that their pantheon was always expanding.

The Aztec worldview was based on the concept of opposite but complementary halves, somewhat like the Chinese concept of yin and yang. The Gods were dualities, both male and female, good and evil. The same god could create and destroy, tempt a man to sin and forgive him for sinning. Everything had its opposite, and these two opposing forces were in constant conflict.

This duality ruled the cosmos, which was divided horizontally in half, with nine celestial levels above and nine underworld levels below. The levels above were the kingdoms of the sun, who is the father of us all. His realms were light, hot, and dry, and ruled by fire. The underworld levels were the kingdoms of the earth, who is the mother of us all. Her realms were dark, cold, and wet, and ruled by water.

Man lived on four earthly levels that were visualized as a great disk surrounded by water, suspended between the nine upper and nine lower realms. This earthly plane was the kingdom of the four directions, divided into four quadrants corresponding to the four cardinal points ruled by the four sun gods. The black sun ruled the north, the blue sun the south, the white sun ruled the west, and the red sun the east. Four immense ceiba trees supported the sky, one in each of the four quadrants. The fifth direction, a vertical up and down, was located in the center of the quadrant. It was the very center of the universe.

Like the Aztecs themselves, the cosmos was always at war. Nature was violent. The Aztecs believed that each night the earth swallowed the sun. And each morning as the sun rose in the sky, it killed off the moon and stars. The very survival of the world was in constant jeopardy, dependent on the mood of the gods. For the cosmos to remain intact, for the sun to continue to rise and set, the opposing forces of light and dark and day and night had to be kept in balance, through ritual, prayer, and sacrifice.

An invisible conveyor belt moved through the cosmos, carrying the gods and the forces of nature that they controlled from level to level. Gods traveled from the heavenly and underworld levels to converge on the earthly plane, bringing blessings or harm. Man had to be ever vigilant, protecting himself from the displeasure of these invisible invaders.

THREE CENTERS OF THE SPIRIT

These levels, the celestial, earthly, and underworld planes, were manifested in the human body and informed the Aztec method of diagnosing illness. The Aztecs believed that the spirit resided in three centers of energy, which, like the universe itself, must be maintained in a state of balance.

The *tonalli*, corresponding to the celestial levels, was located in the head. Its name comes from the Nahuatl word for heat, *tonal*. Its patron is *Tonatiuh*, one of the names for the sun god. Loss of *tonalli* resulted in death. A corpse is cold, a living body warm, so the warmth of *tonalli* was the essence of physical life.

Tonalli could be strengthened or weakened. Illness, drunkenness, and excessive behavior weakened *tonalli*; bravery in battle strengthened it. Since *tonalli* was temporarily lost during sexual intercourse, celibacy made it stronger. *Tonalli* could also be strengthened by inhaling fragrances. Aztec doctors prescribed pleasant odors to relieve melancholy, stress, and fatigue, making them forerunners of today's aromatherapists.

Members of the nobility, the *pipiltin* class, believed that they had been born with greater *tonalli* than commoners. They increased their *tonalli* even more by postponing sexual activity until a relatively late age. For noble and commoner alike, *tonalli* increased with age, wisdom, and circumstance. The very old were held in high esteem, since they were full of strong *tonalli*.

Aztec shamans, called *nahualli*, under the influence of hallucinogenic plants, had the power to send *tonalli* out of their bodies and into the bodies of animals.

The second center of the spirit, the *teyolia*, was located in the heart, corresponding to the earthly plane. Thought, personality, and creativity were in the *teyolia*. Artists and poets had particularly powerful *teyolia*. Like *tonalli*, the *teyolia* could be harmed by carnal excess or immoral behavior. It could be strengthened through confession and penance, which was permitted only once in a lifetime.

The *teyolia* was the spirit that survived in the afterlife. The fate of a person's *teyolia* depended on the manner of death. The *teyolia* of a person who was sacrificed to the gods enjoyed the best fate of all. It shot straight up to a magnificent heaven. Next best was the fate of the *teyolia* of a warrior who bravely died in battle. His *teyolia* accompanied the sun on its journey from daybreak to noon for four years, after which it was reincarnated as a butterfly or a hummingbird. The *teyolia* of a woman who died during the birth of her first child was also honored. Her *teyolia* accompanied the sun from noon to sunset for four years, after which she became a powerful ghost who haunted the earth on certain days.

The *teyolia* of those people whose death was caused by the water god Tláloc—by accidents such as drowning or being struck by lightning, or through diseases related to excess water in the body such as rheumatism and dropsy—were sent on an arduous journey to the watery paradise of Tláloc and his female counterpart Chalchiuhtlicue. The *teyolia* of an infant who died while still nursing was returned to the heavens where it awaited another chance at life on earth. The *teyolia* of everybody else went to Mictlán, the underworld.

The third energy center was the *ihiyotl,* located in the liver, corresponding to the lower plane of the underworld. It was the center of vigor, of the breath, of all sorts of passions—envy, anger, carnal desire. An ill or damaged liver exuded a dangerous gas that spread disease. Laziness was associated with a weakened *ihiyotl.* Just as we say of a cowardly person, "Oh, he doesn't have the guts," the Aztecs would say of a lazy person, "Oh, he doesn't have the liver."

Since these three centers of the spirit were located in the body, diagnosis of an illness was spiritual as well as physical. A head injury or a chill could result in loss of precious *tonalli.* Certain emotional traumas could result in damage to the *ihiyotl,* causing liver problems. A Nahuatl definition of rage was "swollen liver," which could explain the Mexican-American folk disease *bilis,* a liver-related ailment caused by *coraje,* excessive anger.

MAGIC AND MEDICINE

The Aztecs believed that just as the balance of the opposing forces in the cosmos must be maintained, imbalances in the human body led to disease. Since human beings were created from the opposing elements of heaven and earth—the blood of the gods and the crushed bones of a former race—it was essential to maintain balance in the body. Bodily imbalance could be caused by excessive behavior, by infractions of the strict Aztec moral code, or by poor eating habits. An accident of any kind could unbalance the body, resulting in illness.

Disease could be inflicted by one of the many gods, as punishment for bad behavior, or it could be inflicted by a person with special powers. It was believed that some people, through no fault of their own, could involuntarily cause disease simply by looking at someone. Disease could also be caused by the malicious machinations of mortal sorcerers and witches.

These ideas have persisted over the centuries. Many people still believe that immoral or excessive behavior can lead to illness. Markets and *botánicas* still sell amulets to protect against the *ojo fuerte* or *mal de ojo*, the strong or evil eye. To this day in some Mexican-American neighborhoods it is commonly believed that anyone who looks admiringly at a child must also immediately touch that child, to negate the risk of accidentally inflicting the *mal de ojo*. And there still are professional *brujas*, good witches, who are hired to undo the evil spells of sorcerers.

The Aztecs knew that disease could also be caused by uncleanliness. Long before the invention of the microscope revealed the existence of microbes, they realized that disease could be passed invisibly from one person to another, by touch or through the air.

Aztec doctors were highly trained professionals. Like other trades, the practice of medicine was passed from father to son, mother to daughter, just as this gift of healing is handed down among generations of *curanderos* today. There were two kinds of Aztec doctors; all were specialists, each with an area of expertise patronized by one or more of the gods. The *tepati* treated illness on the physical level. The *tictli* treated illness on the spiritual level and were often trained in schools maintained by the priests. The services of both types of doctors might be required to remedy an illness.

The *tlamatepatli* were herbalists who treated gastrointestinal illnesses, respiratory and genito-urinary infections, and cardiac problems. Aztec dentists used herbs to treat inflamed gums, pulled teeth, and also did their share of cosmetic dentistry, setting precious gems into the teeth of the wealthy.

The midwives, forerunners of the *parteras* of today, were known as *tlamatquiticitl*, meaning doctors who tap with their hands, because of their skill at palpating the bellies of their pregnant patients. They provided an excellent

level of prenatal care, and partly because of their insistence on absolute clean-
liness, the Aztec rate of survival in childbirth substantially exceeded that
which prevailed in Europe where women routinely died from infections.

Aztec military surgeons were far more advanced than their European counterparts. Amazingly, Cortés and his men arrived in Mexico with a friar on
board but no professional physician. The conquistadors dressed their battle
wounds by searing them with hot oil. When they had no oil available, they cut
the fat from the body of a slain opponent and melted it down to use as a
dressing. If the wound began to ooze pus, they considered it a sign of healing.

The Aztec military surgeons first cleaned battle wounds with some sterile
liquid; if nothing else was available, the urine of a healthy warrior would do
fine for this purpose. Then they dressed the wound with maguey sap or pine
oil, which discouraged infection. They stanched the bleeding with the herb
coapatli (*Commelina pallida*), an effective styptic. They reduced swelling by applying the juice of the papaya or the prickly pear.

While European surgeons had no anesthetics to ease the suffering of their
patients, the Aztec surgeon could choose from a selection of narcotic plants.
They made their incisions with razor-thin obsidian knives and sutured them
with human hair. Some Aztec doctors were highly skilled at setting bones, using feathers and the sap of a tree called *liquidámbar* to make a plaster.

But perhaps the most important of these specialists were the *papiani* or
panamacani, the pharmacists who dispensed herbs and advice from their stalls
in the *tianguis*, the great marketplaces. Cortés wrote to the king of Spain that
in the great market at Tlateloco he had seen "herbalists selling all the many
roots and medicinal plants that are found in the land. The apothecaries have
houses of a sort there, where they sell medicines made from these herbs, for
drinking and for ointments and salves." He could have been describing Mexico City's Sonora Market today.

BODY AND SOUL

Since the Aztecs treated the body and spirit as one inseparable entity, they
were, in a sense, holistic healers. In making a diagnosis, the Aztec doctor
looked for the spiritual as well as the physical source of an illness. For example, if a man were to fall ill after having been exposed to a cold wind, the

Aztec doctor, the *teopati*, might treat the symptoms caused by the chill. The spiritualist, the *tictli*, might try to discover which of the gods had inflicted the cold wind. He might divine the source of the illness by tossing corn kernels on a mat or into a vessel of water. Or he might ingest a hallucinogenic plant to put himself in an altered state so that his spirit, his *tonalli*, could travel through time and space to find the root of the illness.

In accordance with the Aztec dualistic worldview, the same god who caused an illness had the power to cure it. The doctors would treat the patient's physical symptoms, but they might also find it necessary to appease the god who caused them. In this way doctors and patient worked complicitously to remedy the illness through their shared belief system. The patient, believing that the appeased god would remove his illness, was psychologically primed to aid in his own recovery. This combination of the pharmaceutical and the spiritual added up to very effective medicine.

But these were no mere psychosomatic cures. We know this because the physical aspects of the treatment worked on the Spanish, who were firm nonbelievers. The sixteenth-century Spanish chronicles abound with tales of the Aztecs' medical superiority. The Franciscan friar Toribio Motolonía wrote, "Some of the Indians are so experienced that they have cured many old and serious infirmities which the Spaniards have suffered many days without finding a remedy." And Cortés reputedly wrote to King Carlos I telling him not to bother sending any physicians to New Spain, as the native ones there were far better than those he knew at home.

THE GODS MUST BE DEAD

The Aztecs feared that their gods had abandoned them. Huitzilopochtli, the sun god who had led them to victory after victory, now permitted them to be defeated and humiliated by the Spanish. Nanáhuatl, who had protected them from loathsome diseases, now allowed them to suffer the horrors of a lethal and disfiguring scourge, as smallpox swept through every household in the capital of Tenochtitlán. Tonantzín, the grandmother, the earth goddess, goddess of medicine, who had watched over and nurtured them, now allowed them to be impoverished and enslaved. Still, they were unwilling to relinquish their will and their lives to the god of the Spaniards.

After the initial fury that resulted in the destruction of the ancient archives, the Church realized that the tactics of the Inquisition were not serving their purpose. Despite the public floggings and burnings of heretics, forced conversion was not going well at all. The specter of physical torture had done little to enhance the appeal of Christianity. In 1538, King Carlos I issued a decree that suspended the jurisdiction of the Inquisition over the "Indians" and limited the corporeal punishments that could be inflicted on them. A more tolerant approach was called for if the glad tidings of Christianity were to be received.

In 1524, twelve Franciscans from Cortés's home region of Extremadura had sailed into Vera Cruz harbor and walked barefoot from there to the colonial capital of Mexico City. When they arrived, Cortés, who was known to have been fanatically religious, astonished the emperor, Cuahtémoc, and the assembled Aztec nobility by kneeling and kissing first the tattered habit of their leader, Martín de Valencia, and then the hands of each friar.

The first friars to arrive in the colony were humanists. They were resolutely determined to root out the ancient Aztec ways and to convert the heathens, but within the limits prescribed by their mission, they championed the cause of the natives. The friars immediately applied themselves to the mastery of Nahuatl and other native languages, realizing that they would need to communicate with the people they aimed to convert.

In the interest of creating a "civilized" society, the Franciscans established schools where they taught Spanish, Latin, ecclesiastical music, and painting to the children of the fallen Aztec nobility. They taught the students to write in their native Nahuatl, using the alphabet in place of phonetic glyphs. (The Aztecs were not always delighted with these new educational opportunities and often hid their favorite sons to avoid having to send them to the friars' schools, or they sent the children of servants in their place.)

The aptitude of the native Mexicans astonished the Franciscans. In his *Historia de los Indios de Nueva España*, Fray Toribio Motolonía devoted an entire chapter solely to the brilliance of these students. He claims that they learned to write the alphabet in only a few days and were quickly able to speak Spanish and Latin, composing "long and well-written essays in hexameter and pentameter."

The Franciscans' admiration was not always shared by the secular Spaniards, many of whom thought it was an outrageous idea to educate these "heathens" whom they preferred to use as beasts of burden. Don Jerónimo López, an adviser to the first viceroy of Mexico, actually wrote in outrage to Carlos I, complaining that there were Aztec boys in the Franciscan schools "who speak Latin as elegantly as Cicero."

Fortunately, the viceroy, Antonio de Mendoza, ignored his adviser. He wrote a different sort of letter to the court, requesting funds to establish a college of higher learning for Aztec boys. Mendoza supplemented these funds from his own purse, designating that the income from some of his lands should be used to support the college. In 1536 the Colegio de Santa Cruz was established at Tlateloco, which at that time was the suburban "Indian quarter" of Mexico City. In addition to Latin, philosophy, logic, mathematics, and music, the curriculum included a course in Aztec medicine, taught by native doctors.

THE FRIARS' LEGACY

The earliest surviving record of Aztec medical knowledge was produced at the college. The *Libellus de medicinalibus indorum herbis*, the Little Book of Medicinal Herbs of the Indies, popularly known as the Aztec Herbal of 1552, was probably intended as a gift for the Spanish king. It was created at the request of the viceroy and sent to the court at a time when royal interest in the school had waned and funds were dwindling. It must have been hoped that the little book would impress the crown with the value of keeping the college open.

Its author was an Aztec physician, a convert, who had taken the Christian name Martín de la Cruz. His text, written in Nahuatl, was translated into Latin by another convert, Juan Badianus, probably a teacher at the college. The book was completed under the watchful eye of the Franciscan rector, who would have deleted the least hint of heresy, so all of the Aztec medical theory is missing. The authenticity of the remedies themselves is suspect, since they include elements of sixteenth-century European medical practice. They involve elaborate combinations of herbs, stones, and animal parts, which was the custom of European physicians of the time, who liked to impress their patients by cooking up complicated remedies using lots of ingredients, whereas Aztec medicines more often involved the use of only a single herb.

Another teacher at the college, Fray Bernardino de Sahagún, bequeathed to posterity the purest record of Aztec medicine. Long before modern anthropologists began traveling around with tape recorders, Fray Sahagún used a series of questionnaires to take testimony from a group of aged informants who could still remember pre-Cortesian life. Working with a team of students over the course of forty years, Sahagún laboriously recorded many aspects of Aztec culture.

His *Historia general de las cosas de la Nueva España*, General History of the Things of New Spain, included eighty pages on the uses of medicinal plants, which he said were taken from the testimony of native doctors. Other sections dealt with Aztec ideas about the human body and illness. The volumes, which were illustrated by native artists, were organized in double columns, with the original Nahuatl testimony side-by-side with a paraphrased Spanish version.

The books were completed in 1569. A year later the Holy Inquisition was established in Mexico. Sahagún's work was deemed heretical, and all of his papers were confiscated. He was able to return to the project a decade later, but this time he made a number of judicious changes. In 1585 he completed a revised version, which was sent to Madrid.

By the end of the sixteenth century the hierarchy of the Church included the first generation of *criollos*, Mexican-born Spaniards, who were considerably less sympathetic to the "Indians." The eager idealism of the early friars had been dampened by a growing cynicism as the ancient Aztec religion proved to be a stubborn and insidious foe.

The *tictli*, the Aztec spiritual healers, were considered witches or sorcerers who had made a pact with the devil and must be routed out. One *criollo* priest, Hernando Ruiz de Alarcón, was so zealous in performing his duties that in 1614 he was investigated by the tribunal of the Holy Inquisition in Mexico City for conducting autos-da-fé and public floggings. Three years later he was appointed an ecclesiastical judge. In performing his duties as an informant to the Inquisition, he unwittingly preserved the very rituals he was so fanatically determined to eliminate. In his *Tratado de las supersticiones y costumbres gentilicas que oy viven entre los indios naturales desta Nueva España*, Treatise on the Heathen Superstitions That Today Live Among the Indians Native to This New Spain, Ruiz de Alarcón placed the medicinal uses of the herbs in context, describing the entire ritual and including the invocations in the original Nahuatl. He recorded not only a selection of the Nahuatl prayers he deemed most offensive but also his own haughty attitude toward these "wretched people," "these mangy sheep."

TRAFFICKING IN HERBS

Meanwhile, back in Madrid, the royal court was hearing about the amazing vegetation of New Spain. For some time Europe had been intrigued with the possibility of finding miracle cures in the Americas. Columbus had set sail in search of a route to the land of herbs and spices. When he found instead a whole new world of plants he couldn't identify, he decided to come back with an expert. On his second voyage he brought along one of the royal Spanish physicians. Reports from expeditions such as that one, and the news that was now filtering back from Mexico, led the crown to realize that the medicinal plants of the colonies were yet another natural resource to be exploited.

Felipe II, who had succeeded Carlos I on the throne, decided to commission a botanical survey. He appointed one of the most esteemed scientists in all of Spain to do the job. Francisco Hernández, a physician to the court, was named *protomédico* of the Indies and sent off across the seas, charged with the gargantuan task of cataloging all the flora and fauna of New Spain.

Accompanied by his son, Hernández sailed in 1570, half a century after the fall of the Aztecs. For the next seven years he traveled throughout the colony with a team of native interpreters and artists, asking everywhere about the properties and medical benefits of the plants. He endured freezing cold and blistering heat; he crossed treacherous mountains and rivers. He had to overcome the jealousy and distrust of the Spanish doctors in New Spain and the trickery of his interpreters and of the native healers, who were by now very old and often reluctant to give him good information. He spent a great deal of time in the former imperial botanical gardens at Huaxtepec, cataloging the medicinal plants and interviewing the Aztec doctors there. He was astounded by the knowledge of these native herbalists who, he said, knew how to use everything that grew—just as an expert Mexican-American *yerbera*, today will tell you that every plant heals something if you know how to use it. Hernández was a relentless and conscientious researcher, often trying out remedies on himself. In 1577 he presented the court with his monumental *Historia natural de la Nueva España*, eleven volumes in which he listed some 3,076 plants, most of which were used for medicinal purposes.

The Spanish practiced the most advanced medicine in the Western world, having benefited from the legacy of the ancient Arabs and Hebrews, courtesy of the recently expelled Moors and Jews. But European medicine hadn't made much progress since the ancient Greeks and Romans. Throughout the

Middle Ages, medicine had been dispensed primarily by the Church. Pre-Christian ideas had been discarded as "heathen." But renaissance Europe re-embraced the medical theories of Hippocrates, Aristotle, Dioscorides, Pliny, and Galen, and the profession of learned physicians flourished again.

THE FOUR HUMORS

Because Francisco Hernández was an enlightened scientist of his day, he was an expert on the humoral theory of medicine. Hippocrates first put forth the idea that the four elements—earth, wind, rain, and fire, were present in the human body. Illness was caused by an imbalance of the four humors that related to these four elements: blood, which was hot and moist; yellow bile, which was hot and dry; black bile, which was cold and dry; and phlegm, which was cold and moist. When we say today that someone is in a foul humor, we are referring to this ancient theory.

Hernández was trained in the accepted medical theory of his time, based on the teachings of Galen, a second century Alexandrian physician who had developed a method for characterizing diseases and their remedies based on the four humors. Medicines were analyzed by the degree to which they were hot, cold, moist, or dry. An illness caused by an excess of phlegm, which is cold and moist, would be cured by administering a treatment that was hot and dry to correct the imbalance.

Hernández classified the plants he found in New Spain in accordance with his Galenic training. This scientific analysis gave the New World plants credibility in Europe. We do exactly the same thing today, analyzing the chemical constituents of the ancient medicinal plants to determine whether they work and explain why. We look for corroborating evidence according to our own modern science, just as Hernández did.

THE MYSTERY OF THE LOST VOLUMES

In one of the stranger turns of history, all the volumes of de la Cruz, Sahagún, and Hernández disappeared for centuries. The de la Cruz Aztec herbal never reached the hands of the king for whom it was so carefully created. It was received instead by his son, who immediately consigned it to the royal archives where it was forgotten for 377 years. An American professor came upon it completely by accident in 1929 while doing research for the Smithsonian Institution at the Vatican library. In the same year an Italian translation of the manuscript was discovered in the English Royal Library at Windsor. How the book ended up in these two libraries remains a mystery.

A similar fate befell the volumes of testimony that Fray Sahagún had so patiently and meticulously collected. When the manuscript reached Madrid, it was quickly confiscated. The Church was working hard to obliterate the very practices and ideas that Sahagún had written down in Nahuatl, the Aztecs' own language. Considered dangerous and subversive, his work was hidden under lock and key. The volumes were not published until 1829, 240 years after they were sent to Spain.

Poor Francisco Hernández, who had labored so arduously and so long to complete his mammoth encyclopedia, died without seeing his work published. By the time he returned to Spain, the mood of the court had shifted. Under the influence of certain Italian advisers, the king decided the work was too long to be useful. Hernández was cast aside, and an Italian court physician was assigned to reorganize his work and edit it down to a more manageable length. The original illustrations, drawn by native artists, were replaced by more "appropriate" European drawings. This butchered and inaccurate version was published in 1615. To add insult to injury, Hernández's work was plagiarized by other authors for years, and the original manuscript, which had been stored in the Escorial, outside of Madrid, was lost when the building caught fire in 1671. More than a century later a copy was found in the Imperial College of Madrid. But his prodigious work was largely unknown and ignored until the 1940s when it was published by the Universidad Autónoma de México (Mexico's national university with campuses all over the country), in Mexico City.

Although Felipe II had cooled toward Hernández, he was still intent on exploiting the natural resources of his American colony. Between 1579 and 1585 a questionnaire was sent to each of the 177 *cabeceras de poblados*, the regional capitals, asking for detailed information on the flora and fauna. Two of the fifty questions referred specifically to medicinal plants and their uses. As the completed questionnaires made their way back to Spain, interest in the healing herbs of the New World became intense. New World plants began arriving by the boatload in Spanish ports. And in Seville, a physician named Nicolás Monardes wrote a book that became an international bestseller.

JOYFUL NEWS FROM THE NEWFOUND WORLD

Monardes completed the three volumes he called *Historia Medicinal de las Cosas que se traen de nuestras Indias Occidentales que sirven en Medicina* in 1574. The work was "Englished" by John Frampton in 1596, who published it under the much snappier title *Joyfulle Newes Out of the Newe Founde Worlde*. Eventually the book was published in twenty-six editions and translated into Latin, French, Italian, and other languages.

Like Hernández, Monardes had been educated at the esteemed University of Alcalá. Both men were renaissance scientists who rejected the superstition and magic of the Middle Ages in favor of experimentation and the more enlightened science of Hippocrates and Galen. Monardes backed up his descriptions of the medicinal plants with what today might be called case studies, stories of the cures he had witnessed. And he included detailed instructions on how the plants should be used in treatments. His remedies appropriated the New World plants and adapted them to Old World medical practices. The cultural context in which the plants had been so effectively used didn't concern him. He would have tossed all that aside as paganism.

Monardes was an entrepreneur as well as a doctor, importing medicinal plants from the New World. His book must have been good for business. With the New World medicinal plants now backed up by science, their use exploded in Europe. Plants from the Americas began to be included in standard herbal texts as a whole new repertoire of herbal remedies transformed European medicine.

MESTIZO MEDICINE

Soon after the conquest, European plants began arriving in Mexico. In one of his letters to the king, Cortés requested that every ship that set sail for New Spain be required to carry a specified number of European seeds and plants. The vegetation of Mexico, which may have been the most varied in the world when Cortés arrived, soon became even more diverse.

In the early days of the colony, the Spanish had been forced to look for native plants that would substitute for those they had used in Europe. They were motivated to stay close to Aztec doctors and to learn from them. But when

European herbs became available, they reverted to these more familiar medicines.

The friars were health practitioners, administering European herbs to their parishioners. Native Mexicans soon integrated the friars' herbs into their own traditional remedies. European medicinal herbs escaped from mission gardens and have been growing wild throughout Mexico and the American Southwest ever since. More than half the plants used in traditional Mexican-American medicine today are of European origin, including many of the most commonly used and beloved herbs such as *manzanilla, yerba buena, ruda,* and *romero*—chamomile, spearmint, rue, and rosemary.

In 1691, Johannes Steinhoffer, a young Moravian lay-Jesuit who was trained as a pharmacist and physician, was sent to the colony to administer to the medical needs of his fellow missionaries. The Jesuits had been latecomers to the New World, preceded by the Franciscans, the Augustinians, and the Dominicans, so they were assigned the less desirable territories of northwestern New Spain. Jesuit botanists and pharmacists like Steinhoffer began to catalog the medicinal herbs of this arid terrain and to learn about their uses from native healers.

In 1712, near the end of his life, Steinhoffer completed a book that was to remain a standard text for centuries. Writing under the more "politically correct" name of Juan de Esteyneffer, he compiled his *Florilegio medicinal de todas las enfermedades,* Anthology of Medicines for All Illnesses. Although the book concentrates on European herbs, thirty-five indigenous medicinal plants are included among the remedies listed. Because the book was not intended for medical professionals but for missionaries who were stationed in remote areas, far from the services of a doctor or pharmacist, it was written in an accessible language that could be followed easily. The *Florilegio* became a household reference, passed down from mother to daughter throughout northern Mexico and what is now the southwestern United States. Many of the traditional Mexican-American remedies still used today can be found on its pages.

The friars brought European medical theories with them to the New World. Medical texts by Pliny and Galen were on the shelves of the library at the Colegio de Santa Cruz and other Franciscan schools. The humoral theory of hot and cold, wet and dry was close to the ancient Aztec notion of duality in the cosmos, of the opposing forces; the heat of *tonalli* versus the cold loss of the spirit; the heat of the sun's kingdom versus the cold of the underworld. Native Mexicans incorporated some of the humoral theory into their own remedies, and these ideas, merged with the hot and cold Aztec concept of duality, have persisted over the centuries.

In his book *The Virgin's Children*, anthropologist William Madsen reported that in the village of Tecospan, not far from Mexico City, people continue to classify everything in the world. Alka-Seltzer is "fresh" (a degree of cold), iodine is hot, movies are cold. The world continues to be understood as a struggle to maintain the balance of opposing forces.

In Las Cruces, New Mexico, an elderly woman asks for *yerba de víbora*, a "hot" herb, because she is suffering from a "cold" stomach. In East L.A., a *yerbera* instructs her daughter to let the herbs soak in alcohol for nine days, and in San Antonio, a *curandera* tells her patients to massage their bellies nine times to the right, then nine times to the left, invoking the Aztec mystical number—the nine celestial levels and the nine levels of the underworld. This is the legacy of Mexican-American medicine, the persistence of ancient ideas.

Aztec medicine had been demolished in every way possible. The medical texts had been destroyed in the burning of the codices. The fragments of ancient knowledge preserved by de la Cruz, Sahagún, Hernández, and others had been buried and forgotten. The relentlessly vigilant Mexican Inquisition had forced the native healers to abandon their practices or continue them in secret under peril of death. Even the most secular Aztec herbalists were persecuted by Spanish doctors whose very credibility was threatened by the remarkable effectiveness of these "heathen" remedies. The Aztecs used plants for ritual as well as medicine. Herbs such as the Mexican marigold, *cempoalxóchitl*, which had been used in ceremonies honoring the old gods, were banned by the Church and replaced with "Christian" substitutes such as rosemary.

Still the old knowledge persisted. Native healers quietly passed the legacy from mother to daughter, father to son, just as they had always done, just as they continue to do. Aztec medicine had been infected with the ways of Europe. It had become a *mestizo*, but it had survived. What had been a mainstream, professionally practiced medicine went underground and became the "folk medicine" still practiced today, the medicine called *curanderismo*.

AZTEC REVIVALS

Near the dawn of the nineteenth century, as science began to replace religion as the source of absolute truth, the Aztec herbs attracted a new interest. In 1786 the king of Spain, Carlos II, issued a decree that unearthed a copy of the original manuscript of Francisco Hernández's botanical encyclopedia. At the same time he ordered the establishment of a royal botanical garden in Mexico City and sponsored expeditions to study New World plants.

Two Spaniards, Martín Sesse and Vicente Cervantes, sailed for Mexico. A second expedition was conducted by the Mexican botanist José Mariano Mociño. These scientists collected and studied the flora of Mexico from a new perspective, using the newly developed Linnean method of classifying plants with Latin names according to genus and species. The expeditions brought more than thirty-five hundred species to the herbarium in Madrid. Twenty-five hundred of them had been previously unknown in Europe.

In 1801, Mociño, working with Dr. José Montaña, initiated hospital studies in Mexico City to determine whether the indigenous Mexican plants really had curative properties. Using the best science of the era, they classified the plants as effectively astringent, corrosive, aromatic stimulant, or narcotic. They were able to show why each of the plants would have worked in the Aztec remedies. In their report Mociño and Montaña made the same arguments that are echoed by proponents of herbal medicine today. They said that the herbs they had studied were safer, less expensive, and more effective than many of the mainstream treatments in use at the time.

Although science was beginning to pay attention to the Aztec plants, *curanderos*, the native healers who used them, gained no such respect. There were very few doctors in Mexico, and fewer still who were willing to treat poor indigenous people. In rural areas, access to mainstream medical care was virtually nonexistent. More than half the population relied solely on the local medicinal herbs and services of *curanderos*. But the practice of *curanderismo* was outlawed. *Curanderos* were sentenced to a hefty fine and exile if they were caught practicing their craft. The punishment increased each time the *curandero* was apprehended. This law was not repealed until 1842, two decades after Mexico had won its independence from Spain. The new law that replaced it was not much better, labeling *curanderos* and *yerberos* as vagrants, quacks who should be punished by being pressed into military service. To this day if you look up *curandero* in a Spanish-English dictionary, you will find the word defined as "quack" or "witch doctor."

After the revolution of 1910 that overthrew dictator Porfirio Díaz, Mexico began to look back, searching for its pre-Hispanic identity. For the first time since the chronicles of the early friars an effort was made to salvage remnants of the lost Mesoamerican civilizations. The National Institute of Anthropology and History founded in 1939 by President Lázaro Cárdenas, continues to do important archaeological and ethnobotanical work throughout Mexico. Mexico's national university in Mexico City established the Seminar on Nahuatl Culture in 1957 and the Institute of Anthropological Research in 1973.

In 1989, under the auspices of the National Indigenous Institute, an extensive research project was begun, working pueblo by pueblo with local *curanderos* to record the old herbal remedies. The result is an immense computer-driven database, the *Atlas de la Plantas de la Medicina Tradicional Mexicana*, which catalogs the names and uses of medicinal plants throughout Mexico. Still, the old knowledge continues to disappear. As researchers Arturo Argueta and Abigaíl Aguilar have written, "With each indigenous wise man who dies, it is as if a library of sixteenth-century books goes up in flames."

Today almost everyone in Mexico uses the traditional herbal remedies to some extent. The old medicines have never fallen out of use in rural areas where, despite the efforts of the government to send doctors into the field, herbs are still the most readily available form of treatment. Urban Mexicans use both ancient herbs and modern pharmaceuticals. The effectiveness of the old herbal remedies is generally accepted as fact, and in some sophisticated circles it has become fashionable to know a certain marvelous *curandero* you can recommend to your friends.

CURANDERISMO EN EL NORTE

In the United States, Mexican nationals crossed the border looking for work, bringing their knowledge of the ancient healing ways to *el norte*, where a new tradition of Mexican-American folk medicine began to evolve.

Traditional medicine is very regional in Mexico. The Tarascans of Michoacán have their own legacy of herbal knowledge. In Oaxaca the heritage is Zapotec. In the Yucatán it's Maya. In Sonora and Chihuahua it's the legacy of the Tarahumara, Yaqui, and other tribes. Each region has the legacy, too, of the friars who were missionaries there—the Franciscans in the central valley of Mexico and the Jesuits in the northwest. Each pueblo uses the plants that grow nearby. The names of the plants, and sometimes their uses, differ from pueblo to pueblo.

But in Mexican-American neighborhoods, all these regions meet. The Chávez family from Jalisco find themselves living next door to the Alvarado family from Sonora and the Flores family from Morelos. At times the differences within the Mexican-American community itself can result in an herbal tower of Babel. In his encyclopedic *Catálogo de Nombres Vulgares y Científicos de Plantas Mexicanas,* the great twentieth-century Mexican botanist Maximino Martínez listed eleven different plants called *mirto.* In Nuevo León, *mirto* is a species of sage, *Salvia coccinea.* In Oaxaca it's a different sage, *Salvia microphylla.* In Durango it's another plant altogether, *Bouvardia ternifolia.* And *Bouvardia ternifolia,* meanwhile, has at least eleven other regional names in addition to *mirto.* In Sinaloa its called *yerba del indio;* in Hidalgo it's *trompetilla.* But there are other plants called *yerba del indio* and *trompetilla* in different parts of Mexico. Communicating with your neighbors about the herbs can be a challenge even if you're all speaking Spanish.

The Mexican herbal remedies were also influenced by other neighbors in the United States. There are Spanish families who have lived in the Southwest since the sixteenth century when the territory was still *Nueva España,* long before California, Arizona, and New Mexico became part of the United States. These families have their own *mestizo* medicine that integrates sixteenth-century Spanish medicine with the medicinal herbs native to the Southwest, including a few healing herbs such as *oshá* and *cota* (Navajo tea) learned from local North American tribes.

In south Texas many *botánicas* sell traditional herbs of two cultures side-by-side, accommodating both their Mexican-American and African-American customers.

The traditional remedies continue to evolve. Like their wandering Aztec ancestors, Mexican Americans are resourceful people, learning to make use of whatever is available. Patent medicines such as aspirin and castor oil have been added to the pharmacopoeia. Barrio *botánicas* sell Chinese ginseng and tiger balm along with Mexican *palo azul* and *tlachichinola.*

Aztec doctors treated the mind and body as one. They understood the value of touch, of massage. They empowered their patients by requiring them to participate in their own recovery. They spent time with members of the patient's family, enlisting their help in the cure. Modern *curanderos,* the descendants of the Aztec *tepati* and *tictli,* practice healing in these same ways. In this era of the HMO and the fifteen-minute consultation, it's no wonder they continue to find patients.

Distrust and inadequate access to the established medical system, the cost of visits to the doctor and expensive prescription drugs, the language barrier, the isolation of rural areas and urban barrios are all reasons why recently arrived immigrants from Mexico continue to resort to traditional herbal medicines. But many educated, assimilated Mexican Americans, professionals with excellent health care plans, also continue to take infusions of *barba de maíz* for cystitis, *passiflora* for insomnia, or *gordolobo* for a chest cold. If you ask why, they will tell you that these remedies work, that the herbs are gentle, safe, cheap, and effective. They may also tell you that these remedies worked safely for their mothers and grandmothers and great-grandmothers, and that they don't need the approval of the U.S. Food and Drug Adminstration in the face of such irrefutable proof.

Most Mexican-American herbal remedies are dispensed at home, like grandmother's chicken soup. If an illness can't be cured within the family, a more knowledgeable neighbor may be consulted. In some cases the family may turn to a professional *curandero* for help. *Curanderos,* like the Aztec doctors, tend to specialize. *Parteras,* traditional midwives, still practice their craft along the border. Some have studied modern medical techniques and become licensed. *Sobradoras* specialize in massage. *Yerberas* are expert in the uses of the herbs. Like the Aztec doctors, *curanderos* can also be spiritual specialists. Some are *brujas,* good witches. Some are diviners who use tarot cards and other tools to see the unseeable. Mexican Americans may turn to the medical establishment only as a last resort, or they may turn to a *curandero* when the doctor's medicine fails to help.

This has been a problem for professional health care workers. In the Southwest, where doctors and nurses often treat patients newly arrived from Mexico, medical schools teach their students something about Mexican culture and the traditional remedies so they'll know what they are up against. A "Handbook for Public Health Nurses Working with Spanish-Americans," issued by the U.S. Department of Health, Education and Welfare in New Mexico in 1964, outlined the problems faced by the medical establishment, including the fact that for some Spanish Americans "the conviction that scientific practitioners or medicines are clearly superior to traditional ones may be lacking."

While some doctors and nurses recognize the value of *curanderismo* in treating psychological problems and psychosomatic aspects of illness, the use of medicinal herbs has caused difficulties. Since many patients are embarrassed to admit to doctors that they are also taking herbal remedies, double dosing and drug interaction is always a danger. The herbs have rarely been considered a potentially useful form of treatment.

But now that herbal medicine is becoming a big business, the medical establishment in the United States is beginning to take a more serious look at alternative remedies. Major pharmaceutical companies, anxious to cash in on this multibillion-dollar industry, have begun to enter the market, producing their own brand-name herbal preparations. Since most medical research in the United States is funded by the drug companies, this should mean that more money will be directed toward studying the traditional herbs.

In Mexico the medicinal herbs have been under investigation since the founding of the Instituto Médico Nacional in 1888 and have continued to be studied under the auspices of Mexico's national university and other organizations. These studies analyze the phytochemistry of the herbs, looking for a chemical explanation of their uses. There have been some animal studies, as well, but very few human clinical trials.

The Germans have been leaders in the field of phytochemistry. It was in Germany that St. John's Wort was legitimized as an alternative treatment for depression. Medicinal herbs are taught in German medical schools, and doctors there frequently prescribe them. German scientists have begun to join their Mexican counterparts in studying the medicinal plants of Mexico.

In the United States, the University of Illinois School of Pharmacy maintains a database known as NAPRALERT, which stands for Natural Products Alert. It contains information on the chemistry and activity of plant and animal extracts relating to more than forty thousand organisms, using sources that date back to 1650.

But while exotic kava kava from the South Pacific and ginseng from China are herbal superstars, the hundreds of medicinal plants growing in our own southwestern backyards continue to be all but unknown outside the Mexican-American community—and rarely explored by the scientific establishment.

We can assume that these plants are useful remedies, based on the empirical evidence of hundreds of years of continuous use. But we haven't done many studies to find out *why* they work. And in some cases it may not be possible to find a rational, twenty-first century scientific explanation. There is always the possibility that a remedy may not be effective outside its cultural context.

Native herbalists have a profound knowledge of the herbs, passed down through many generations. They know exactly when to pick an herb and how to store it, prepare it, and administer it. It may not be possible to simply isolate the active chemical component of every healing plant and transform it into a standard-dosage, easy-to-swallow capsule.

But the herb business is booming, and as more big companies get into the market, they inevitably look for the next big herbal superstar. Eventually, for better or worse, they may begin to focus on the hundreds of indigenous herbs used every day in Mexican-American neighborhoods throughout the country. The legacy of Aztec medicine may be coming soon to a supermarket or pharmacy near you.

LOS SANTOS CURANDEROS

The tradition of the Aztec healer, the *tepati*, or *tictli*, continues to this day in rural villages and urban barrios. In modern *curanderismo*, San Martín de Porres, San Judas Tadeo, and la Virgín de Guadalupe have taken the place of Tláloc, Quetzlcóatl, and Tonantzín. The Ave Maria and the Apostles' Creed have replaced the ancient Aztec incantations. The Greco-Roman theories of the four humors have been fused with the medicines of the Toltecs, Mixtecs, Olmecs, and Tarahumara, Spanish, Moors, and Jews. The modern *curandero* heals with Aztec *toloatzin*, German chamomile, and Vick's Vaporub.

From this potent blend of traditions, legendary faith healers have arisen— miracle-working *curanderos* whose followers place them among the pantheon of the Catholic saints.

Santa Teresa de Cabora

Teresa Urrea was born in 1872 or 1873. Her father was the son of a wealthy Sinaloa rancher; her mother was a fourteen-year-old Yaqui girl who briefly satisfied his youthful lust. Teresa became a legend not only for her miraculous healing powers but because of the role she inadvertently played in the revolt against Mexican dictator Porfirio Díaz.

Although her father, Tomás Urrea, eventually fathered seventeen more children, he decided to acknowledge her, perhaps because she grew up to be lovely looking and charming, accomplished at singing and playing the guitar. At the age of sixteen she moved out of her mother's hut and into the great house at Rancho Cabora.

According to the legend, in her father's house Teresa met an old Yaqui *curandero* with whom she began her *desarollo,* her apprenticeship in the art of *curanderismo,* learning how to use the traditional remedies. Like many *curanderas,* she discovered her extraordinary healing power while in an altered state.

When a suitor whom she had rebuffed attempted to rape her, Teresa became severely traumatized. She was catatonic, her heartbeat imperceptible. Assuming she was dead, her family prepared to bury her, but at the wake, while the mourners held their vigil, Teresa suddenly sat up in her coffin and spoke. Three days later the old Yaqui *curandero* who had been Teresa's teacher died and was buried in the same coffin.

Teresa had come back to life, but for three months she was lost, distracted, and strange. She seemed to be seeing apparitions and speaking to God. During this time it was somehow discovered that she had a healing touch. The word of her miraculous gift spread quickly. So many pilgrims came from all over Mexico that her father was forced to open a cantina to sell food to the throngs of followers.

Porfirio Díaz had seized control of the country, canceled elections, and begun to systematically wipe out his opponents. He had struck a deal with the Church, in which he agreed to leave their holdings untouched, so in order to reward his allies, he seized lands from the native Mexican tribes, using any excuse to confiscate them. Soon the Tarahumara, Yaqui, and Mayo rose up against the Díaz regime. The rebels chose Teresa, the legendary half-Yaqui healer, as their patron. *¡Viva la Santa de Cabo de Cabora!* became their battle cry. Díaz was not amused. Teresa and her father were summarily escorted to the border at Nogales.

In Arizona they were welcomed by the Mexican-American community and given a house. They moved from Nogales to El Bosque, to Solomonville, to El Paso. Wherever they went, the crippled and ill came in droves for Teresa's miracle cures.

Teresa never said a word in public that would implicate her in the rebellion, and she tried in vain to deny any involvement. In an open letter to the *El Paso Herald* in 1896 she wrote, "I am not one who encourages such uprisings, nor one who in any way mixes up with them. . . . I have noticed with much pain that the persons who have taken up arms in Mexican territory have invoked my name in aid of the schemes they are carrying through."

To avoid any further implication in the politics of the rebellion, the family moved to the quiet mining town of Clifton, Arizona. A physician there, observing Teresa's work, began sending patients to her. Validated by at least one member of the medical profession, her reputation spread. She was hired by a medical company to tour the United States on a promotional "curing crusade."

In 1906 a terrible flood washed over Clifton, Arizona. Teresa was on the front lines night and day, dragging people out of the raging waters and mud slides, administering to the sick and dying. She herself became gravely ill. Knowing that the end was near, she sent for her Yaqui mother, whom she had not seen in seventeen years. The newspapers reported her death as the passing of a saint. In Clifton, where she is buried in exile beside her father, her grave is known as the shrine of Santa Teresa de Cabora.

Don Pedrito

In any south Texas *botánica* you can find a selection of statues, medals, and photographs depicting the legendary *curandero* Don Pedrito Jaramillo, a formidable looking man with a long white beard and a round-brimmed black hat. But in each of his portraits there is a flaw: a funny line across the nose in his photograph, a cracked nose on the plastic statuette. The scar on Don Pedro's nose is never retouched or omitted, because the accident that left him with this scar showed him the way to his gift of healing.

Pedro Jaramillo was born near Guadalajara in 1829. He spent most of his life in the countryside working as a shepherd. When his beloved mother fell ill, he prayed to God, vowing that if she didn't get well, he'd leave Mexico. But his prayers went unanswered, and after his mother's death, Pedro Jaramillo made good on his threat. He loaded up his saddle bags and headed north for the border. He was fifty-two years old and determined to start over in Falfurrias, Texas, near Los Olmos creek. One day he fell off his horse and landed on his nose. The pain was terrible. Then something compelled him to bathe his poor nose in the mud of a lagoon. For three days he kept his nose covered in mud. On the third night God spoke to him in a dream, telling him that he had *el don,* the gift of healing, and that he must now devote his life to helping others. The next day the pain in his nose was gone.

In those days the few doctors in rural south Texas were Anglos with little interest in treating poor Mexican Americans. Pedro Jaramillo became Don Pedrito, the healer of Los Olmos, savior of the sick and the poor. His good works are legendary. He never charged for his services, but with the donations he received, he fed the pilgrims who came to see him. During the drought of 1903 he opened his barn and gave away his stock of grains and groceries to feed the hungry. He financed the travel expenses of those who couldn't afford to come to Falfurrias, and he toured south Texas, visiting those who were too ill to come. When the railroad came to Falfurrias, Don Pedrito's fame grew. Patients came from all over the Southwest and Mexico.

At the heart of *curanderismo* is the belief that healing can take place only with the help of God, a legacy from the ancient Aztec belief that illnesses were inflicted by the gods and that only the gods could cure them, and from the early Catholic friars who taught the notion of God's will and the power of prayer. Don Pedrito never took credit for his cures. He said that he was only able to heal by releasing the power of God through the faith of his patients. Carrying out his remedies often required a leap of faith, and he always insisted on prayer.

He used the traditional herbs, but many of his remedies were unique. He would instruct his patients to drink a glass of warm water or take a certain number of baths. He prescribed black coffee, whisky, canned tomatoes. His therapies often involved sequences of nine, the Aztec mystical number, or three, evoking the Holy Trinity. He might tell a patient to take a walk every day for nine days or to take three sips of water.

After his death in 1907, many of his followers believed that he would continue his healing work from the spirit world. A little chapel was erected over his grave in Falfurrias. Inside there are two altars, side by side, one honoring Jesus Christ, the other Don Pedrito. The walls of the chapel are plastered with notes, photographs, messages, and even driver's licenses left by the faithful. Pilgrims still visit every day, lighting candles, bringing fresh flowers, praying for help, believing that Don Pedrito hears their prayers and has the power to answer them.

El Niño Fidencio

Twice a year, in October and March, thousands of people descend on the tiny northern Mexico town of Espinazo, near Nuevo León. They come from both sides of the border, driving recreational vehicles, pickup trucks, and minivans. They crowd the narrow, dusty streets and the tiny train station. They are pilgrims commemorating the birthday and saint's day of a strange young man who died in 1938.

José Fidencio Sinotra Constantino was born near Guanajuato. In 1925, when he was twenty-seven years old, he moved to Espinazo to work as a housekeeper on the hacienda of Don López de la Fuente. According to the legend, he had been healing people since childhood. In Espinazo he became the most famous *curandero* in history.

There are varying accounts of the incident that transformed El Niño Fidencio from a humble rural healer to a national legend. It was a difficult time in the history of Mexico. The Catholic Church, which had held enormous influence over the country since the arrival of the first friars, was engaged in a power struggle with the government of President Pultarco Elías Calles, who had severely restricted the political influence of the Church and secularized the schools. When the clergy protested, he deported two hundred priests back to Spain, igniting the guerrilla war known as the Guerra Cristero.

In 1928, at the height of the conflict, President Calles astonished the country by paying a visit to El Niño Fidencio. That a president would consult a *curandero* was big news. That Calles took the time, in the midst of a national crisis, to travel to a remote village to see an uneducated mestizo spiritual healer put the story over the top. It was the mountain coming to Mohammed. And by publicly demonstrating his own faith in the folk religion of the lower classes even as he fought to undermine the Catholic establishment, Calles gave yet another slap to the Church.

Some say that Calles had a daughter, whom he had kept hidden, and that El Niño had amazed the president by telling him all about her. Others say that this daughter was ill and that the president traveled to Espinazo hoping to find a cure for her. Still others say that El Niño Fidencio cured the president himself of a chronic ailment.

Whatever the *curandero* did for President Calles, he earned his continued gratitude. The patronage of the president made the humble *curandero* a superstar. Dressed in white robes, his feet bare, he held court under a big pepper tree at the edge of the village. The sick and the crippled began to make the difficult trip to Espinazo by the thousands. El Niño worked the crowd, reaching out to touch thousands of outstretched hands. He believed in the healing power of laughter, good food, good times, and music. His miraculous cures became legendary.

All his life he was called El Niño, Niñito—names usually reserved for children—not out of disrespect, but affection. He is remembered as a gentle soul, an innocent, childlike man with the high-pitched voice of a young boy.

The circumstances of his death are a mystery. He told his followers that he was going away, leaving for a place where no one could follow him. He said he needed to be alone for three days. Some say he went into a trance and that by the third day he was dead. Some say his throat was slit by jealous doctors. Others say the doctors performed an autopsy before he was really dead. He was forty years old.

Thousands of mourners came to Espinazo for the wake. And as they made their way up the dusty road toward the hacienda of Don López de la Fuente, they turned in awe when they heard the familiar high-pitched voice of El Niño Fidencio coming from the mouth of a woman standing with her arms outstretched beneath the pepper tree.

That woman was the first of a cult of *materias,* men and women who carry on El Niñito's work by channeling his spirit. They call themselves *cajonitas,* little boxes, or *vasos preferidos,* chosen vessels, the physical conduits through which he continues to reach his followers here on earth. Each *materia* heads a *misión,* a congregation of devoted Fidencistas, and holds weekly healings called *curaciónes.* Tens of thousands of Fidencistas continue to make the twice-yearly pilgrimage to Espinazo. By all accounts their numbers are growing.

The ritual begins at *el pirulito,* the now sacred pepper tree, which each pilgrim must circle three times before proceeding up the hill toward the tomb where El Niñito is buried. Some pilgrims make the journey on their knees; others carry the burden of a heavy wooden cross on their shoulders. They are penitents, repaying El Niñito for some goodness he has brought them or simply making themselves worthy of his consideration and care. Abandoned crutches, canes, and jars with tumors preserved in formaldehyde crowd the shrine that is still maintained at the López de la Fuente hacienda.

Because he attracted the attention of the press, El Niñito's life and work were memorialized in photographs, collectors' items now treasured and traded among the Fidencistas. Dapper in a suit and tie or dressed humbly in his white robes, his dark-rimmed eyes stare out from framed photos on the walls and shelves of *botánicas* in Mexican-American communities throughout the United States. His image, surrounded by rays of light, appears on boxes of El Niño Fidencio soap, votive candles, incense, cologne, and medallions.

All three of these folk saints administered to the poor, the disenfranchised. None of them ever charged a fee. Santa Teresa died while trying to save lives. Don Pedrito lived in a simple shack and gave away whatever he received. The gifts El Niño Fidencio received from President Calles and other wealthy clients were distributed among the needy. These *curanderos* are as famous for their generosity as they are for their miracle cures. They are the people's saints—poor rural Mexicans who found the power to impact thousands of lives. not through force but through compassion.

PROFILES: *LAS ABUELAS*

Ofelia Esparza, Concha Talavera, Fidela Gutiérrez— *Yerberas* (East L.A., California)

The barrio doesn't benefit from the Pacific breezes that cool the affluent west side. In August the sidewalks of East L.A. are empty until dusk. Even the dogs are too hot to patrol the yards, and lie listless and indifferent on porches, panting feebly. Radios tuned to Spanish-language stations spill *norteños* and *rancheras* out of open doors. Most of the modest, well-kept homes, set back from the street by tidy gardens, have been occupied by the same families for fifty years.

One of Ofelia Esparza's sons lives with his family in the house where Ofelia's mother once lived. Ofelia's house is behind it, on the far side of a patio furnished with an assortment of umbrella-shaded tables. Potted herbs are clustered under the old trees and rosebushes that frame her front door.

Her living room, crowded with the artifacts of a long life and a big family, has the musty comfort of an *abuela*'s house where generations of children have been running through the rooms for decades. The well-worn furniture is camouflaged with layers of Mexican blankets and hand-crocheted afghans. A pot of *pozole* simmers on the stove, perfuming the still air with chiles and onions.

Ofelia Esparza has an innate elegance and grace that never leaves her even when she is relaxed and at home in an old T-shirt and a cotton skirt, her copious gray-and-white hair tied behind her neck. She settles into the depths of her Barcalounger with the quiet dignity of a queen ascending her throne.

She is a respected artist who makes elaborate altars on important occasions such as Christmas and the Day of the Dead. She is also a third grade teacher who put herself through college, going back to school when the youngest of her nine children was only two years old. And she is a *yerbera*, an herbalist, who has agreed to tell me what she knows about the healing plants and to introduce me to her mentors. But first I want to learn about her life.

"I was born in East L.A. I've lived all my life within five blocks of this house. I've lived a long time. Sixty-five is a lot of years. I have fourteen grandchildren and three great-grandchildren. I'm never alone. I've been alone maybe three months in my whole life. I got married when I was nineteen and stayed married for forty years.

"My mother was raised by my great-aunt, whom we called Mamá Pola. She was a little Mayan lady, born in 1907 in the village of Guanimero in the state of Guanajuato. She told us such stories!

"Once in Guanimero, Mamá Pola got called to attend a woman who was dying in childbirth. She told my mother to stay home, but my mother followed Mamá Pola and snuck into the woman's hut. Mother had to crouch down, so she could only see the woman's feet. She watched Mamá Pola brush the woman with branches of herbs and heard her mumble Mayan chants. Then Mamá Pola lit three bunches of herbs that smoked around the bed, and massaged the woman's stomach. The next morning when my mother asked Mamá Pola about what she'd seen, Mamá Pola told her, 'Oh, that's not for you, m'ija.' Mamá Pola went back to *México* during the repatriation. She said she didn't want to die in this barbarous country.

"About fifteen years ago, I started to do my own research, reading up on herbal remedies. Of course, I recognized certain things my mother used to do, and I used mentors in the neighborhood."

One of her mentors is Concha Talavera, a great-great-grandmother of ninety whom she addresses respectfully as *maestra*. *La maestra* has lived down the street from Ofelia since 1942, but she was born in rural Arizona. The herbs she remembers grew wild along the arroyo and *en los campos,* in the fields of her father's big ranch.

Señora Talavera's East L.A. garden is lush and overgrown—knobby old trees and scruffy hedges entangled with unruly vines. In her kitchen, bunches of newly harvested herbs hang upside down, drying.

She is a willing teacher, happy to share anything she can remember, even with a gringa who barely speaks Spanish. Yes, the dried *popotillo* is still potent as long as it has retained its aroma. Only use two or three *boldo* leaves in your cup, or the tea will be too strong. Heat the *golondrina* leaves a little before applying them to an insect bite. There is so much to learn.

Another of Ofelia's neighborhood mentors is her *comadre,* Fidela Gutiérrez. They are in-laws; Ofelia's son is married to Fidela's daughter. Dark-haired and slender, Fidela Gutiérrez is a vivacious seventy-three, constantly moving, talking, gesturing, laughing. She was born in El Salto, near Guadalajara. No one in that tiny town missed the presence of a doctor because Fidela's grandmother was able to cure all their ailments, using the old herbal remedies. Continuing a long unbroken line, her grandmother passed this knowledge of the remedies to her mother, and her mother passed them to Fidela.

At the late age of thirty-three she met and married a man who had come from the States to visit relatives in El Salto. Now widowed, she shares her home with one of her daughters, her son-in-law, and two grandchildren. They have recently been prettying up the house. Garlands of silk flowers are draped over the curtain rods. Needlepoint throw pillows are carefully arranged on the freshly upholstered couches.

Standing at her kitchen stove, Fidela expertly pats *masa* between her palms, turning out *gorditas* and *quesadillas* while her two daughters and I sit at the table, happily consuming plateful after plateful. Fidela keeps one eye on the skillet and the other on her grandchildren who whiz past her feet in pursuit of the family dog. All the while she volleys *remedios* at me like tennis balls. A fork in one hand, a pen in the other, I scribble madly, trying to keep up with her.

Her daughters have become interested in their mother's *yerbas* and pay close attention, helping to translate when Fidela's rapid Spanish leaves me in the dust. *"Tome yerba buena con manzanilla y un poquito de miel para cólico."* Take spearmint with chamomile and a little honey for colic. *"Y la ruda. Todo eso cura la ruda."* And rue, rue cures everything. Take *cedrón,* lemon-scented verbena, for gas pains and dizzy spells; *borraja,* borage, for bleeding after childbirth; *orégano para la tos,* oregano for cough. When she can't instantly remember a remedy I ask for, she wrinkles her expressive face, and for a moment her mind flies back to El Salto, searching for a certain plant that grows along the riverbank. Then she lights up and resumes wagging her hands at me. *Berro,* watercress, for the liver. It grows by the *río* Santiago.

She is so animated and moves about with such apparent ease that I am astonished to hear she suffers from arthritis. Her daughter tells me that in the morning Fidela is bent over and stiff. As soon as she wakes up, she treats herself with a liniment she makes with *florifundio,* angel's trumpet flowers. Within a few minutes she has recovered enough to be out in the garden, tending her herbs and flowers.

A good *yerbera* can make anything grow from a cutting; she trades with other women and snitches samples from neighbors' gardens. Fidela is always prepared to take a cutting wherever she finds an interesting plant. She has even been known to pilfer a stem or two from the nearby Cavalry Cemetery, where she goes every morning to attend the chapel mass.

One morning a strange woman appeared at the chapel. She was well dressed and not terribly old. Without saying a word, she picked Fidela out of the crowd, pressed some papers into her hands, and then disappeared. The papers listed *remedios* allegedly given to a Señora Margarita Ramirez by the Blessed Virgin herself during a divine apparition that took place in October 1993. Fidela doesn't know why the woman chose her, who she was, or how she got there. Hoping to thank her, every morning she looks for her at mass, but she has never seen her again.

According to the papers, after a fervent admonition to prayer and repentance, the Virgin Mother dictated *remedios* for everything from vaginal inflammation to cancer and AIDS. For heart problems, pregnancy, or to purify the blood of a baby, put five red rose petals in a cup with boiling water and sweeten with bee's honey. The five petals signify the wounds of *Nuestro Señor Jesucristo.* The bees are blessed creatures because their wax illuminates the altars. For typhoid fever take a stalk of celery liquefied in a glass of water. While drinking it, pray, *"En el Nombre del Padre, del Hijo, y del Espíritu Santo."*

It's impossible to be sure how much credence Fidela gives these holy papers, but I think I detect an extra twinkle in her eye.

She follows me to my car, still hurling remedies at me. Dry the blossoms of the lemon tree to make a tea for stomachache and insomnia. Pineapple juice is good for the kidneys. *La fruta de guayaba* for insect bites. And just as I'm about to pull away, she catches me at the curb with a plant she has pulled up by the roots. *Es altamisa.* She thinks I'll need it to get me through the coming fall. *Para los resfriados, para la gripe.* For colds, for flu.

After I met Ofelia Esparza and her mentors, a corner of my kitchen was devoted to herbs. I learned to take infusions of *gordolobo* for chest congestion; *ruda* for menstrual cramps; *cola de caballo* and *barba de maíz* for water retention; *yerba mansa* and *malva* to soothe inflamed tissues, *yerba buena, poleo,* and *manzanilla* to soothe the stomach; *passiflora* to soothe the nerves.

Inspired by Fidela Gutiérrez, I planted a *florifundio* bush in my front yard. When the flowers bloom, I put them in jars and cover them with alcohol so I'll always have some of the liniment available to hand out to a friend suffering from arthritis or a strained muscle. Everyone who has tried it has told me how well it works.

Simple remedies for simple ailments, the herbs of *las abuelas* have become a part of my life.

PART II

PLANTAS QUE CURAN:
HEALING PLANTS AND THEIR USES

INTRODUCTION

A big part of writing this book has been the intricate task of unraveling the web of names given to each of the Mexican-American medicinal plants. Many times, I had to become a detective to discover the true botanical identity of a medicinal plant with numerous aliases.

No matter which part of Mexico she comes from, or where she lives in the United States, to a Mexican American, *romero* is always rosemary and *ruda* is always rue. Plants of European origin with Spanish names are easy to identify. But a medicinal plant of American origin can have dozens of names.

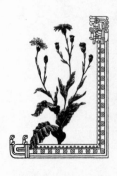

In Mexico, each region—even each pueblo—may have its own local names for the medicinal plants that grow in the area. And the same name can refer to many different plants. For example, the name *yerba del golpe*, which literally means herb of the wound or bruise, can refer to any number of plants used regionally to treat banged-up flesh.

This confusion extends over the border to the southwestern United States. Take the creosote bush, that most common of desert plants, popularly known as chaparral. In California, where I live, Mexican Americans often call chaparral *gobernadora*, a female form of the Spanish word for governor, perhaps because it reigns over the desert. In New Mexico, chaparral's fetid odor has earned it the name *hediondilla*, from the Spanish word *hedionda*, meaning stinky. In northern Mexico, chaparral is also sometimes called *goma de Sonora*, meaning Sonora rubber, for its sticky resin. But according to the binomial Latin botanical system, chaparral is always *Larrea tridentata*, no matter what anybody calls it. So for purposes of positive identification, I have included the two-part Latin botanical names of all the plants cataloged in this section.

Modern researchers estimate that there are more than 2,500 medicinal plants in use in Mexico today. Even more medicinal plants, native to the southwestern United States, have been incorporated into the traditional medicine of Mexican Americans. From this vast pharmacopoeia, I have cataloged more than two hundred plants, choosing to include herbs one might find in a *botánica*, herb store, or market in the United States. I have cross-referenced all the most-commonly used names I found for each plant, so that if you are looking for your grandmother's *yerba del cancér*, you can easily find it, although it's listed under *cancerina*, the name somebody else's grandmother called it. Most, but not all of the plants have English names, and I've listed those for reference. And to place the plants in the context of their rich history, wherever applicable I've included the native Nahuatl or Maya names as well.

I have included medical warnings and contraindications whenever I found them, referring particularly to the research published in *The Complete German Commission E Monographs—Therapeutic Guide to Herbal Medicines,* the American Herbal Products Association's *Botanical Safety Handbook,* and the publications of the American Botanical Council and the Herb Research Foundation.

Herbs can have active chemical properties that function just like drugs. In fact, many prescription drugs are plant derivatives. **It is absolutely critical that you tell your doctor if you are using an herbal medicine.** If you take both an herb and a prescription or over-the-counter medication, you may be double-dosing. Conversely, some herbs may work against a prescription drug, lessening or negating its effect.

Medicinal plants should not be used for prolonged periods of time or in excessive quantities. A little nutmeg sprinkled into a cup of tea or over a dish of custard is usually harmless. But nine heaping spoonfuls of ground nutmeg taken in one day would be toxic.

Many medicinal plants should not be used during pregnancy. This is particularly true of any of the herbs used to treat menstrual cramps, as well as laxatives and diuretics. But it's also dangerous for pregnant women to take therapeutic doses of common herbs like rosemary and basil, which are perfectly safe if used in smaller amounts for cooking.

Remember, too, that anybody can be allergic to a plant.

So how safe are the traditional medicinal plants? Consider that although few of these plants have ever been subjected to strictly controlled scientific studies they have been in continuous use for centuries, hundreds of years longer than any prescription medicine. They have a good safety record when used prudently.

INSTANT AZTEC: THE NAHUATL SYSTEM OF IDENTIFYING PLANTS

To the untrained eye Nahuatl plant names can look like a long string of indecipherable letters. Actually, they are scientific botanical names.

The Aztecs had developed a highly sophisticated system of identifying plants, not unlike the Linnean system of binomial Latin nomenclature used universally today. Just as modern botanists classify plants first according to kingdom, then family, genus, and species, the Aztecs divided all plants into two natural orders, then divided them again by type and finally by characteristics. Plants of the *quah* order are woody—a tree or bush. Plants of the *xiuh* order are herbaceous—an herb or plant. Within these two orders a plant was named first according to type. Nahuatl plant names are likely to include one of these words:

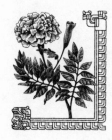

ayotl—gourd
capac—cane
etl—bean
huaxin—pod bearing
mecatl—vine

metl—maguey
nochtli—nopal cactus
patli—medicine
quahuitl—tree
quilitl—edible plant
tollin—reed
tomatl—tomato
xihuitl—inedible plant
xiuh—plant
xóchitl—flower
xocotli—sour fruit
zacatli—grass
zapotl—sweet fruit

Prefixes and suffixes were then added to these names to further define the plant. These modifiers referred to some characteristic of the plant.

Color

coztic—yellow
itzac—white
matlatic—cobalt blue
tlapalli—red
tlitlic—black
xoxoctic—green

Texture

cutli—sticky
huitz, hoitz—spiny or twisted
tzitzicaztli—thorny
tzontli—hairy

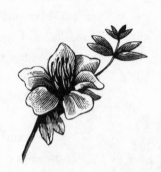

Taste

chichi—bitter
cococ—savory

Size

> *tlaco*—medium
> *tlal*—low
> *tontli*—small

Where the Plant Grows

> *atoya, atl*—brook, water; becomes the prefix *a*
> *quahtla*—forest; becomes the suffix *quah* or *cua*
> *tepe*—mountain
> *texcal*—rock; becomes the prefix *te*
> *xal*—sand

What the Plant Is Used For

> *amate*—paper
> *amolli*—soap
> *chichiz*—sleep
> *totonqui*—fever medicine

An Identifying Property or Concept

> *ahuiyac*—fragrant
> *coatl*—snakelike; becomes the prefix *coa*
> *iyac*—foul-smelling
> *nenepilli*—tongue, looks like a tongue
> *papalotl*—butterfly, attracts butterflies
> *quetzal*—rare plume, looks feathery
> *teo*—sacred
> *tletl*—fire, burning

Several qualifiers attached to a plant name can add up to a feature-length word. But once the word is broken down into its components, it is not so hard to decipher.

For example, the Nahuatl botanical name for artichoke, *quahtlahuitzquilitl*, looks imposing until you break it down:

quahtla = forest
huitz = spiny
quilitl = edible plant

Quahtla-huitz-quilitl is a spiny edible plant that grows in the forest.

Quahtlatehuitzquilitl, which we know as *cardo santo* or Mexican thistle, is differentiated from the artichoke by the addition of just two letters, "te," rock.

quahtla = forest
te = rock, rocky
huitz = spiny
quilitl = edible plant

Quahtla-te-huitz-quilitl is a spiny edible plant that grows in rocky places in the forest.

Tepepapaloquilitl, the Nahuatl name for the plant we know as *yerba del venado* or deerweed, breaks down like this:

tepe = mountains
papolo = butterfly
quilitl = edible plant

Tepe-papalo-quilitl is an edible plant that grows in the mountains and attracts butterflies.

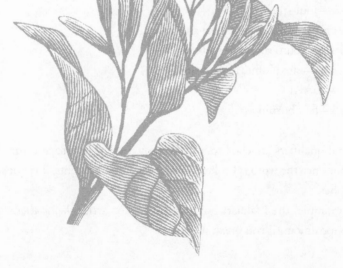

THE PLANTS

Abedul
Birch

Botanical Names: *Betula alba, Alnus acuminata, Betula pubescens*
Other Names: *Alamo Blanco*, White Birch
Nahuatl: *Aylin, Tepeylin*

This tall, graceful tree is often found growing near water, so the Nahuatl name for the birch, *ylin*, is modified to become *aylin*, birch growing by the water, or *tepeylin*, birch growing in the mountains. The Aztecs used the leaves in a formula for an enema to treat dysentery. They used the bark in a liquor to "clear the bowels" and in a salve to heal wounds. In Sonora the plant is still used for wounds and indigestion. Mexican Americans use the leaves in a diuretic tea. A German study published in the *Commission E Monographs* indicated that the leaves were useful in treating bacterial and inflammatory diseases of the urinary tract.

Parts Used: Young leaf, resin, bark
Property: Diuretic
Used to Treat: Disorders of the kidneys and urinary tract

Should not be used by persons with impaired heart or kidney function.

Abrojo
Puncture Vine

Botanical Names: *Tribulus cistoides, Tribulus terrestis*
Other Names: *Abrojo Rojo*, Jamaica Feverplant
Maya: *Chanixnuk, Punah-ki*

Touted as a magical macho herb, *Tribulus* is marketed on the Internet and in health food stores as a testosterone booster, fertility drug, and natural steroid for body builders. One website lists the top ten reasons for taking *Tribulus* capsules, including muscle building, anti-aging, aiding sperm production, urinary tract infections, increasing circulation to the eyes, and even menopause.

A creeping vine, *Tribulus* grows wild in tropical climates throughout most of the world and is commonly found on Mexican beaches. The Spanish name, *abrojo*, which could be roughly translated as "eye-opener," and the English name "puncture vine" refer to the thorny pods that are no pleasure to step on with bare feet.

The plant has long been used in the Aryuvedic medicine of India as a diuretic, an aphrodisiac, and a remedy for male impotence. When it was discovered that Bulgarian athletes were taking *Tribulus* supplements to increase lean body mass, the plant began to be marketed as the herbal alternative to steroids.

In traditional Mexican and Mexican-American medicine, an infusion of the leaves is used as a kidney cleanser.

Parts Used: Leaf, fruit
Properties: Diuretic, anti-inflammatory
Used to Treat: Kidney and liver problems

Acacia
Gum Arabic

Botanical Name: *Acacia senegal*
See also: *Espino Blanco, Huizache, Uña del Gato*

The huge *Acacia* genus includes more than twelve hundred species of flowering trees and shrubs, many of them used medicinally for their soothing properties. *Acacia senegal*, as its name suggests, is an African native exported to the Americas. A low, spreading tree, its spikes of small ball-shaped yellow flowers give way to dark brown or purple pod-shaped fruit. The stems produce a gum that is collected and used as a medicine after being dissolved in water. Mexicans and Mexican Americans use the flowers, leaves, and roots to make soothing teas and washes.

Parts Used: Flower, leaf, root
Properties: Soothing, anti-inflammatory
Used to Treat: Headache, skin irritations, diarrhea, dysentery, sore throat, coughs

Aceitilla
Burr Marigold

Botanical Names: *Bidens pilosa, Bidens* spp.
Other Names: *Té de Coral, Té de Milpa,* Beggar's Ticks, Tickseed, Spanish Needles
Nahuatl: *Acocohxihuitl*
Maya: *Chichik-kul, K'an-mul*

These daisylike flowers grow wild from the western United States through Mexico and south to Argentina. The plant gets its English names from the burry seeds. It contains properties that are particularly soothing to the mucous membranes, which make it useful in treating digestive tract inflammations such as colic and acid indigestion, as well as irritations of the respiratory and urinary tracts.

Parts Used: Leaf, stem, flower
Properties: Anti-inflammatory, astringent
Used to Treat: Colic, intestinal inflammations, sore throat

Aceitunillo
Chaste Tree

Botanical Names: *Vitex mollis, Vitex agnus-castus*
Other Names: *Uvalama, Ahuilote*

Species of this small flowering tree are found in subtropical climates throughout much of the world. The ancient Greeks believed that it had anaphrodisiac properties, so ladies who did not wish to be disturbed draped their couches with garlands of the leaves to dampen the ardor of suitors. The tree is not widely used in Mexican-American healing, but it has received a lot of attention in the past few years as a remedy for menstrual ailments. A 1997 German study showed that daily use of *Vitex* in capsule form was an effective treatment for symptoms of premenstrual syndrome.

In Mexico, *aceitunillo* is traditionally used to treat menstrual distress as well as a variety of unrelated problems including scorpion bites, diarrhea, and respiratory infections.

Parts Used: Leaf, fruit, stem
Properties: Expectorant, normalizes female hormonal balance
Used to Treat: Pulmonary ailments, menstrual problems, diarrhea

Not be be used during pregnancy.

Achiote
Annatto

Botanical Name: *Bixa orellana*
Other Name: Lipstick tree

Nahuatl: *Achiotl*
Maya: *Ku-xub*

This beautiful tree, native to the American tropics, is cultivated in gardens for its clusters of roselike flowers. The spiny lipstick-red fruits were used by the indigenous people of Mexico and South America to make a body paint, a pigment for mural painting, and an ink. The fruit pulp is still used to color butter and cheese. *Achiote* is a classic flavoring in the cuisines of the Caribbean and the Yucatán peninsula. The seeds are ground, then fried with crushed garlic, pepper, and sometimes a little vinegar and oregano to make a paste that is added to soups, stews, and other dishes.

Medicinally, *achiote* is a topical treatment for bites, sores, rashes, and burns. In parts of Mexico it is also used as an insect repellent.

Part Used: Leaf
Properties: Astringent, soothing
Used to Treat: Skin inflammations, insect bites

Aguacate
Avocado

Botanical Names: *Persea americana, Persea gratissima*
Other Name: *Ahuacate*
Nahuatl: *Ahuacatl*

Aguacate was widely used throughout the Aztec empire for both food and medicine. All parts of the avocado tree are used medicinally. The leaves, bark, and even the pit and peel of the fruit are used in treating a full spectrum of ailments from skin problems and muscle pains to chest congestion, wounds, and diarrhea.

Parts Used: Leaf, fruit, seed, bark, peel
Properties: Astringent, emollient, diuretic (leaf), antibiotic (seed)
Used to Treat: Menstrual cramps, headache, muscle strain, rheumatism, cough, parasites

Ahuehuete
Montezuma Cypress

Botanical Name: *Taxodium mucronatum*
Other Name: *Sabino*
Nahuatl: *Ahuehuetl*

These magnificent trees, native to Mexico, look a little like giant cypresses and have brown bark, brilliant blue-green foliage, and conical fruit. The name comes from the Aztec words for "old one of the water," and they can indeed live for hundreds of years. Legend has it that Cortés knelt and wept under an *ahuehuete* tree outside Tenochtitlán during the historic *Noche Triste,* June 30, 1520, after his brutal—albeit temporary—defeat at the hands of the Aztec forces. The ancient *ahuehuete* of Tule near Oaxaca, a tourist attraction, is more than 144 feet high and 160 feet in circumference.

The Aztecs used a tea of the leaves and bark to bathe wounds, and they placed a piece of burned bark directly on sores, burns, and ulcerations of the skin. Packets of *ahuehuete* twigs and needles are commonly found in *botánicas* and markets in Mexican-American neighborhoods today. Some people consider the fruit an aphrodisiac.

Parts Used: All of the tree
Properties: Astringent, vasoconstrictor, mild antiseptic
Used to Treat: Hemorrhoids, varicose veins, chest congestion, scabies, wounds

Ajenjo
Wormwood

Botanical Name: *Artemisia absinthium*
Other Names: *Artemisia, Yerba Maestra*
See also: *Altamisa, Estafiate*

Throughout Mexico a number of plants are referred to as *ajenjo, artemisia,* or *estafiate* and used somewhat interchangeably. This leads to a great deal of confusion and arguing among Mexican Americans who disagree about which is the true *estafiate,* which is the true *ajenjo,* and so on. The plant commonly known as wormwood in English and as *ajenjo* in Morelos and other parts of Mexico is *Artemisia absinthium,* a feathery-leafed plant with pale gray foliage. This ancient and respected European herbal remedy was brought to Mexico by the Spaniards and began living a wild life in the New World, where it is now a weed. It's one of the bitter-tasting herbs immortalized in the Bible: "For the lips of a strange woman drop honey, and her mouth is smoother than oil; but her end is bitter as wormwood, sharp as a two-edged sword" (Proverbs 5:3,4).

Although the several species of *Artemisia* are used routinely in home remedies, large doses can be toxic. This species is used to flavor the liquor absinthe, which was once outlawed in France because habitual drinkers became brain-damaged. But it is considered safe to use the herb in moderation as a simple tea. A German study published in the *Commission E Monographs* reported no known side effects or contraindications.

Parts Used: Leaf, stem
Properties: Anti-inflammatory, antiseptic, insecticide
Used to Treat: Indigestion, heartburn, stomach gas, menstrual cramps, gallbladder, intestinal parasites

Dangerous in large doses or if taken for a prolonged period of time. Should not be used by women during pregnancy.

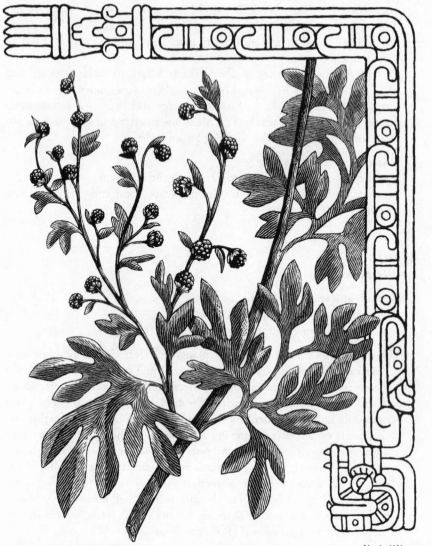

Ajenjo / Wormwood

Ajo
Garlic

Botanical Name: *Allium sativum*

Garlic, a native of Asia, is now grown extensively all over Europe and the Americas. The ancient Aztecs used an indigenous variety of garlic as a seasoning and remedy. In traditional Mexican-American medicine it is used for circulation and respiratory ailments, for digestive problems, and to expel intestinal parasites. A clove of garlic crushed against the gum is used as a temporary remedy for a toothache. Garlic is widely regarded today as one of nature's great remedies, a natural immune system booster.

Part Used: Root
Properties: Disinfectant, stimulant, diuretic, antiflatulent, antispasmodic
Used to Treat: Toothache, indigestion, stomach gas

Alacrán
Plumbago

Botanical Names: *Plumbago pulchella, Plumbago scandens, Plumbago* spp.
Other Names: *Yerba del Alacrán, Yerba del Pescado, Cola de Iguana, Pañete,* Leadwort, *Dentallaria*
Nahuatl: *Tlepatli, Tlachichinolli*

These flowering shrubs or climbers are native to warm climates. They are cultivated for the sprays of five-petaled blue, white, or red flowers that bloom from late spring through early fall.

The juice of the leaves has been used for centuries in both Europe and the Americas to alleviate dental pain. In France the plant is called *dentelaire.* The Aztecs used it for "fever in the mouth" and tooth decay. The mashed leaves are still used as poultices for toothache, wounds, and sores. The name *alacrán* is Spanish for scorpion, referring to the plant's use as an antidote for poisonous insect bites.

Part Used: Leaf
Properties: Antiseptic, astringent
Used to Treat: Toothache, wounds, poisonous insect bites

For topical use only. Can be toxic if taken internally.

Alamo
Cottonwood

Botanical names: *Populus angustifolia, Populus alba, Populus wislizeni, Populus* spp.
Other names: Poplar

These tall trees grow in temperate climates all over Europe and North America. In early eighteenth-century New Spain, the Jesuit physician Juan de Esteyneffer prescribed the buds in an ointment for hemorrhoids. He used a charcoal made from the bark as a remedy for digestive problems and applied the leaves to small skin ulcers. Mexican Americans today use the bark to make a tea for fever and arthritis, and chew a fresh twig or leaf for gum disease or loose teeth.

Parts Used: Inner bark, leaf, twig
Properties: Anti-inflammatory, fever reducer
Used to Treat: Arthritis, diarrhea, dental problems

Albahaca
Common Basil

Botanical Names: *Ocimum basilicum, Ocimum* spp.
Other Names: *Albahacar, Albácar*
Maya: *Kha-kal-tun*

Like other herbs whose Spanish name begins with the Arabic prefix *al*, basil was probably introduced to Spain by the Moors. The herb has long been associated with death in many cultures. Basil was planted on graves in ancient Persia and Malaysia, and basil blossoms were scattered over the tombs of ancient Egypt. The Hindus, who regard the herb as sacred to the gods Krishna and Vishnu, place a basil leaf on the breast of the recently departed.

Mexican Americans sometimes plant basil in front of their houses to ward off evil or carry lucky basil in a pocket or purse. As a medicinal herb it has many of the same properties as its cousins, spearmint and peppermint, and is similarly used as a digestive aid and calmative. The essential oils have properties that are effectively anti-inflammatory, absorb stomach gas, and inhibit some of the microbes that cause dysentery.

Parts Used: Leaf, stem
Properties: Anti-inflammatory, antimicrobial, antispasmodic
Used to Treat: Digestive disorders, dysentery, nervousness, menstrual cramps, fevers, stomach gas

Should not be used in large doses by pregnant or nursing women, or by infants or toddlers.

Alcachofa
Artichoke

Botanical Name: *Cynara scolymus*
Nahuatl: *Quahtlahuitzquilitl*

The flowers and leaves of the vegetable we know as "artichoke" are used for medicinal purposes. Its primary usefulness is as a diuretic, but these properties are diminished during heating, so although it's traditionally used as a tea, a cold infusion of the leaves is more effective. A tea of the boiled flowers and leaves is used as a treatment for adult-onset diabetes in northern and western Mexico.

Parts Used: Flower, leaf
Properties: Mild diuretic, appetite stimulant
Used to Treat: Liver problems, diabetes

Persons with gallstones should not use the plant medicinally without consulting a physician.

Alcancér
(see *Cancerina*)

Alcanfor
Camphor Tree

Botanical Name: *Cinnamomum camphora*
See also: *Plumajillo*

Those smelly white crystals we use to keep moths away are the gummy sap of a tall evergreen tree with longish, spade-shaped leaves, clusters of small white flowers and red berries. Marco Polo may have brought the tree to Europe from China. It found its way to the New World after the conquest. The Spanish name for the plant comes from the Arab *al kafur*, which suggests that it was part of the Spanish/Moorish medicine chest.

Mexicans and Mexican Americans use the sap as a counter-irritant to relieve aches and pains. It has slight antiseptic properties.

Part Used: Gummy sap
Properties: Analgesic, antiseptic
Used to Treat: Aching muscles, wounds

Should not be used on broken skin or on the face of infants or small children. Not to be used during pregancy.

Alegría
Amaranth

Botanical Name: *Amaranthus* spp.
Other Names: *Chile Puerco*, Pig Weed, Cockscomb, *Chichilquiltic*
Nahuatl: *Tlanepaquelitl, Quílitl, Huauhtli*
Maya: *Kix-xtez*

Amaranth was a major food source in the Aztec empire. The seeds were ground into a grain, and the young leaves were boiled and eaten as a vegetable. It is a highly nutritious plant and easily cultivated. Because a dough made with amaranth seeds was sculpted into representations of the Aztec gods for use in religious festivals, this very important food source was banned by the Spanish clergy after the conquest.

Today it is a common crop in Mexico where the seeds are used to make porridge, pastries, and small tamales called *huaquiltamales*. During the celebration of the Day of the Dead, a paste made from the seeds is formed into sugary skull-shaped candies, a holdover from Aztec times.

Amaranth cereal, rich in iron and fiber, can be found in health food stores. Elderly Mexican Americans who suffer from geriatric feebleness drink amaranth tea as a tonic, to "strengthen the heart." And some Mexican Americans add a handful of amaranth flowers to the bathwater to turn it red, in the belief that bathing in rosy waters will lift the spirits.

Some species are ornamental garden plants with clusters of droopy red flower spikes and showy leaves.

Parts Used: Flower, leaf, stem, seed
Property: Tonic
Used to Treat: Geriatric heart problems

Alfalfa
Alfalfa

Botanical Name: *Medicago sativa*
Other Names: Purple Medic, Lucerne

Alfalfa was brought to Spain by the Moors. Its Arabic name, *al-fasfasah*, became *alfalfa* in Spanish. A member of the pea family, it is a low herb with small, hairy, cloverlike leaves and clusters of purple flowers. For centuries it has been cultivated primarily to feed cattle, although in recent years health food aficionados have begun adding the vitamin-rich sprouts to salads.

Mexican Americans treat a variety of disorders with alfalfa tea. The plant loses most of its potency when dried, so it's important to use fresh leaves, crushing them slightly before infusing them in boiling water.

Parts Used: Leaf, seed
Properties: Anti-inflammatory, detoxifier, restorative, blood purifier
Used to Treat: Kidney and urinary tract disorders, indigestion, arthritis, rheumatism

Not to be used during the first trimester of pregnancy.

Alferillo
Fillery

Botanical Name: *Erodium cicutarium*
Other Names: *Alfilaria,* Storksbill, Heronsbill

A member of the geranium family but smaller than the true geranium, alferillo is a low-growing flowering ground cover. One of the many Moorish herbs to reach the New World by way of Spain, its Arabic name, *al-filal,* means "stork fingers," referring to the cupped, five-petaled blooms.

Parts Used: Leaf, flower
Properties: Diuretic, anti-inflammatory
Used to Treat: Urinary disorders, sore throat, wounds, arthritis

Alhucema
Lavender

Botanical Names: *Lavandula spica, Lavandula angustifolia, Lavandula* spp.

The popular garden herb, prized for its fragrance since ancient Phoenicia, came to the New World with the Spanish. Because the Romans used the herb as we do, to perfume bathwater, we call it lavender, from the Latin verb *lavare,* to wash. The Spanish name, however, is derived from the Arabic.

Over the centuries lavender has been touted as a remedy for a wide variety of problems from snakebite to epilepsy. Because of its soothing effect on the digestive system, it is still used as a seasoning in cooking, and lavender conserve was served as a condiment in medieval Europe.

Mexican Americans use the tea for indigestion and burn it as a kind of aromatherapy. Smudge sticks made with bundles of dried lavender are burned to fumigate sick rooms, and new mothers are purified with the scent of burning lavender after childbirth.

Parts Used: Stem, leaf, flower
Properties: Sedative, absorbs intestinal gas, antiseptic, topical stimulant, insect repellent
Used to Treat: Colic, indigestion, nerves

Altamisa
Mountain Mugwort

Botanical Name: *Artemisia franserioides*
See also: *Ajenjo, Estafiate*

This species of *Artemisia* is a mountain-loving cousin of the popular herb *estafiate.* Both species are called *ajenjo, estafiate,* or *altamisa,* depending on whom you talk to and where they are from. In parts of the southwestern United States this particular little plant is often referred to specifically as altamisa.

Parts Used: Leaf, stem, flower
Used to Treat: Colds, flu, indigestion, diarrhea

Altamisa Mexicana
Feverfew

Botanical Names: *Tanacetum parthenium* syn. *Chrysanthemum parthenium*
Other Names: *Santa Maria, Yerba de Santa María,* Featherfoil

This hardy herb, two to three feet tall, has feathery leaves and small, daisylike white flowers with yellow centers. Introduced to the New World from Europe, it's a garden escapee, often found growing wild throughout temperate regions of the United States and Mexico.

In recent years feverfew has become famous as a remedy for migraine headaches. British studies in the 1980s showed that an infusion of the herb, sipped three times a day, diminished the frequency of migraine attacks and eased arthritic symptoms.

Mexican Americans take sitz baths spiked with *altamisa* tea for menstrual cramps. The herb is burned in smudge bundles and sometimes used in the spiritual "sweepings" of *limpias*.

Parts Used: All
Properties: Anti-inflammatory, antispasmodic, insecticide
Used to Treat: Migraines, stomachache, menstrual cramps, colds and flu

Not to be used during pregnancy.

Amapola
Field Poppy

Botanical Name: *Papaver rhoeas*
Other Names: *Adormidera*, Corn Poppy, Flanders Poppy

Poppies are mostly natives of Africa and Eurasia and are cultivated as ornamental bedding plants. *Amapola*, or field poppy, is a small red flower with a black center. Like its cousin, the opium poppy, it has sedative qualities, but it is much milder and non-narcotic. If you grow it at home, the blooms should be picked in summer, dried, and kept in a tightly closed jar.

Part Used: Flower
Properties: Antispasmodic, sedative
Used to Treat: Nerves, insomnia, cough

Amarilla
(see *Maravilla*)

Amate
(see *Higueroa*)

Amole
(see *Palmilla*)

Anacahuite
Little Trumpet

Botanical Name: *Cordia boissieri*
Other Names: *Trompillo, Camichín, Zalate*
Nahuatl: *Amatl, Amaquahuitl*

Clusters of small trumpet-shaped flowers give this tree its English-language name. In Mexico it is cultivated for the small, sweet, white fruit that turns red-brown as it ripens. The wood contains a resin and a balsamic substance that is used to soothe inflammations of the mucous membranes. Its tonic action may come from the calcium and potassium in the plant's essential oil. The Nahuatl name *amatl* means paper. The Aztecs made paper from the inner white bark of both the *anacahuite* and *higueroa* (fig) trees.

Parts Used: Wood, resin
Properties: Anti-inflammatory, diuretic, general tonic
Used to Treat: Laryngitis, bronchitis, cough, kidney problems, cystitis

Angélica
Angelica

Botanical Names: *Angelica archangelica, Angelica atropurpurea*
Other Name: *Raíz de Angélica*

Angelica was held in high esteem by medieval physicians, who particularly prized it as an antidote for poison and a cure for infectious diseases. According to one story, the plant was given its lofty name by a doctor who had a dream in which an angel proclaimed that it was the much-sought-after cure for the plague.

The whole plant has a lovely aroma and a sweet taste. In France it is used to make candies and to flavor liquors such as Chartreuse. In Morelos a tea made with the root is used for digestive problems and to promote the flow of milk in nursing mothers.

Part Used: Root
Properties: Digestive, antispasmodic, expectorant, induces perspiration
Used to Treat: Intestinal inflammation, indigestion, menstrual cramps, bronchial congestion

Not to be used during pregnancy or by persons suffering from peptic ulcers.

Añil del Muerto
Crownbeard

Botanical Name: *Verbesina encelioides, Verbesina crocata*
Other Names: *Capitaneja*, Goldweed

Añil, a Spanish word for indigo dye, can refer to several plants. In the southwestern United States, *añil del muerto* usually refers to some species of *Verbesina*. These nasty-smelling, scrawny weeds with tooth-edged leaves and yellow flowers crowd along roadsides and cover hillsides in the spring throughout the southwestern United States and northern Mexico.

Parts Used: Leaf, flower
Properties: Anti-inflammatory, antiflatulent
Used to Treat: Stomach gas, hemorrhoids, chapped lips, spider bites

Anís
Anise

Botanical Name: *Pimpinella anisum*
See also: *Pericón*

Garden-variety anise is a medicinal herb dating back to the ancient Greeks and Romans who used it to treat bad breath, flatulence, and indigestion. The Arabs brought it to Spain, and the Spanish in turn planted it in the New World.

In early eighteenth-century New Spain, the Jesuit physician Juan de Esteyneffer prescribed *anís* for stomach gas, bad breath, hiccups and fainting spells.

Many supermarkets stock oil of anise among the spices used for baking. The oil can be used as a digestive aid by adding it to a cup of hot water along with a little brown sugar. Sambucco, the popular Italian after-dinner drink, a *digestivo,* gets its distinctive flavor from anise.

Pericón, the Mexican marigold, is sometimes called *yerba de anís* because of its peculiar aniselike aroma.

Part Used: Seed
Properties: Digestive aid, expectorant, antibacterial, antispasmodic
Used to Treat: Stomach cramps, sore muscles, cough

Not to be used during pregnancy.

Anís de Estrella
Star Anise

Botanical Name: *Illicium verum*

This small tree is an Asian native cultivated in the southwestern United States. The packets of dry little brown stars often found in Mexican-American markets are actually the fruit of the tree, which is used as a digestive aid.

Part Used: Fruit, dried
Properties: Antispasmodic, digestive
Used to Treat: Upset stomach

Apio
Celery

Botanical Name: *Apium graveolens* var. *dulce*

Celery has been cultivated in Asia and Europe for centuries. It grows wild in central Mexico and was used medicinally in New Spain. The Jesuit pharmacist Juan de Esteyneffer reported in the eighteenth century that *apio* was good for melancholy, liver obstruction, urine retention, rheumatic pains, and gout. Celery juice is still used as a diuretic today. Drinking the juice is believed to loosen the excess mucus of a chest cold. And the leaves are used as poultices on the eyelids to soothe irritation.

Parts Used: Leaf, flower, stalk
Properties: Tonic, diuretic, anti-inflammatory, expectorant
Used to Treat: Kidney problems, cough, colds

Aquiche
(see *Guázima*)

Arbol de las Manitas
(see *Flor de Manita*)

Arnica
Arnica

Botanical Name: *Arnica montana*

Arnica Mexicana
Camphor Weed

Botanical Names: *Heterotheca inuloides, Heterotheca* spp.
Other Names: *Falsa árnica, Arnica del país,* Telegraph Weed
Nahuatl: *Tlályetl*

Arnica montana is a wildflower native to Europe and western Asia. *Heterotheca,* or false arnica, a plant native to Mexico and southwestern United States, is put to similar use as a topical ointment or liniment. Both plants have small yellow or orange daisylike flowers.

In Mexican-American markets you are more likely to find *Arnica mexicana,* but it's very important that you know which plant you are buying if you intend to take it internally. Unless it is used in extremely diluted doses, true arnica, *Arnica montana,* can raise blood pressure and have a toxic effect on the heart. It should not be used on broken skin and causes dermatitis in some people.

It is fine to take mild teas of *Arnica mexicana,* but *this plant should also be used with caution. It should not be taken internally in large doses or for more than a few consecutive days.*

Parts Used: Entire plant and root
Properties: Anti-inflammatory, topical disinfectant, antimicrobial
Used to Treat: Wounds, hemorrhoids, bruises, toothache, sore muscles, bronchitis, stomachache, diarrhea, menstrual cramps

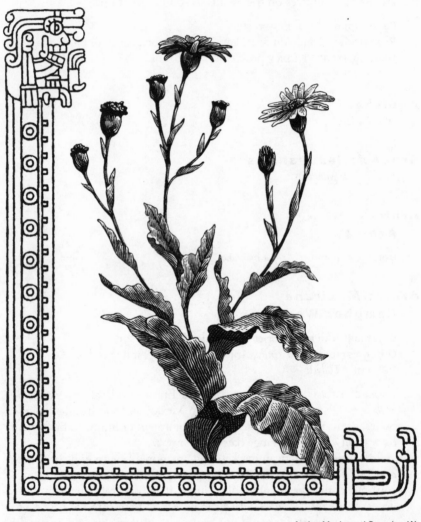

Arnica Mexicana / Camphor Weed

Ayoyote
Yellow Oleander

Botanical Name: *Thevetia thevetioides*
Other Names: *Yoyote, Narciso Amarillo,* Be Still Tree, Giant Oleander
Nahuatl: *Yoyotli*

Not really an oleander but a relative from tropical America, this small tree is very showy when in bloom, with fragrant yellow flowers that give way to fleshy green fruits. The milky sap and seeds are poisonous if ingested but can be safely used topically to make analgesic liniments and salves. The sticky sap is also applied to pimples to bring them to a head.

The Nahuatl name refers to rattles made with the seed pods, which were used in ceremonial dances. In the sixteenth century Francisco Hernández reported that indigenous Mexicans used the mashed leaves as a topical analgesic to calm toothaches.

Parts Used: Juice of the fruit, pit, seed
Property: Analgesic
Used to Treat: Arthritis, rheumatism, hemorrhoids, pimples

Azafrán
Safflower

Botanical Name: *Carthamus tinctorius*
Other Names: American saffron, false saffron

A prickly relative of the thistle, with small yellow-orange blooms topping two- to three-foot stalks, safflowers are Mediterranean natives that were introduced to the New World by the Spanish. They are cultivated for their seeds, which produce the popular oil, and are ground as a substitute for expensive saffron threads.

Part Used: Flower petal
Properties: Fever reducer

Not to be used during pregnancy or by persons with peptic ulcers or hemorrhagic diseases.

Azahares
Orange blossoms

Botanical Names: *Citrus sinensis, Citrus aurantium*
Other Names: *Azahar de Naranjo*
See also: *Naranja, Límon*

Azahar simply means "citrus blossom" in Spanish, but when used to describe a tea, it almost always refers specifically to dried orange blossoms, a popular sedative. Citrus fruits are not native to the Americas but were brought to Europe from Asia and introduced to the New World by the Spanish. Sour orange, *naranja agria (Citrus aurantium)*, which is grown for marmalades, syrups, and colognes, is often specified in herbal remedies.

Parts Used: Flower, leaf
Properties: Sedative

Azumiate
(see *Sáuco*)

Bálsamo
Tolu Balsam

Botanical Names: *Myroxylon balsamum* var. *Pereírae, myroxylon* spp.
Other Names: *Bálsamo de las Indias, Bálsamo Negro del Perú, Bálsamo de Cartagena*
Nahuatl: *Huitziloxitl*

The balsam of Tolu is a tall tree, native to central and southern Mexico. In its blooming season, it is covered with stalks of fragrant tiny white flowers. The crushed bark produces a thick balsam that is used commercially for cosmetics, perfumes, and medicines.

The Aztecs cultivated these balsam trees in their royal gardens. They made compresses with the mashed leaves to speed the healing of wounds. The balsamic sap was highly valued by the Spanish clergy who used it in sacramental ointments. Papal bulls of 1562 and 1571 forbid the destruction of balsam trees.

In his *Joyfulle Newes Out of the Newe Founde Worlde*, the sixteenth-century Spanish physician Nicolás Monardes described the way in which indigenous Mexicans collected the balsam on wax dishes held under incisions cut into the bark. Writing enthusiastically about its wondrous effect on a wide variety of ailments, he deemed this medicine with a lemony aroma and a sweet taste one of the best to come from the Americas.

Parts Used: Sap, bark, seed, leaf
Properties: Antiseptic, antibacterial, antiparasitic, speeds healing, mild laxative

May cause allergic skin reactions in some people.

Barba de Chivo
Clematis

Botanical Name: *Clematis virginiana, Clematis lasiantha, Clematis* spp.
Other Names: Virgin's Bower, Old Man's Beard
Nahuatl: *Cocotemecatl*

This pretty climber adorns trellises and arbors with its bell-shaped flowers. The Spanish name, meaning "goat's beard," was probably inspired by the fluffy white seed heads that replace the blossoms. The showy cultivated varieties are mostly natives of Asia, but wild clematis vines grow throughout the southwestern United States and Baja California, wrapping themselves around tree trunks or covering the chaparral.

In the sixteenth century, Francisco Hernández described a plant the Aztecs called *cocotemecatl,* "pungent vine," which was probably a species of *Clematis.* He reported that a handful of the crushed leaves cured dysentery and that the plant was useful for ringworm and as an aid in childbirth, although none of these remedies appears to have survived to the present day.

Part Used: Leaf
Properties: Diuretic, counter-irritant, promotes healing
Used to Treat: Headaches, sore throat, colds, skin sores, scratches

Because clematis is an irritant, it should be used with caution. Not to be used internally during pregnancy.

Barba de Maíz
Corn Silk

Botanical Name: *Zea mays*
Other Names: *Barba de Elote, Cabello de Elote, Estilos de Maíz*
Nahuatl: *Elotl*
Maya: *Ix-im*

Common, supermarket-variety corn silk makes a wonderful tea for treating cystitis. It seems to work both as an anti-inflammatory and a diuretic, so it takes care of the whole problem. It is also effective for the water retention of premenstrual syndrome and is used as a treatment for the incontinence associated with old age. Because of its anti-inflammatory properties, it is used topically to wash spider bites.

Parts Used: Silky hairs of unhusked corn
Properties: Diuretic, anti-inflammatory, antispasmodic
Used to Treat: Cystitis, incontinence, PMS, spider bites

Barbasco
Texas Croton

Botanical Names: *Croton texensis, Croton corymbulosus;* also *Discorea densiflora, Discorea floribunda*
Other Names: *Pionillo, Palillo,* Dove Weed

Barbasco is the name given to a number of plants used by indigenous Mexicans to poison fish so they'll be easy to catch. In the southwestern

United States the name may refer to a local species of *Croton*, but all the herbs called *barbasco* are toxic. If they can kill a fish, what can they do to a human? *Barbasco* is safe to use externally; just don't swallow any. It is used in ointments for inflammatory conditions such as rheumatism. Despite its potential toxicity, some people make a laxative tea with the leaves.

Texas croton is a low, silvery gray shrub with small white flowers and a nasty smell. It is used as an insecticide by burning it to fumigate a room, possibly on the theory that its smell is so foul even bugs can't stand it.

Other plants also sometimes called *barbasco* are species of *Discorea*, the "Mexican yam" that has attracted so much attention recently as a natural alternative to hormone replacement therapy for postmenopausal women.

Part Used: Leaf, fresh or dried
Properties: Analgesic
Used to Treat: Rheumatism, swollen joints, headache, earache

For topical use only. Can be toxic if taken internally.

Bejuco
(see *Tripa de Judas*)

Bellota de Sabina
(see *Enebro*)

Berro
Watercress

Botanical Names: *Nasturtium officinale* syn. *Rorippa nasturtium-aquaticum*

Common salad-variety watercress is used medicinally to stimulate the lymph system, cleanse the kidneys, and clear the throat of mucus. A watercress compress is used to reduce the inflammation of gum problems such as gingivitis.

The plant loses its potency when heated, so it should always be used fresh in salads, as a juice or cold infusion.

Parts Used: Leaf, stem
Properties: Anti-inflammatory, stimulates lymph glands and liver
Used to Treat: Kidney problems, gum problems

Boldo
Bold

Botanical Name: *Peumus boldus*

This tall tree, a native of Chile, bears clusters of white flowers that give way to an edible fruit. The aromatic leaves are used to flavor foods, and the bark was once used to cure leather. *Boldo* has been used for medicinal purposes since prehistoric times. It has become one of the more popular Mexican-American remedies, used as a tea or a compress to treat a wide variety of illnesses.

Part Used: Leaf, dried
Properties: Digestive aid, kidney cleanser, tonic after a long illness, laxative
Used to Treat: Headache, common cold, liver problems, sore muscles

Should not be used without consulting a physician by persons suffering from severe liver disease, obstruction of the bile ducts, or gallstones.

Borraja
Borage

Botanical Name: *Borago officinalis*

Borage, a native of the Mediterranean region, was brought to the Americas where it became a popular garden herb. The whole plant is very hairy, with hollow stems and large, fleshy oval leaves. Borage is used as a seasoning by the Italians, who make a very good risotto with the blue star-shaped flowers. In traditional medicine it is used in a tea to treat colds, particularly if there is cough and fever.

Parts Used: Leaf, flower
Properties: Anti-inflammatory, soothes mucous membranes, diuretic, fever reducer
Used to Treat: Fever, cough, sore throat, kidney and bladder problems

Potentially toxic in large doses. Do not use on broken skin. Not to be used by nursing mothers.

Brasil
Brazilwood

Botanical Name: *Haematoxylum brasiletum*
Other Names: Logwood, *Palo del Brasil, Palo Rojo, Palo de Tinto, Brasilillo, Marismeño*
Nahuatl: *Quamóchitl, Hoitzquánhuitl*
See also: *Tabachín*

This small tree is commonly found in Brazil, hence its name, but it also grows wild in many parts of Mexico. Rural Mexicans tint yarn for blankets with a dye made from the reddish brown bark. The bark is also used industrially to make a pigment for paint.

The Aztecs used the bark as a treatment for diarrhea. In Sonora the twigs are chewed for dental problems, and the bark is boiled to make a tea for kidney ailments and fever.

Part Used: Bark
Properties: Antibiotic, astringent, tonic
Used to Treat: Diarrhea, rheumatism

Brionía
(see *Jalapa*)

Bugambilia
Bougainvillea

Botanical Names: *Bougainvillea glabra, Bougainvillea spectabilis*
Other Names: *Camelina*

Throughout the southwestern United States and Mexico, trees, walls and rooftops are covered with the vibrant pink, red, or orange flowers of these rapidly growing climbers. The petals are usually used in combination with other herbs to make an expectorant tea for treating coughs and chest congestion.

Parts Used: Flower, leaf
Properties: Expectorant
Used to Treat: Cough, bronchitis, asthma

Cabellitos de Angel
(see *Tabachín*)

Cabello de Elote
(see *Barba de Maíz*)

Cachana
Gayfeather

Botanical Name: *Liatris punctata*
Other Name: Blazing Star

Native to the mountainous regions of Colorado and New Mexico, this flowering plant has pretty stalks of blue to purple flowers that give way to fluffy seed balls. In addition to its medicinal uses, the plant is believed to have protective powers. The roots are carried to ward off the influence of witches and the "evil eye."

Parts Used: Root, flower
Used to Treat: Sore throat, tonsillitis

Calabacita
Buffalo Gourd

Botanical Name: *Cucurbita foetidissima*
Other Names: *Calabazilla Loco, Calabacilla Amarga, Chilicoyote*
Nahuatl: *Chilicayotli*

In Mexico the seeds of this gourd, a relative of yellow squash and pump-kin, have been used for centuries to treat intestinal worms. They are eaten, either toasted or raw, on an empty stomach along with a few leaves of *yerba buena* (spearmint). The leaves and roots are also used to make a lax-ative tea, but it can be a very strong purgative.

Part Used: Seed
Used to Treat: Intestinal parasites

Calavera
(see *Cancerina*)

Caléndula
English Marigold

Botanical Name: *Calendula officinalis*
Other Names: *Mercadela, Coronilla, Virreyna Caléndula,* Pot Marigold
See also: *Cempasúchil, Pericón*

The *Calendula* genus, a native of the Mediterranean region, is the Euro-pean version of the flower we call marigold. The native American marigold, which looks very similar, belongs to the *Tagetes* genus. One of the great medieval remedies, European marigold was transplanted by the Spanish to Mexican soil.

In medieval times it was called Mary Gold, after the golden blossoms the Virgin Mary was believed to have worn in her hair. Legend had it that adulterous women would find it impossible to enter a church if even a sin-gle marigold were present. A marigold gathered in the month of August and wrapped in a bay leaf along with a wolf's tooth was thought to be an amulet so protective that no one could speak a word against the bearer.

In the second century, the extraordinary German abbess Hildegard von Bingen, who was a brilliant poet and composer as well as a pioneer-ing physician, used the blossoms to treat impetigo and skin blemishes. Marigolds were even thought to prevent the plague when steeped in wine or ale. On the battlefields of the American Civil War, marigold blossoms were pressed against wounds to stanch bleeding.

Today the essential oil of the calendula blossom is a well-regarded anti-inflammatory and an ingredient in commercial ointments. In tradi-tional Mexican-American medicine the flowers are used in infusions and salves whenever something soothing is called for.

Part Used: Flower petal
Properties: Anti-inflammatory, promotes healing, mildly antiseptic
Used to Treat: Eye infections, sore throat, fever, burns, wounds, insect bites, rheumatism, earache

Not to be used internally during pregnancy.

Campana, Campanilla
(see *Florifundio*)

Cañafistula
(see *Hojasen*)

Cañaigre
Red Dock

Botanical Name: *Rumex hymenosepalus*
Other Names: *Cañagria, Yerba Colorada*, Pie Plant, Wild Rhubarb, American Ginseng
Nahuatl: *Mámaxtl*
See also: *Lengua de Vaca*

Cañaigre grows plentifully throughout the desert regions of southwestern United States and northern Mexico. Its big, fleshy leaves and small green flowers give way to rosy, heart-shaped seed pods. The long tubers, similar to sweet potatoes or yams, are not good for eating but are high in tannin, a natural astringent. Dried and boiled they make a mouthwash for gum problems or to "tighten the teeth," a lotion to dry up pimples, and a wash for skin irritations.

Part Used: Tuber
Property: Astringent
Used to Treat: Diarrhea, sore throat, skin and gum problems

Cancerina
Mexican Heather

Botanical Names: *Cuphea aequipetala, Cuphea jorullensis, Cuphea* spp.; also *Hemiagium excelsum*
Other Names: *Yerba del Cáncer, Alcancér, Calavera, Chanclana, Yerba del Coyote*
Nahuatl: *Ayauhtona*

There are more than two hundred species of *Cuphea* in the Americas. Ninety of them are found growing wild in central and southern Mexico from Durango to Chiapas. Like its English counterpart, Mexican heather grows profusely on hillsides and in fields. The small bushy plants, covered with tiny tubular orangy-red to purple flowers, make attractive flowering garden ornamentals, and various cultivated species are sold in nurseries. The Spanish name comes from the plant's traditional use as a treatment for tumors.

Parts Used: Stem, leaf, flower
Properties: Promotes healing, anti-inflammatory, astringent
Used to Treat: Indigestion, dysentery, wounds, bruises, muscle pain

Candelilla
(see *Inmortal*)

Canela
Cinnamon

Botanical Name: *Cinnamomum zeylanicum*

This most popular spice, which comes from a tree native to Sri Lanka, is now grown in tropical climates of the Americas. The part we use in cooking is the inner bark of the young shoots, which rolls up to become the familiar cinnamon stick.

In early eighteenth-century New Spain, the Jesuit physician Juan de Esteyneffer highly valued cinnamon as a medicine. He believed that sudden blindness could be cured by chewing a stick and then blowing it into the eyes. If the ears were subjected to the same treatment, sudden deafness could also be cured. Then as now, it was used in teas for upset stomach and fever.

Part Used: Inner bark of young branches, dried
Properties: Digestive, astringent, stimulant, antimicrobial, antifungal, antiflatulent
Used to Treat: Cough, colds, fever, rheumatism, indigestion, nausea, hangover

Cantaris
(see *Trompetillo*)

Cantue, Cantuesa
(see *Salvia Real*)

Cañutillo del Llano, Cañutillo del Campo
(see *Cola de Caballo, Popotillo*)

Capitaneja
(see *Añil del Muerto*)

Capulín
Wild Cherry

Botanical Names: *Prunus serotina, Prunus capuli, Prunus virginiana*
Other Name: Black Cherry
Nahuatl: *Capolinquahuitl, Capulxihuitl*

These little cherries, along with the fruits of the prickly pear cactus, figs, and corn, were the foods that the conquistadors found to sustain them during the siege of Mexico. The trees, native to North America, have fragrant small white flowers and small but very sweet and delicious fruits that are used today in jellies and jams. The juice or fruit is baked in cakes called *capultomal.*

The leaves, which have antispasmodic and astringent properties, are infused in a tea to treat dysentery. They should be used fresh because the essential oils are very volatile and lose their potency when dried. The simmered bark is used traditionally to treat coughs and colds. An extract of the bark is an ingredient in some over-the-counter cough syrups.

Parts Used: Bark, leaf
Properties: Sedative, expectorant, antispasmodic, astringent
Used to Treat: Cough, diarrhea, fever, dysentery

The seeds can be toxic. Bark should not be used in large doses or for prolonged period of time.

Cardo Santo
Mexican Thistle

Botanical Names: *Cirsium undulatum, Cirsium mexicanum*
Other Names: *Sueldo, Chicalote*
Nahuatl: *Quauhtlatehuitzquilitl*

The Aztecs used this spiny plant with big brushlike red flowers in remedies for fevers and melancholy.

In his *Joyfulle Newes Out of the Newe Founde Worlde,* the sixteenth-century Spanish physician Nicolás Monardes told the tale of a friar whose chronic stomach distress was cured by a native Mexican doctor who prescribed drinking *carlo santo* [sic] teas at lunch and dinner. This treatment relieved the charming friar not only of his stomach pains but of his bad breath and flatulence as well. Monardes also reported that *"carlo santo"* profited women in the hard labor of childbirth when given with wine or water infused with orange blossoms and that it strengthened the gums and preserved the teeth from "eating of worms."

In traditional Mexican-American medicine, *cardo santo* is used to remedy many of these same ills. The roots are boiled to make a tea for stomach inflammation, to hasten labor during childbirth, and to quiet the pain of a toothache or earache. The roots or the flowers are used to make a tea for diarrhea. In Michoacán, a little piece of the root and a little piece of *tejocote* (Mexican hawthorn) are brewed in a tea for severe urinary tract inflammations.

Because the Spanish name for the herb means "sacred thistle," it is sometimes confused with the European holy thistle, or blessed thistle *(Cnicus benedictus)*, which has different properties.

Parts Used: Root, flower
Properties: Anti-inflammatory, astringent
Used to Treat: Diarrhea, stomach inflammation, urinary tract inflammation, toothache, earache, protracted labor in childbirth

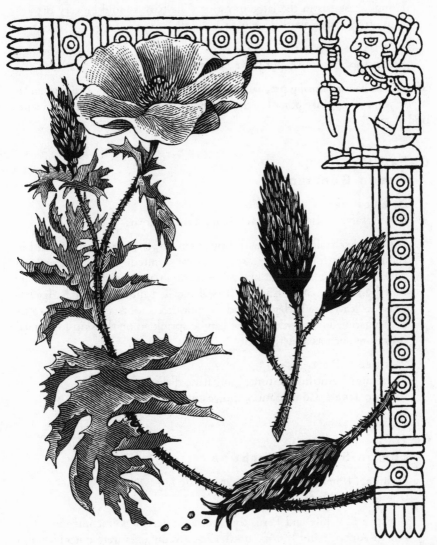

Cardo Santo / Mexican Thistle

Cáscara Sagrada
Bearberry

Botanical Names: *Rhamnus purshiana, Rhamnus californica*
Other Name: Buckthorn

Aztec healers introduced the bark of this tall shrub to the conquistadors, who were so impressed by its effectiveness that they gave it its exalted name, which means "sacred bark." The Aztecs used *cáscara sagrada* as a remedy for many ailments, but its effectiveness as a gentle laxative has kept it in constant use to this day. Many commercial laxatives sold over the counter include *cáscara sagrada* as an active ingredient. It works by stimulating peristalsis in the large intestine. The bark should be very dry because fresh bark can cause nausea.

Part Used: Bark, dried
Properties: Laxative, purgative, tonic, antibacterial

Should not be used during pregnancy, by nursing mothers, or by children under twelve years of age. Like other laxatives, it should not be used for a prolonged period of time.

Cebadilla
Green Gentian

Botanical Name: *Swertia radiata*
Other Names: Indian Caustic Barley, Deer's Horn

A tall, single stalk covered with tiny green flowers, *cebadilla* grows wild in the mountain forests of the southwestern United States and northern Mexico. Because it is used like yellow gentian as a tonic, it is commonly called green gentian in English. It is also called Indian caustic barley because its leaves are barleylike, and the powdered roots are used as a caustic purgative. The powdered root can be sprinkled on the skin for fungal infections such as athlete's foot

Part Used: Root
Properties: Antifungal, tonic, purgative, digestive
Used to Treat: Constipation, indigestion

Cedrón
Lemon-Scented Verbena

Botanical Name: *Aloysia triphylla,* formerly *Lippia citriodora*
Other Name: *Yerba Luisa*

A native of Chile and Peru, this aromatic herb was not introduced to North America and Europe until 1784. Many uses were quickly found for it. The fragrant leaves scent potpourri, bath oils, soaps, and perfumes.

They add a lemony flavor to marinades, garnish salads and cold drinks, and are preserved in jellies. The tea, hot or iced, is a favorite beverage on its own or blended with other leaves.

The little bushes add a lovely aroma to gardens and are easily grown indoors as pot herbs. It is a pretty plant with lance-shaped leaves and stalks of delicate, light purple flowers. Medicinally, it's used primarily as a soothing tea or added to a bitter herbal tea to mask the taste.

Part Used: Leaf
Properties: Soothing, sedative
Used to Treat: Upset stomach, menstrual cramps, restlessness

Cempasúchil
Aztec Marigold

Botanical Name: *Tagetes erecta*
Other Names: *Flor de Muerto*, African Marigold, American Marigold
Nahuatl: *Cempoalxóchitl*
Maya: *Ix-ti-pu*
See also: *Caléndula, Cincollagas*

Surely when the Spanish discovered the Aztec marigold they must have thought they were looking at the plant they knew as *caléndula* at home because the flowers are very similar. In fact, they are cousins—both members of the *Asteraceae* family. Both are used for medicinal purposes. The native Aztec marigold, ubiquitous in gardens on both sides of the border, has shiny dark green leaves and yellow-and-orange many-petaled flowers.

Cempasúchil was highly esteemed in pre-Hispanic Mexico for its ability to heal many infirmities. In the sixteenth century, Francisco Hernández reported that the juice of the leaves cured a variety of stomach ailments, reduced fever, and relaxed the nerves, and that the mashed leaves taken with water or wine promoted menstrual flow, urine, and sweat.

The flower was associated with sacred rituals. In his *Historia general de las cosas de la Nueva España*, Fray Bernardino de Sahagún described the Aztecs carrying armloads of *cempasúchil* in ceremonies honoring the god Huixtocíhuatl. And Mayan priests wash their hands and face with a tea of the leaves and flowers before calling the spirits. The petals of these marigolds are still used during celebrations of the Day of the Dead when they are strewn over graves and home altars.

Cempasúchil also serves a more mundane purpose in modern Mexican life. The plants are grown industrially to produce a chicken feed that is a major export. Eating the feed gives a yellow color to the skin of the chickens and to the yolks of their eggs.

Parts Used: Leaf, flower
Properties: Anti-inflammatory, antiseptic, induces perspiration
Used to Treat: Fever, stomachache

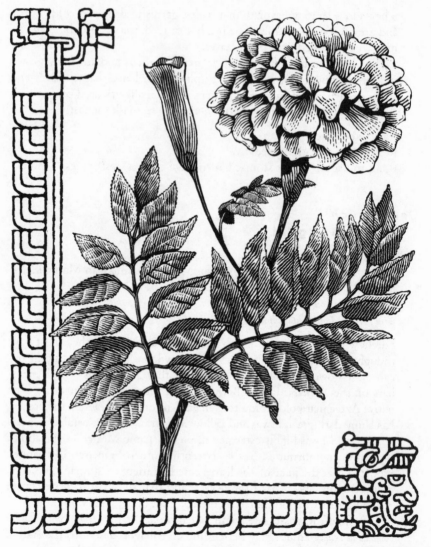

Cempasúchil / Aztec Marigold

Cenizo
Purple Sage

Botanical Names: *Leucophyllum laevigatum, Leucophyllum texanum, Leucophyllum frutescens*
Other Names: *Flor de Ceniza, Palo de Ceniza,* Chihuahuan Rain Sage, Texas Ranger, Silverleaf
See also: *Chamiso*

The desert that stretches for hundreds of miles along the United States–Mexico border is covered with all sorts of plants called "sage."

Some are related to true sage, members of the *Salvia* genus, but many are not even distant cousins. *Leucophyllum* is native to the long, dry corridor shared by Texas, and the Mexican state of Chihuahua. It is completely unrelated to *Salvia officinalis*, the common garden sage we use in cooking, which is a member of the mint family. The plant we call sagebrush in English and *chamiso* in Spanish is from yet another family, the *Compositae*, or sunflower. But if you ask a *botánica* owner what she is selling in those little packets labeled *cenizo*, she may answer simply, "It's sage."

The problem is that *cenizo* is the Spanish word for ash-colored, so any gray-leafed sagelike plant could be given that name. In Texas and New Mexico, *cenizo* often refers to some species of *Leucophyllum*. (Look for small egg-shaped gray-green leaves and perhaps a few tiny pale purple flowers.)

Parts Used: Leaf, flower
Properties: Sedative, induces perspiration
Used to Treat: Colds, fever, colic

Cerillito
(see *Trompetilla*)

Chacate
(see *Crameria*)

Chamiso
Four-Wing Saltbrush

Botanical Name: *Atriplex canescens*
Other Names: *Chamizo, Costilla de Vaca, Cenizo*
See also: *Cenizo, Chamiso Hediondo*

A low shrub with spikes of greenish flowers, *chamiso* is called saltbrush in English because it likes saline soil. Reputedly good for grazing cattle, it is also a well-regarded medicinal herb frequently found in southwestern *botánicas*. Purple sage *(Leucophyllum laevigatum)* and basin sagebrush *(Artemisia tridentata)* are also sometimes called *chamiso*.

Part Used: Leaf
Used to Treat: Fever, stomachache, diarrhea

Chamiso Hediondo
Basin Sagebrush

Botanical Name: *Artemisia tridentata*
Other Names: *Chamizo*, Big Sagebrush

This big gray-green bush, which proliferates throughout the Great Basin, is the "purple sage" immortalized by novelist Zane Grey. Its curved stems stand up like the bristles of a giant brush. The long leaves end in a scalloped tip, the three "teeth" that give the species its Latin name, *tridentata*. Both the leaves and the greenish yellow flowers, which are used to scent bath water, have a heavy camphor odor. The tea is used to ease postchildbirth discomfort.

Parts Used: Leaf, flower
Used to Treat: Rheumatism, aches, pains

Chanclana
(see *Cancerina*)

Chaparro Amargoso
Crucifixion Thorn

Botanical Names: *Castela emoryi, Castela texana, Holacantha emoryi*
Other Names: *Chaparro Amargo, Corona de Cristo*

Considered a highly effective treatment for amebic dysentery, this nearly leafless desert bush appears to be little more than a dense mass of thorns growing wild throughout the arid zones of Mexico and the southwestern United States. Its Spanish name means "bitter oak," referring to the flavor. Be warned.

Part Used: Dried bits of stem
Properties: Astringent, tonic, liver cleanser
Used to Treat: Dysentery

Chapote
(see *Zapote Blanco*)

Chayote
Vegetable Pear

Botanical Name: *Sechium edule*
Other Name: *Choyotl*

This native Mexican vine bears fruit that looks like a cross between a cucumber and a pear. Chayote were cultivated by the Maya and Aztecs, and are used in contemporary Mexican cuisine. All parts of the plant are useful. The fruit, available in some U.S. supermarkets, is an interesting addition to stews and salads. The roots are cooked like potatoes, and the leaves make a diuretic tea.

Part Used: Leaf
Properties: Diuretic
Used to Treat: Kidney disorders, high blood pressure

Chía
Sage

Botanical Names: *Salvia hispanica, Salvia columbariae*
Nahuatl: *Chianzotzolli*
See also: *Salvia*

The Aztecs used the seeds of this species of sage as food—toasted, ground into flour, and added to cooked cornmeal to make a thick drink called *chianzotzolatolí. Chía* is still used today to prepare cold beverages with lemon and sugar.

The little round black seeds, sold in markets and *botánicas,* are chewed as a digestive aid. A single seed placed in the eye before going to sleep is said to collect excess mucus.

Part Used: Seed
Used to Treat: Indigestion, eye irritations

Chicalote
Prickle Poppy

Botanical Names: *Argemone mexicana, Argemone* spp.
Other Names: *Cardo Santo,* Thistle Poppy, Mexican Poppy
Nahuatl: *Chicálotl, Chillazotl*

This Mexican desert poppy has weedy, prickly stems and leaves, big, brilliant yellow or white flowers, and thorny seed pods. The plant was sacred to Tláloc, the Aztec god of rain and water. Following the Aztec belief that certain illnesses were caused by the wrath of a displeased god, the plant was used to treat diseases considered to be water related, such as rheumatism and palsy. The physical damage caused by accidents induced by the rain god, such as being struck by lightning or nearly drowning, were also treated with Tláloc's herbs.

The Chinese who arrived in Mexico in the nineteenth century to work on the railroads, discovering that *chicalote* shared some of the properties of its relative, the opium poppy, used it to produce an opium substitute. In parts of Mexico the dry leaves are smoked as an aphrodisiac, although this practice can produce very unsexy side effects such as vomiting and diarrhea.

In traditional medicine a pinch of the ground seeds is eaten or mixed with water to make a laxative drink. An infusion of the leaves is used as a sedative. The sap, which oozes from the cut flower stems, is used as a topical analgesic.

Parts Used: Seed, leaf, sap
Properties: Sedative, antispasmodic, analgesic, laxative

Used to Treat: Skin irritations, burns, scrapes, cough, migraine headache, aches, pains

The seeds can be toxic.

Chichiquelite
(see *Yerba Mora*)

Chicória
(see *Diente de León*)

Chícura
Canyon Ragweed

Botanical Name: *Ambrosia ambrosioides* syn. *Franseria ambrosioides*
Other Name: *Yerba del Sapo*

Ragweed, the infamous blue-green bush that plagues the allergy prone with stuffy noses and runny eyes, is a remedy as well as a cause of discomfort. It is primarily used to treat "women's problems." In Sonora the leaves and roots are brewed in a tea for menstrual discomfort and the expulsion of the placenta after childbirth. Mexican Americans use an infusion of the leaves for menstrual cramps or in a vaginal douche after menstruation.

Part Used: Leaf
Used to Treat: Menstrual cramps

Chile
Various chiles

Botanical Name: *Capsicum* spp.
Other Names: *Tlachili, Chiltecpin, Max-ic*

Since pre-Hispanic times chiles have been used as a condiment and remedy. In traditional medicine they are used internally as a respiratory decongestant and externally to stimulate circulation. A little chile powder mixed with cold cream, petroleum jelly, or olive oil is a good, cheap homemade liniment. Because chiles lower the body temperature by inducing perspiration, they are eaten in hot climates throughout the world. Chile peppers contain substances that help lower cholesterol levels and reduce deposits of fat in the liver. Chile is a general stimulant, aiding digestion and blood circulation. Eating chiles is also thought to release endorphins, and capsaicin, which gives chiles their hot bite, may help ward off cancer.

Part Used: Fruit, fresh or dried
Properties: Counter-irritant, anti-inflammatory, induces perspiration

Chile Puerco
(see *Alegría*)

Chincona
(see *Quina Roja*)

Chinita
(see *Diente de León*)

Chirimoya
Custard Apple

Botanical Name: *Annona cherimola*
Other Names: *Chirimolla, Cheremoya*
Nahuatl: *Quahtzapotl*

Lumpy, dark yellow, ugly but delicious *chirimoya* fruit is sold as a delicacy in some U.S. supermarkets. The tree, a native of the Peruvian Andes, was transplanted to Mexico in the sixteenth century by the Spanish. One or two of the seeds, crushed and fried in a little lard to make an ointment, is an old remedy for ringworm and other skin infestations.

Part Used: Leaf
Properties: Astringent, disinfectant
Used to Treat: Sore muscles, diarrhea, ringworm

Seeds may be toxic if ingested.

Chuchupate
(see *Oshá*)

Chuparrosa
(see *Espinosilla, Muicle*)

Cilantrillo
(see *Hinojo*)

Cilantro
Coriander

Botanical Name: *Coriandrum sativum*

The name *cilantro* is used to describe the leaves of the same plant whose seeds are called "coriander." Cilantro is such a staple of Mexican cuisine that it is hard to believe it's not indigenous to the Americas but a native of southern Europe and Asia. It is used in Indian curries and Thai soups as well as in Mexican salsas.

It is one of the most ancient medicinal herbs. Coriander seeds were found in Egyptian tombs, and we know that the plant has been used medicinally at least since the time of Hippocrates. In traditional Mexican-American medicine the leaves or seeds are used to make a soothing bedtime tea for children and a mouthwash to treat gum disease. In Mexico a tea of coriander seeds and rose petals is used as a remedy for menstrual discomfort. Because of its strong but pleasant flavor it is often used to mask the taste of bitter herbal teas.

Part Used: Seed
Properties: Sedative, soothing, diuretic
Used to Treat: Inflamed gums, earache, menstrual cramps

Cinco Negritos
Common Lantana

Botanical Name: *Lantana camara*
Other Names: *Siete Negritos, Yerba de Cristo, Confiturilla, Alfombrilla,* Shrub Verbena
Nahuatl: *Piltzinteuhxochitl*
Mayan: *Pet-k'in*

"Common" is the right word to describe this spreading shrub. It's a ubiquitous weed, growing wild along roadsides in the warm climates of Mexico and the southern United States. But it's a pretty plant, covered from spring to fall with delicate flowerheads composed of tiny yellow and orange blossoms. Cultivated varieties are useful in gardens for their hardiness and rapid growth, and the leaves have a lovely minty aroma. *Cinco negritos,* five little black ones, may have gotten its name from the little black berries that were used medicinally in pre-conquest Mexico.

Toxic varieties of the plant poison animals who graze on it, so it is probably a bad idea to take it internally, although some people use it as a stomach tonic. Used topically, it serves as a remedy for symptoms of rheumatism, muscle pains, snakebites, and insect stings. The Maya apply the powdered dried leaves to itchy skin or wash the skin with an infusion of the leaves.

Part Used: Leaf
Properties: Antibacterial, antivenom
Used to Treat: Rheumatism, snakebite, insect bites

For topical use only. Can be toxic if taken internally.

Cirián
Gourd Tree

Botanical Name: *Crescentia alata*
Other Names: *Cuatecomate, Tecomate, Ayal,* Calabash

These small trees, native to the warmer regions of Mexico, bear large hard-shelled green fruit. The leaves have a strange cross shape that gave the Spanish missionaries the idea that the tree had some religious significance. In traditional medicine the fruit pulp is used to make a poultice for wounds and an expectorant syrup for coughs; the leaves are boiled to make a tea for diarrhea, and the shells are carved or painted to make vases, drinking cups, and maracas.

Parts Used: Leaf, fruit pulp
Properties: Expectorant, emollient, astringent
Used to Treat: Diarrhea, cough, chronic asthma

Not to be used during pregnancy.

Clavo
Clove

Botanical Name: *Syzygium aromaticum* syn. *Eugenia aromatica*

The common clove, used in cooking and baking, is the flower bud of a pretty tree native to Southeast Asia, Australia, and Africa. The eighteenth-century Jesuit physician Juan de Esteyneffer reported that the tree was cultivated in New Spain and that the flower buds were used as an aphrodisiac and stomach tonic as well as a condiment. He also recommended cloves in remedies for wounds, ulcers, and vomiting. Today it is used as an effective emergency anesthetic for toothache, and a tea of cloves in combination with other soothing herbs is a remedy for nausea.

Part Used: Flower bud, dried
Properties: Anesthetic, antiseptic, digestive
Used to Treat: Toothache, nausea

Coahtli
(see *Palo Azul*)

Cocolmeca
Greenbrier

Botanical Name: *Phaseolus* spp.
Other Names: *Gotoko, Cocolmecate,* Kidney Bean Vine
Nahuatl: *Etl, Ayacotli*
See also: *Zarsaparilla*

Cocolmeca and *zarsaparilla* refer to similar climbing vines, and even botanists disagree about which is which, so the two herbs routinely get confused. The name *cocolmeca* refers to plants of the *Smilax* genus in some parts of Mexico, while in others it refers to some species of *Phaseolus.* In the United States, *cocolmeca* will usually be some species of *Phaesolus,* commonly known in English as greenbrier.

Part Used: Root
Used to Treat: Kidney pain, infertility

Cola de Borrego

(see *Santa Rita, Siempreviva*)

Cola de Caballo
Horsetail

Botanical Names: *Equisetum arvense, Equisetum hyemale, Equisetum* spp.
Other Names: *Cañutillo del Llano, Carricillo,* Shave Grass, Scouring Rush

A perennial plant found growing near water in higher elevations, *Equisetum* is one of the oldest plants on the planet, dating back to prehistoric times. The surviving species are dwarf versions of the enormous reedlike ferns that once covered the earth. In rural Mexico the plant's leafless stalks are tied together to make scouring brushes used in cabinet-making to finely sand wood, and by housewives for cleaning pans. Children make whistles from pieces of the hollow stems. The herb was once considered a remedy for gonorrhea because it relieved the burning urination that is a symptom of that disease. Divergent cultures throughout the world use it to treat kidney problems. The plant is high in silicone and makes an effective diuretic. *Cola de caballo* is one of the most popular Mexican-American home remedies, carried by most *botánicas* and markets. It has a mainstream following as well, and many health food stores now sell a commercially packaged "horsetail tea." A 1994 Spanish study of the effects of this and other herbs commonly used to relieve kidney stones concluded that in addition to its diuretic and antiseptic qualities, it may contain saponins (toxic substances that occur in plants) which could have some solvent action.

Part Used: Stem
Properties: Diuretic, antiseptic, astringent
Used to Treat: Kidney stones, water retention, wounds, skin diseases

Excessive use should be avoided, particularly during pregnancy, and by young children.

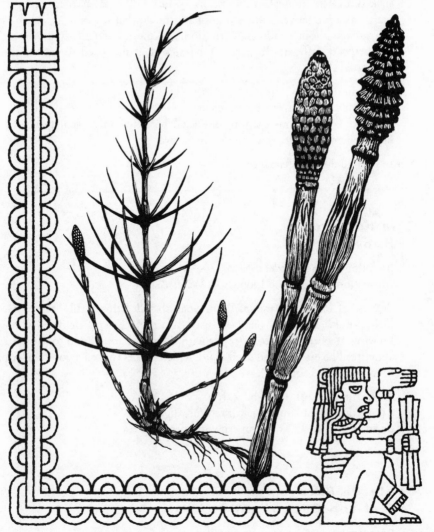

Cola de Caballo / Horsetail

Cola de Iguana

(see *Alacrán*)

Cola de Zorra

Botanical Name: *Perezia* spp.
Other Names: *Pipichaguí, Mata Gusano, Yerba del Zopilote*
Nahuatl: *Coatl, Coapatli*

The Aztecs called this plant "snake medicine" (*coapatli*—from *coatli,* snake; *patli,* medicine) because they used the roots in a remedy for

103

snakebites. (Its Spanish name means "skunk tail.") Today it is used primarily as a purgative. Some studies have shown that it can be effective as a laxative without producing irritation, making it particularly useful for hemorrhoid sufferers. In parts of Mexico it is also used to induce the menstrual flow.

Part Used: Root
Properties: Purgative, abortifacient
Used to Treat: Constipation, intestinal parasites, menstrual problems, male venereal problems, wounds, sores, fever

Not to be used during pregnancy.

Cola de Zorrillo
Hop Tree

Botanical Name: *Ptelea trifoliata*
Other Names: Swamp Dogwood, Wafer Ash

Because of its unpleasant smell, the Spanish called this shrub "tail of the little skunk." The fruit has been used as a replacement for hops in the brewing of beer, and a tonic made with the root bark is used to promote appetite. The essential oil is alkaloid, which makes the tea a good remedy for acid indigestion.

Parts Used: Leaf, fruit, bark, root
Properties: Anti-inflammatory, tonic, digestive
Used to Treat: Lack of appetite, indigestion

Colita de Rata
Flat-top Buckwheat

Botanical Name: *Eriogonum fasciculatum*

The *colita de rata*, which in Spanish means "little rat's tail," belongs to a large genus of shrubs native to the mountains and deserts of western North America. This species has silvery white leaves and white or red flowers. In Sonora the entire plant is used to treat colds. In New Mexico, it is brewed to make a topical wash for wounds and a tea for various irritations involving the mucous membranes. The flowers are used to make a soothing diuretic tea for urinary tract inflammations, and the stems are used to clean the teeth.

Parts Used: Entire plant
Properties: Diuretic, astringent, antiseptic
Used to Treat: Bladder problems, wounds, diarrhea, sore throat

Colorín
Whistle Tree

Botanical Names: *Erythrina americana, Erythrina flabelliformis*
Other Names: *Pito, Chilicote, Zompantil,* Coralbean
Nahuatl: *Patolli, Tzompatli*
Maya: *Chacmolcé*

Indigenous Mexicans carved amulets from the stems of this spiny little tree, and they tossed its red beanlike seeds in a game similar to dice. Although the beans are toxic enough to make an effective rat poison, Aztec holy men ingested them to induce a state of hypnotic clairvoyance. The bark has such a strong paralyzing property that Aztec fishermen threw it into the water in order to stun their prey.

The flowers, on the other hand, are perfectly edible and can be cooked as a vegetable or added to salads. The medicinal properties are in the roots, which are believed to lower fevers, and in the juice of the stems, which is squeezed onto scorpion stings. In Sonora some people eat the seeds as a treatment for diarrhea, but don't try this at home.

Part Used: Root
Used to Treat: Fever

Bark and seeds can be toxic if taken internally.

Collálle
(see *Escoba de la Víbora*)

Comino
(see *Yerba del Indio;* also refers to the spice cumin)

Consueldo
(see *Jarilla, Sueldo*)

Contrayerba
Arizona Poppy

Botanical Names: *Kallstroemia californica, Kallstroemia grandiflora;* also *Dorstenia contrajerva*
Other Names: *Varbulilla,* Caltrop, California Poppy, Summer Poppy
Nahuatl: *Coanenepilli*
Maya: *Kabal-hau*

Contrayerba is just a way of saying "antidote" in Spanish, so a number of plants have been given that name. In Mexico the name often refers to a species of the genus *Dorstenia*, used as an antidote for snakebites and a remedy for skin diseases and fevers. *Contrayerba*, or *contrayerba blanco* (see below), can also refer to the of root of a species of *Psoralea*. Other plants called *contrayerba* include some species of milkweed *(Asclepias stetosa)* and bouvardia *(Bouvardia terniflora).*

This *contrayerba*, the Arizona poppy *(Kallestroemia)*, is a pretty little plant cultivated in gardens for its bright orange flowers that give way to prickly fruits. It is not really a poppy, but it looks a bit like one. The genus is found from the southern United States to Argentina.

Parts Used: Root, peeled and powdered
Property: Astringent
Used to Treat: Eye irritations, sore throat, swollen gums, diarrhea

Contrayerba Blanco
Drake's Foot

Botanical Names: *Psoralea pentaphylla, Psoralea glandulosa, Psoralea tenufolia*
Other Name: Prairie Potato
Nahuatl: *Yolochiahitl*

These native American shrubs have needlelike leaves and white or blue-and-white flowers that look almost like sweet peas. The root is curved and, when peeled, reveals a white flesh so that it resembles a foot. Because the root of *Psoralea glandulosa* contains a substance that can provoke vomiting, it was used as an antidote to food poisoning, but in smaller doses it does not have this effect. The powdered root should be mixed with cool water, not brewed as a tea.

Part Used: Root, peeled and powdered
Used to Treat: Food poisoning, fever, chills, stomach flu

Copal
Elephant Tree

Botanical Names: *Bursera jorullensis, Bursera microphyllia, Bursera* spp.
Other Names: *Palo Mulato, Torote, Cuajiote*
Nahuatl: *Copalquahuitl, Xochicopal, Tepecopalquahuitl*

The curvy branches of this strange-looking tree are covered with a papery bark, so they look a little like an elephant's trunk. With its twisted foliage spreading low to the ground, the tree stands out against the stark desert landscape of southwestern Arizona, Baja California, and Sonora.

The Nahuatl name *copalquahuitl* means "incense tree." The aromatic resin, which oozes from the stems when they are broken, has been used as a ceremonial incense since before the conquest of Mexico, and it continues to be used today in Day of the Dead ceremonies and in the spiritual cleansings called *limpias.*

The resin was also an Aztec remedy. In the sixteenth century, Fray

Bernardino de Sahagún wrote that a little ground *copal*—the size of a small fingernail—added to water and drunk only once a day on an empty stomach would cure diarrhea.

In traditional medicine today, the brewed bark, or a cold infusion of the mashed leaves, is considered a remedy for fever. The gum, bark, and leaves are used for toothache, animal bites, sore throat, and catarrh; and a tea of the leaves or the leaves and bark is used as a tonic to fortify the immune system.

Parts Used: Bark, resin, leaf
Properties: Expectorant, analgesic, astringent, antibiotic, tonic
Used to Treat: Fever, gum problems, scorpion stings, spider bites

Copalchí
Copalchí

Botanical Name: *Coutarea latiflora;* also *Croton niveus, Croton tiglium, Croton reflexifolius*
Other Names: *Copalchín, Quina Blanca, Falsa Quina, Garañona*
Nahuatl: *Chichiquáhuitl*

This small semitropical tree with large white flowers is native to Mexico. The Aztecs used it in infusions to treat infectious diseases such as typhoid fever and as a general tonic. The tree's leaves are somewhat breast-shaped, and they exude a milky sap. According to an Aztec religious myth, the souls of babies who died while they were still nursing were sent to a special heavenly waiting room where they nursed on *copalchí* leaves until their souls could be reincarnated. In Tabasco the juice of the leaves was actually used to augment an inadequate supply of mother's milk.

Both the leaves and the bark are used medicinally, but the bark is more potent. It is used to treat symptoms of adult-onset diabetes and may have some hypoglycemic effect. Some species of *Croton* are also called *copalchí* and are used to treat fever.

Parts Used: Leaf, bark
Properties: Diuretic, hypoglycemic
Used to Treat: Kidney ailments, diabetes, fever

Coralillo
(see *Pingüica*)

Cordoncillo
(see *Hoja Santa*)

Cosahui
(see *Crameria*)

Cota
Navajo Tea

Botanical Name: *Thelesperma gracile*
Other Names: *Té de Cota, Indian Tea, Hopi Tea*

A wildflower with blue-green leaves, yellow-gold flowers, and a pleasant aroma, *cota* grows plentifully throughout the desert Southwest. Native Americans use it to cleanse the kidneys and soothe the stomach. It is also a favorite of Spanish New Mexicans who use it as a diuretic. It makes a refreshing iced tea, flavored with cinnamon or mint.

Parts Used: Leaf, flower
Properties: Diuretic, kidney cleanser, digestive

Crameria
Rhatany

Botanical Names: *Krameria lanceolata, Krameria cytisoides, Krameria parviflora*
Other Names: Cramer Plant, *Chacate, Cosahui, Mezquitillo*
Aztec: *Chacatl*

These low shrubs with red or purple flowers and spiny fruit grow wild in parts of Mexico, Baja California, and the southwestern United States. The indigenous people of Baja California used the plant as a red dye for wool and leather, and as a remedy for diarrhea and dental problems. It is still a staple of Mexican and Mexican-American traditional medicine and can be found in markets and *botánicas*. The flowers and stems are sometimes used in remedies, but the root bark is more potent.

Parts Used: Root, bark, flower with stem
Properties: Astringent, decreases mucous secretions, tonic
Used to Treat: Diarrhea, hemorrhoids, sore throat, sore gums, sore nipples

Cuachalalate
Juliana

Botanical Names: *Juliana adstringens, Amphyterigum adstringens*
Other Names: *Cuachalate, Cuachalalote*
Nahuatl: *Cuauchalalaltl*

In the eighteenth century the Spanish throne sent prominent botanists on extensive expeditions to study the plant life of the New World. Stopping at a primitive rural inn at Carrizal, near Mexico City, Arcadio Pineda and his fellow scientists met a native healer who taught them to wash the wounds of their horses with the bark of *cuachalalate*. Mexican Americans today use the herb to cleanse their own wounds as well, in a tea combined with *Arnica mexicana*. The herb has astringent properties that make it a useful cleanser. It's also included in remedies for infertility and stomach problems.

Part Used: Bark
Property: Astringent
Used to Treat: Wounds, gum problems, infertility

Cuahulote
(see *Guázima*)

Cuajiote
(see *Copal*)

Cualaldulce
(see *Palo Azul*)

Cuasia
Quassia

Botanical Name: *Quassia amara*

Cuasia is a tree native to Jamaica that has found its way into traditional Mexican medicine. *Botánicas* and markets in Mexican-American neighborhoods sell packets of white wood chips cut from its branches. The chips are used to make a bitter-tasting tonic that is used primarily to aid digestion and increase appetite. As a tonic it is considered especially useful in building up the bodies of those who are wasting away from a debilitating disease. As a digestive aid it is particularly recommended for those whose digestion has been ruined by a major emotional upset such as anger.

Parts Used: Wood chips
Properties: Tonic, digestive, appetite stimulant
Used to Treat: Amebic dysentery, *bilis*, indigestion, lack of appetite

Not to be used during pregnancy.

Cuautecomate
(see *Cirián*)

Culantrillo
Maidenhair Fern

Botanical Names: *Adiantum pedatum, Adiantum* spp.

Culantrillo is a familiar fern popularly cultivated as a house plant. A native of moist, warm climates throughout North America and Asia, it has been used since the time of the ancient Greeks as a remedy for chest congestion. In eighteenth-century New Spain the Jesuit Juan de Esteyneffer used the fern to make a syrup or tea for colds and bronchitis as well as other ailments. Today the dried leaves are sold in *botánicas* primarily as a remedy for menstrual cramps.

Part Used: Leaf
Properties: Emollient, expectorant
Used to Treat: Menstrual cramps, bronchial congestion, sore throats

Not to be used during pregnancy.

Curucumín
(see *Pericón*)

Damiana
Damiana

Botanical Names: *Turnera diffusa* var. *aphrodisiaca, Turnera ulmifolia*
Other Names: Mexican Damiana, *Agüita de Damiana, Yerba del Pastor, Pastorcita*

This fragrant flowering shrub is one of the most popular Mexican-American medicinal herbs. It is used to treat all kinds of sexual dysfunction from impotence to frigidity and infertility—although its effectiveness has yet to be scientifically proven.

The ancient Mexicans used it as a tonic to increase the appetite and as a digestive aid, but today it is better known as a love potion for temporary male impotence caused by "overdoing it" or excessive drinking.

Because it is such a popular cure for a hangover, it's a little ironic that the plant is also used to flavor a liquor made in Guadalajara called Damiana.

Parts Used: Leaf, stem
Properties: Diuretic, aphrodisiac, anti-inflammatory, antidepressant, tonic
Used to Treat: Chronic bed-wetting, hangover, impotence

Long-term use may interfere with the body's ability to absorb iron. Not to be used during pregnancy.

Datilla
(see *Palmilla*)

Diente de León
Dandelion

Botanical Name: *Taraxacum officinale*
Other Names: *Chicória, Chinita,* Wild Endive

This common weed tenaciously plagues lawns and gardens, but it redeems itself as a useful food and medicine. An Arab medicinal herb, it was brought to the Americas by the Spanish. In the United States we can probably blame several other European nationalities as well for importing it to our shores. Both the English and Spanish names are derived from the French *dent-de-lion,* or lion's tooth, referring to the toothy-edged leaves. Because of its diuretic qualities, the French also call the weed *pissenlit,* which means wet-the-bed. It is an especially good choice for treating water retention because it contains a lot of potassium.

Mexican Americans take an infusion of the roots to "purify the blood." The leaves, rich in chlorophyll and vitamin A, iron, calcium, potassium, and niacin, are nutritious when added to salads or cooked up as dandelion greens. The flavor becomes increasingly bitter as the leaves mature, so it's best to choose young greens, picked before the flower buds appear. Soaking and boiling them improves the taste. Dandelion wine, a rural favorite in the nineteenth century, is made with the flowers.

Parts Used: Stem, leaf, root
Properties: Diuretic, anti-inflammatory, laxative, appetite stimulant, digestive, tonic
Used to Treat: Liver and kidney congestion, skin eruptions, water retention

Persons suffering from gallstones should not use this herb without consulting a physician.

Dolár

(see *Eucalipto*)

Doradilla
Resurrection Plant

Botanical Names: *Selaginella lepidophylla, Selaginella cuspidata*
Other Names: *Siempreviva, Flor de Piedra, Flor de Rana*
Nahuatl: *Yamanquitexóchitl O, Tapanmimixtin*
Maya: *Much-K'ok*

This little fernlike plant lives in rocky terrains where the climate is wet. It is called the "resurrection" plant because its leaves curl up into balls when the plant is thirsty and then are resurrected, unfurling after the rains. The leaves can also be dried and kept in an airtight jar for years, then "resurrected" by soaking in water.

Doradilla is sold in Mexican-American markets as a remedy for kidney stones and *mal de orín,* urinary tract irritation. It is also among the many herbs used to treat intestinal parasites.

Parts Used: Entire plant
Properties: Diuretic
Used to Treat: Urinary tract disorders, kidney stones, intestinal parasites

Dormilón

(see *Verbena*)

Durazno
Peach Tree

Botanical Name: *Prunus persica*
Other Names: *Hojas de Durazno*

The leaves and bark of the peach tree can be used medicinally. The trick is to find some that haven't been sprayed with chemical insecticides. An infusion of the leaves is used as an expectorant tea and as a douche for menstrual troubles. The bark is boiled to make a tea for treating fever. An infusion of the leaves and flowers is one of the many folk remedies for intestinal parasites.

Parts Used: Leaf, bark
Used to Treat: Intestinal parasites, asthma, menstrual difficulties, fever

Not to be used during pregnancy.

Encino
Oak

Botanical Names: *Quercus gambelii, Quercus* spp.
Other Names: *Encino Blanco, Encino Rojo, Roble*
Nahuatl: *Ahoatl, Ahoapatli*

In Mexico two Spanish names are used to describe the oak tree: *encino* and *roble. Los encinos* are generally smaller trees with smaller leaves and acorns than *los robles.*

Oak bark has been used since the time of the Aztec empire as an effective remedy for diarrhea. The bark has also been shown to be effective in the treatment of inflammatory skin problems and mouth inflammations.

Parts Used: Bark, acorn, leaf
Properties: Astringent, antiseptic, expectorant
Used to Treat: Diarrhea, dandruff, mouthwash, skin abrasions

Not to be used over large areas of damaged skin, such as weeping eczema. Consult a physician if diarrhea persists for more than three or four days.

Enebro
Common Juniper

Botanical Names: *Juniperus communis, Juniperus* spp.
Other Names: *Bellota de Sabina, Sabino, Guata,* Drooping Juniper, Mexican Juniper

These small evergreen trees and spreading shrubs, so familiar in the United States and parts of Mexico, are also found in higher altitudes in temperate climates throughout most of the world. For centuries the trees have been used to make medicine and magic. In the Middle Ages, juniper branches were burned in hearths to drive away evil spirits and ward off the plague. The berries, which are still used to flavor gin, were once boiled to make an aphrodisiac brew. Mexican Americans use *enebro* to treat kidney problems.

Parts Used: Berry, foliage, bark
Properties: Diuretic, urinary antiseptic, tonic, digestive
Used to Treat: Painful urination, colds, fever

Not to be used during pregnancy.

Eneldo
Dill

Botanical Name: *Anethum graveolens*

A native of the Mediterranean area and southern Russia, dill came to the New World with the Spanish. It has been used medicinally since the time of the ancient Egyptians. It is a useful remedy for intestinal gas. Mexican Americans feed mild doses of "dill water" to colicky babies.

Parts Used: Leaf, stem
Properties: Sedative, antiflatulent
Used to Treat: Excess stomach gas, poor lactation in nursing mothers

Not to be used in therapeutic doses during pregnancy.

Epazote
American Wormseed

Botanical Name: *Chenopodium ambrosioides* syn. *Teloxys ambrosioides*
Other Names: *Epasote, Ipazote, Pazote,* Quinoa, Mexican Tea, Goosefoot
Nahuatl: *Epázotl*
Maya: *Lukum-xiu*

Epazote grows wild in the forests of Morelos and the trash-strewn empty lots of East L.A. But it is most easily found in kitchen gardens where pots or patches of the herb are lovingly cultivated for use in both cooking and curing. The Aztecs, who had developed a very sophisticated and refined cuisine, used *epazote* to flavor a variety of dishes. Today it is a staple of Mexican-American cooking, spiking many a pot of beans with its tangy flavor. The whole plant has a pungent aroma; its name comes from the Nahuatl word for skunk, *épatl.*

The Aztecs also used *epazote* medicinally, to treat asthma and dysentery. Mexican Americans consider the herb the first line of defense against intestinal parasites, administering to adults, children, and animals alike. *Epazote* tea is also used for menstrual cramps, fever, and chills.

Parts Used: Entire plant, root
Properties: Antifungal, vermifuge, anti-inflammatory, induces perspiration
Used to Treat: Intestinal roundworms and hookworms, delayed menstruation, dysentery, fever, indigestion, stomach gas

Because it is considered a cardiac stimulant, the herb should not be taken by persons with cardiovascular disease. Not be used during pregnancy.

Epazote del Zorillo
Wormseed

Botanical Names: *Chenopodium graveolens, Chenopodium foetidum* syn. *Teloxys graveolens*
Other Names: *Yerba del Zorillo, Yerba del Perro*

This plant is another species of *epazote,* with a more pungent aroma. (*Zorillo* is the Spanish word for skunk.) Both species are used for menstrual problems and to expel worms. This species is also used to treat nervousness and depression.

Parts Used: Entire plant
Properties: Vermifuge, sedative
Used to Treat: Diarrhea, vomiting, delayed menstruation

Not to be used during pregnancy.

Escoba Ancha
(see *Yerba del Pasmo*)

Escoba de la Víbora
Snake Broom

Botanical Names: *Gutierrezia sarothae, Gutierrezia* spp.
Other Names: *Collálle, Yerba de la Víbora, Yerba de San Nicolás,* Turpentine Bush, Snakeweed
See also: *Yerba de la Víbora*

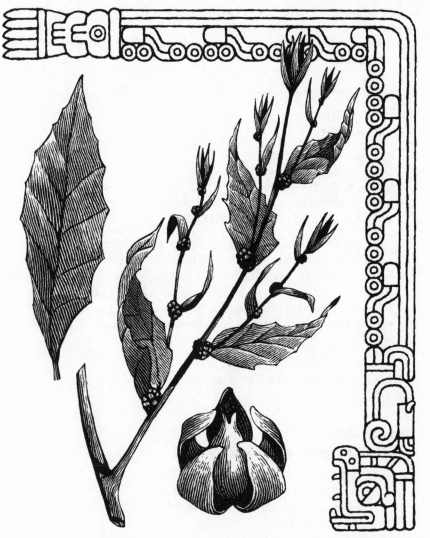

Epazote / American Wormseed

There are many plants with this name. *Escoba* is the Spanish word for broom, so anything that might look vaguely broomlike could be called an *escoba de* something. In the southwestern United States, *escoba de la víbora,* broom of the snake, usually refers to some species of *Gutierrezia,* a low bush with yellow flower heads. But throughout Mexico a number of plants are called *escoba de víbora* or *yerba de la víbora,* presumably because they have all been used to treat snakebites.

115

Parts Used: Branch, flower head
Properties: Anti-inflammatory
Used to Treat: Arthritis, hemorrhoids, excessive menstruation, vaginal inflammation

Espino Blanco
Cockspur

Botanical Name: *Acacia cornigera*
Other Names: *Cornezuelo, Carnizuelo, Velo de Novia, Velo de Viuda*
Nahuatl: *Huitzmamaxalli*
Maya: *Subin-Che*
See also: *Acacia, Huizache, Uña del Gato*

This graceful shrub is native to the tropical Americas and widely cultivated in gardens. Its drooping branches are laden with clusters of yellow, white, or lilac flowers and yellow berries. The lilac varieties are sometimes called *velo de viuda*, widow's veil, while the white are called *velo de novia*, bride's veil. But the plant's more popular name is less poetic. *Espino blanco* refers to the sharp, curved thorns that protect its branches.

Parts Used: Fruit, flower
Properties: Stimulant, fever reducer

Espinosilla
Hummingbird Flower

Botanical Name: *Loeselia mexicana*
Other Names: *Chuparrosa, Huachichile, Huizache*
Nahuatl: *Huitzitzilxóchitl, Cuahuitztzilxóchitl*
See also: *Muicle, Huizache*

The bright red, tube-shaped flowers of this shrubby plant attract hummingbirds. Its Aztec name comes from the Nahuatl words for hummingbird (*huitziz*) and flower (*xóchitl*). The Aztec Herbal of 1552 includes a formula for a restorative footbath using *huitzitzilxóchitl*.

Today a weak infusion of the leaves and flowers is used as a tea to combat fever. In stronger doses it is used as a purgative and can cause nausea. The Aztecs made soap with *espinosilla*, and some people still use it as a shampoo in the belief that it may prevent hair loss. A rinse made with the mashed leaves gives the hair a nice shine.

Parts Used: Leaf, stem, flower
Properties: Purgative, fever reducer

Estafiate
Mugwort

Botanical Names: *Artemisia mexicana, Artemisia filifolia, Artemisia ludovicana, Artemisia frigida*
Other Names: *Istafiate, Ajenjo del País, Romerillo,* Wormwood, Silver Sage, Basin Sagebrush, Sand Sagebrush
Nahuatl: *Iztáuhyatl*
Maya: *Zizm*
See also: *Ajenjo, Altamisa*

According to Aztec religious-medical practice, *estafiate* belonged to the realm of Tláloc, the god of water and rain. It was used to remedy illnesses

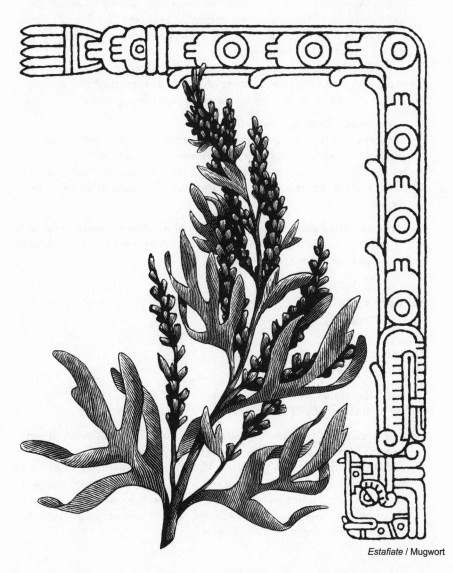

Estafiate / Mugwort

that were considered to have been caused by the gods of this realm, illnesses that involved having too much water in the body. Epilepsy, leprosy, and gout were all illnesses both caused and cured by the water gods. The Aztec Herbal of 1552 listed several remedies using the herb, including one for those who had been struck by lightning.

Estafiate was used in celebrations honoring Tláloc and other water deities. During these rituals children were fanned with the herb to protect them from intestinal parasites. An infusion of the herb is still used to treat intestinal worms today.

Many species of the *Artemisia* genus are known as *estafiate.* They are all little gray-green herbs, no taller than about a foot or two. A species sometimes called long-leaf *estafiate* (*Artemisia mexicana*) has slender lance-shaped leaves. Another species (*Artemisia ludovicana*) has scalloped-edged leaves like a dandelion. An herb known in English as silver sage (*Artemisia frigida*) has feathery leaves. Another feathery-leafed species (*Artemisia absinthium*) is known as both *estafiate* and *ajeno.*

Estafiate, one of the most important of the Mexican-American medicinal herbs, is used to treat a variety of common ailments. Since it is more potent if used fresh, it is often cultivated in kitchen gardens.

Parts Used: Leaf, stalk with flower
Properties: Diuretic, digestive, expectorant, antiseptic (root), induces perspiration, antispasmodic, anti-inflammatory, analgesic
Used to Treat: Fever, asthma, cough, kidney stones, stomach gas, menstrual cramps, intestinal parasites, sprains and bruises, arthritis, hemorrhoids

Estafiate is considered perfectly safe and beneficial if taken in moderation, but it may be toxic if taken in high doses or for a prolonged period of time. Not to be used by pregnant or nursing women.

Estramonio

(see *Florifundio*)

Eucalipto
Eucalyptus

Botanical Name: *Eucalyptus globulus*
Other Names: *Dolár,* Gum Tree

The eucalyptus tree, an Australian native, is widely cultivated in semitropical Mexico. The leaves are used to make various remedies for coughs and colds, although now that Vicks VapoRub has become so widely used by Mexicans and Mexican Americans, it has taken the place of *eucalipto* in many households. In parts of Mexico a tea of eucalyptus leaves is used to decongest the liver, bladder, or kidneys, as a treatment for gastritis, and for symptoms of adult-onset diabetes.

Part Used: Leaf
Properties: Expectorant, liver detoxifier
Used to Treat: Cough, bronchitis, asthma

Not to be used internally in the presence of serious liver disease or inflammation of the gastrointestinal tract and bile ducts.

Fitolaca
Pokeweed

Botanical Name: *Phytolacca americana*
Other Names: Pokeroot, Pokeberry, Inkberry

An effective purge, this plant can be toxic if taken improperly. At one time it was thought to be effective against breast cancer, and the tincture of the fruit is still used by homeopathic practitioners to treat cysts. Some herbalists use the dried root to treat swollen glands. *Fitolacas* are evergreen shrubs, native to the tropics. Their large leaves and clusters of white flowers give way to deep purple-blue berries.

Parts Used: Root, leaf, berry
Properties: Cathartic, laxative, anti-inflammatory

Can be toxic in large doses and should be used with caution.

Flor de Manita
Handflower Tree

Botanical Name: *Chiranthodendron pentadactylon*
Other Names: *Arbol de las Manitas, Mano de Dragón*
Nahuatl: *Macpalxóchitl*

The flowers of this remarkable tree look like decorative cuffs from which slender five-fingered hands emerge, and the flat velvety leaves are so large, they are used to wrap food into packages. The trees were prized by the Aztecs. They were among the rare specimens in the legendary imperial gardens of Huaxtepec, gifts sent to Motecuhzoma II by the cacique of Cuetlaxtla.

The Aztecs used the bark and leaves in a remedy for swelling and pain in the genital organs. The flowers, which the Aztecs used to treat heart ailments, are still sold in the markets of Mexico and the southwestern United States as a heart tonic.

The trees are cultivated for ornamental purposes in frost-free climates in the United States and Mexico.

Parts Used: Flower, fresh or dried; juice of the bark and leaf
Properties: Sedative, analgesic, anti-inflammatory
Used to Treat: Cardiac and nervous system disorders

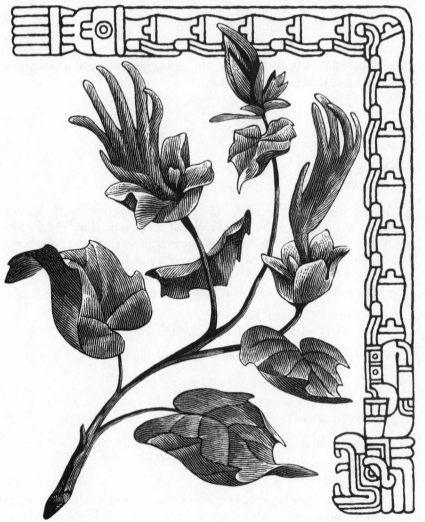

Flor de Manita / Handflower Tree

Flor de Muerto
(see *Cempasúchil*)

Flor de Pascua del Monte
(see *Nochebuena*)

Flor de San Pedro
(see *Tronadora*)

Flor de Santa Rita
(see *Santa Rita*)

Flor de Tila
(see *Tila*)

Flor de Veinte
(see *Pericón*)

Florifundio
Angel's Trumpet

Botanical Names *Datura stramonium; Datura arborea, Datura* spp.
Other Names: *Floripondio, Toloache, Trombita, Estramonio, Campana, Campanilla,* Jimson Weed, Thorn Apple
Nahuatl: *Tolohuaxihuitl, Toloatzin (Datura innoxia) Tlapatli (Datura stramonium)*
Maya: *Tohkú, Mehen-x-toh-ku*

Florifundio is one of the most fascinating of all the traditional medicinal plants used by Mexicans and Mexican Americans. Applied topically, it's a powerful analgesic, providing relief to those who suffer from the pain of arthritis. Taken internally, it can be a dangerous hallucinogen with a long history of ritual use.

Datura species grow in warm climates throughout most of the world. The name of the genus is believed to be derived from a Sanskrit word, *d'hustúra*. Legend has it that in ancient India a band of thugs used a species of the plant *(Datura metel)* to drug their victims, whom they then robbed and strangled as sacrifices to the goddess Kali. Another species was used by the Algonquin tribe in rites of passage from puberty. Witches in medieval Europe used the plant they called "thorn apple" *(Datura stramonium)* in love potions to put their victims into a swoon. In toxic doses the plant paralyzes the central nervous system, inducing a deep comalike sleep, so a thorn apple may well have inspired the poisoned apple fed to Snow White by the wicked witch in the famous Grimm Brothers' fairy tale.

The Aztecs used *Datura* species for both medicine and magic. They called the curved trumpet-shaped flowers *toloazin,* which means "bended head." Aztec soothsayers used the plant to transport themselves into an altered state in which they could visit ancestors, locate stolen property, and divine the future. Criminals were sometimes given infusions of the plant before they were executed in order to alleviate their suffering. Fray Bernardino de Sahagún reported in the sixteenth century that the herb was an effective fever medicine and that it banished pain when used as an ointment. The flowers placed under a pillow were used to induce sleep, and prolonged inhaling of their aroma can, in fact, cause a trance-like state.

All species of *Datura* have tubular flowers and the spiny fruits that earn them the name thorn apple. *Datura stramonium* is a low, common weed with irregularly toothed leaves. Cultivated species of *Datura* can grow to the size of small trees. With their graceful, large white or pastel flowers, they adorn the front lawns of homes throughout the southern United States and Mexico and were among the prized blossoms of the Aztec imperial botanical gardens. The leaves are foul-smelling, especially when crushed, but the flowers themselves, which close in the heat of midday, are sweetly aromatic.

Like its cousin, belladonna, also a member of the nightshade family, *Datura* contains atropine as well as scopolamine, both poisonous hallucinogens when taken in large doses. All parts of the plant are toxic if taken internally. The Internet abounds with messages from teenagers reporting the unfortunate results of *Datura* experimentation, and there have

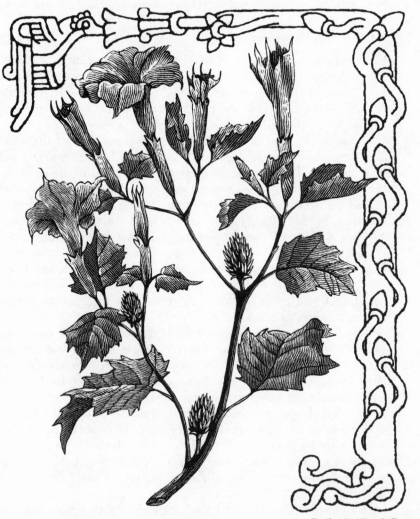

Florifundio / Angel's Trumpet

been cases of fatalities. But used topically as a liniment or salve, it's safe enough and can be extremely helpful in alleviating all sorts of aches and pains.

Parts Used: Leaf, flower, seed
Properties: Analgesic, anti-inflammatory, antispasmodic
Used to Treat: Arthritis, asthma, hemorrhoids, sciatica, pimples, boils, insect stings

This plant is for external use only! Discontinue use if dry mouth, dilated pupils, or blurry vision occur.

Fresno
Evergreen Ash

Botanical Names: *Fraxinus udhei, Fraxinus cuspidata, Fraxinus berlandieriana*

A tea of the leaves or bark and root of these trees is used as a laxative. Because the leaves are considered poisonous to rattlesnakes, some hikers are known to fill their boots with them to avoid being bitten. If they are unlucky enough to be bitten anyway, the leaves are used as a poultice to treat the bite.

Parts Used: Leaf, bark, root
Properties: Tonic, laxative, astringent, diuretic, fever reducer

Garañona
(see *Copalchí, Santa Rita*)

Geranio
Geranium

Botanical Name: *Pelargonium* spp.

The *Pelargonium* genus encompasses nearly three hundred species including the common pot geranium. All the popular scented-leaf geraniums, such as rose, apple, lemon, and peppermint, are members of the *Pelargonium* genus.

The *Pelargonium*, natives of South Africa, were naturalized in Europe and the Americas during the seventeenth century. In the nineteenth century the leaves were popularly used in jellies, baking, and wine making. Many of the traditional Mexican-American remedies are identical to those prescribed by Victorian herbalists. Because of its astringent quality, it was used to treat diarrhea and dysentery. One species is actually called *Pelargonium antidysentericum!*

Parts Used: Leaf, root
Property: Astringent
Used to Treat: Diarrhea, headache, sores, wounds

Girasol
Sunflower

Botanical Name: *Helianthus annus*
Other Names: *Mirasol, Flor de Añil*
Nahuatl: *Acahuale*

The sunflower, now grown as a crop throughout Europe and the Americas, is native to Mexico and Peru where it was used in rituals honoring the sun god. Although some herbals list it as an astringent, Mexican Americans use it primarily as an anti-inflammatory to treat arthritis and sore muscles.

Parts Used: Leaf, stem
Property: Anti-inflammatory
Used to Treat: Arthritis, sore muscles, fever

Gobernadora
Chaparral

Botanical Name: *Larrea tridentata*
Other Names: *Hediondilla, Goma de Sonora,* Creosote Bush

This tall bush is one of the most plentiful inhabitants of the desert. It grows in all the arid areas of Mexico and the southwestern United States. Sometimes planted ornamentally in desert gardens, its yellow flowers give way to fuzzy white fruits resembling cotton balls. The smooth olive green leaves exude a nasty, shiny resin that keeps predators away. This sticky resin is used in folk crafts, as a glue to mend pottery, and as a coating to waterproof baskets. In 1792 the Spanish naturalist José Longinos Martínez observed in his journal that the natives of Baja California used *gobernadora* to induce abortions, to bring on delayed menstruation, and as aid in the expulsion of afterbirth.

Modern herbalists extol the virtues of this desert bush. It is considered a powerful weapon against infection and a useful tea in clearing the lymph system.

Part Used: Leaf
Properties: Analgesic, diuretic, decongestant, expectorant, antiseptic, antiamebic, antioxidant, antiviral, antibiotic, deodorant
Used to Treat: Skin abrasions, insect bite, ringworm, rheumatism, urinary tract problems, body odor

In 1992 four people who were taking large doses of the herb in capsule form developed hepatitis. The resulting scare caused the Herbal Products Association, responding to a press release by the United States Food and Drug Administration, to issue a letter to its members recommending that the sale of the herb be temporarily suspended. After further studies, no scientific basis for the warning was discovered and it was rescinded in 1995.

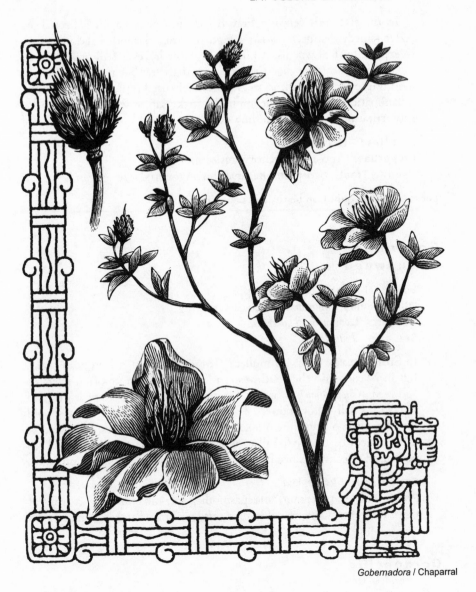

Gobernadora / Chaparral

Golondrina
Spurge

Botanical Names: *Euphorbia prostrata, Euphorbia* spp.
Other Names: *Yerba de Golondrina, Pegahueso, Picachli*
Nahuatl: *Memeya*

There are hundreds of species of *Euphorbia,* many of them low plants with tiny flowers that sprawl across the desert floor. Like its cousin, the poinsettia, the stems of *golondrina* exude a poisonous sticky white sap.

In the sixteenth century; Fray Bernardino de Sahagún collected an Aztec remedy that used *golondrina* roots to treat a distended abdomen and to expel intestinal worms. An infusion of the leaves is still used to treat inflammations of the digestive tract and diarrhea, but it can be toxic if used improperly. The infusion is more safely used topically to treat skin inflammations. Some people apply the sticky sap to warts, but it can be very irritating to the surrounding skin.

Part Used: Leaf
Properties: Anti-inflammatory, antiseptic
Used to Treat: Scorpion bite, snakebite, vaginitis, sores, wounds

For external use only. Can be toxic if taken internally.

Gordolobo
Cudweed

Botanical Name: *Gnaphalium* spp.
Other Names: *Manzanilla del Rio,* Everlasting
Nahuatl: *Tzompotónic, Tlacochichic*
See also: *Punchón*

In Spain *gordolobo* refers to mullein *(Verbascum thapsus),* a European plant. But in Mexico and the southwestern U.S., *gordolobo* more often refers to cudweed *(Gnaphalium),* a native American bush with velvety leaves and stalks of small yellow flowers. If you buy the herb packaged, it should look like little puffy white blossoms with yellowish centers. This *gordolobo* is the remedy of choice for all sorts of respiratory tract problems and has been used effectively since pre-Hispanic times to treat coughs and colds.

Parts Used: Flower, leaf
Properties: Expectorant, antispasmodic, anti-inflammatory, astringent
Used to Treat: Coughs, colds, bronchitis, asthma, diarrhea, hemorrhoids

Gordoncillo
(see *Hoja Santa*)

Gotuko
(see *Cocolmeca*)

Granada
Pomegranate

Botanical Name: *Punica granatum*

The pomegranate tree and its remedies came to Mexico from Spain. Pomegranate seeds have been used since the time of the ancient Greeks to expel intestinal tapeworms. The bark of the tree or the root bark is also used for this purpose, but it can cause nausea, a nasty side effect. The rind of the fruit, which is high in tannic acid, makes a good astringent treatment for sore throat and mouth sores. Mexican Americans treat diarrhea in small children by giving them spoonfuls of a syrup made with pomegranate juice and sugar.

Part Used: Fruit rind
Property: Astringent
Used to Treat: Diarrhea, sore throat, intestinal parasites

Should be used in moderation. Overdoses can cause vomiting. Not to be used by pregnant or nursing women.

Guaco
Rocky Mountain Bee Plant

Botanical Names: *Cleome serrulata, Mikanie guaco*
See also: *Yerba del Indio*

Guaco is an example of the confusion that can result when people from various parts of Mexico get together in the United States. If your family came from southern Mexico, your *guaco* is likely to be *Mikanie guaco*, a semi-tropical tree whose mashed leaves have been used since pre-Hispanic times as a topical anesthetic for painful snakebites, spider bites, and scorpion stings. If your family is from Morelos, you may think of another plant as *guaco*—*Aristolochia*, a flowering vine that is called both *guaco* and *yerba de la víbora*. The *guaco* most likely to be found in the southwestern U.S. is native to the border states of Chihuahua and Sonora. It is *Cleome serrulata*, a common flowering wild herb. Its flowers are notorious for attracting bees, and its leaves are used to remedy bee stings!

Part Used: Leaf
Used to Treat: Skin irritations, insect bites

Guarico
(see *Sáuco*)

Guayaba
Guava

Botanical Name: *Psidium* spp.
Other Name: *Guayabilla*
Nahuatl: *Xaxócotl*
Maya: *Pici*

The Aztecs used the leaves and bark of the guava tree in remedies for dysentery and scabies. In his book *Joyfulle Newes Out of the Newe Founde*

Worlde, the sixteenth-century Spanish physician Nicolás Monardes reported that the indigenous Mexicans used the leaves for washing swollen feet. All those remedies are still recommended in Mexican markets and *botánicas* today.

Parts Used: Leaf, bark, root
Property: Astringent
Used to Treat: Diarrhea, dysentery, wounds, scabies, sore feet

Guayacán

Botanical Names: *Guaicum coulteri, Guaiacum sanctum, Guaiacum officinale*
Other Names: *Palo Santo, Palo del Muerto, Lignum Vitae*
Nahuatl: *Matlaquáhuitl*

When the Spaniards first sent *guayacán* back to Europe, it was proclaimed a cure for syphilis. Columbus and his crew allegedly brought the disease back to Europe from the West Indies, although this theory is now very much in dispute. In his *Joyfull Newes Out of the Newe Founde Worlde,* the Spanish physician Nicolás Monardes tells the story of a sailor who caught the "poxe" from keeping company with an "Indian" woman. His native servant miraculously cured him with the waters derived from boiling down this medicinal wood, and his symptoms were never to recur unless, as Monardes warns, he made the mistake of returning to "tumble in the same bosom where he tooke the firste."

The powdered resin or a tincture, sometimes sold under the name *lignum vitae,* is used in traditional medicine today to treat fever, rheumatism, and water retention.

Parts Used: Bark, wood, resin
Properties: Diuretic, expectorant, antiseptic, induces menstruation and perspiration
Used to Treat: Arthritis, fever, liver problems, sore throat, bronchial congestion

Can have a laxative effect if taken in large doses. Not to be used during pregnancy.

Guázima
Pricklenut

Botanical Names: *Guazuma tomentosa, Guazuma ulmifolia*
Other Names: *Cuahulote, Guasima, Huasima,* West Indian mulberry
Nahuatl: *Ahiya, Cuauhólotl*
Maya: *Aquiche, Pixoy*

Guázima grows along streams and arroyos on both the Atlantic and Pacific coasts of Mexico. It's a bush or small tree with long, oval, serrated-edged leaves, similar to those of an elm tree. The fragrant pale green or cream-colored flowers give way to thorny black fruits that rural Mexicans eat and feed to livestock. Because the fruits are considered to have a tonic effect, they are fed to people recovering from a long illness or suffering from anemia. In Sonora the fruit, flowers, and bark are used for digestive disorders, kidney problems, and fever.

Parts Used: Bark, twig, leaf, fruit
Properties: Antibacterial, diuretic, emollient, astringent, tonic
Used to Treat: Diarrhea and other gastrointestinal infirmities, skin sores and eruptions, bronchial problems, water retention

Hamula
(see *Prodigiosa*)

Hediondilla
(see *Gobernadora*)

Hediondo
(see *Chamiso*)

Higueroa
Common Fig

Botanical Name: *Ficus carica*
Other Name: *Amate*
Nahuatl: *Amatl, Tepe-Amatl, Texcal-Amatl*

The Aztecs painted their important codices on a paper called *amatl,* made with the bark of the fig tree. Each year the subject states were required to deliver thousands of pounds of *amatl* paper to the Aztec capital of Tenochtitlán.

Because the paper was used in religious ceremonies, it was banned by the Catholic Church during the colonial era. But remnants of the old religious traditions have survived in parts of rural Mexico, where *higueroa* bark paper cut into the shapes of crops is planted along with the seeds, an offering to ensure a good harvest. And *brujas,* witches, use the paper for sorcery, making *amatl* paper dolls of a love object or an enemy.

Artisans in the state of Guerrero use brown *amatl* paper as a canvas for the colorful paintings of flowers, animals, and scenes of country life that have become popular souvenirs sold in tourist shops and markets.

The *higueroa* tree is also used medicinally. The rubbery sap is applied topically to scorpion stings, boils, and other skin afflictions such as fungus or ringworm, and it can be used as an emergency bandage to protect wounds. The dried leaves are smoked to treat asthma, and the fruit is eaten for its laxative effect.

Parts Used: Leaf, sap
Properties: Antiseptic, laxative

Higuerilla
Castor Bean Plant

Botanical Name: *Ricinus communis*
Other Name: *Ricino*
Nahuatl: *Asiixa'a*
Maya: *Xcoch*

This tall plant is cultivated as a source of castor oil *(aciete de ricino)*. Red or yellow flowers grow in clusters and give way to the prickly seeds from which the oil is made. A dose of castor oil—or simply a few of the seeds—is popularly used as a follow-up to an herbal treatment for intestinal parasites. The leaves of the tree are also used to make poultices that are placed on the chest for congestion, cough, or fever. In Morelos, this poultice is also placed on the abdomen to treat the acute intestinal distress known as *empacho*. The leaves, which are believed to have an anti-inflammatory property, are used any place that hurts—swollen joints, bruises, and boils.

Part Used: Leaf
Properties: Laxative, anti-inflammatory
Used to Treat: Constipation, colds, fever, bruises, abscesses, neuralgia

Hinojo
Fennel

Botanical Names: *Foeniculum vulgare, Foeniculum officinale*
Other Names: *Hinojo de Castillo, Cilantrillo*

In the Middle Ages, sprigs of *hinojo* were hung over doors to keep away the evil spirits. The seeds, which were considered a hunger suppressant, were eaten by the poor when they had nothing else or on Catholic fasting days. Some people will still tell you that the seeds are an aid in weight loss, while others drink an infusion of fennel to stimulate the appetite.

Mexican Americans use the herb to treat digestive disorders. The infusion appears to be an effective antispasmodic, a remedy for menstrual cramps and baby colic. In Morelos and Oaxaca, fennel tea is used to promote lactation in nursing mothers.

Parts Used: Leaf and flower
Properties: Antispasmodic, mild diuretic, antiflatulent
Used to Treat: Digestive disorders, intestinal gas, menstrual cramps

Not to be used in therapeutic doses during pregnancy.

Hoja Santa
Hoja Santa

Botanical Names: *Piper auritum, Piper sanctum*
Other Names: *Acoyo, Momo, Cordoncillo, Yerba Santa*
Nahuatl: *Mecaxóchitl, Xalquáhutl, Tlanepaquélitl*
See also: *Yerba Santa*

There are more than a thousand species in the *Piper* genus, including ordinary black pepper, the East Indian betel nut known as *kava kava*, and a Peruvian aphrodisiac called *matico* after the Spanish conquistador who brought news of it to the Old World. Some fifty-seven species of the genus are indigenous to Mexico, so it's likely that a variety of plants get packaged with the *hoja santa* label.

The Aztecs called the plant "rope flower" (*mecaxóchitl: meca*, rope; *xóchitl*, flower) because it resembles a little cord. It was one of the herbs used to flavor the chocolate drink reserved for the exclusive enjoyment of the Aztec nobility. And it was used for magical purposes as well. Travelers wore little bags around their necks filled with protective herbs, including *hoja santa.*

Mexican Americans use *hoja santa* primarily in remedies for respiratory afflictions, sore throats, and colds. In southern Mexico it is used as an anti-inflammatory for skin irritations, as a soothing vaginal douche, and to increase the flow of milk in nursing mothers. In the state of Veracruz, *hoja santa* leaves are used to give a peppery flavor to tamales and meat dishes.

Part Used: Leaf
Properties: Expectorant, digestive, diuretic, sedative
Used to Treat: Chest congestion, sore throat, asthma, aches, pains, indigestion

Hojasen
Senna

Botanical Names: *Senna* spp., *Cassia fistula, Cassia amara, Cassia covesii, Cassia tomentosa (retama)*
Other Names: *Cañafistula, Sen, Té de Sena, Retama,* Shower Tree, Monkey Pod Tree
Nahuatl: *Ecapatli, Xiuhecapatli*

These shrubs or small trees with beautiful sprays of delicate pastel flowers are native to most tropical climates throughout the world. The ancient Greeks, the medieval Arabs, and the Aztecs all used infusions of some species of *Cassia* leaves as a laxative.

Mexican Americans know various species of *Cassia* as *té de sena, hojasen,* or *retama,* referring to the leaves, or as *cañafistula,* which refers to the twigs or seed pods. A mild infusion of the leaves or a boiled tea of the twigs or pods is traditionally used both as a laxative and as an anti-inflammatory vaginal douche. Senna is an active ingredient in Ex-Lax and other over-the-counter laxative products sold in drugstores today.

Parts Used: Leaf, twig, seedpod
Properties: Laxative, purgative, anti-inflammatory, increases flow of gastric juices

Should not be used in the first trimester of pregnancy. Should not be used continuously for more than a week.

Huachichile
(see *Espinosilla*)

Huele de Noche
Night-Blooming Jessamine

Botanical Names: *Cestrum nocturnum, Cestrum* spp.
Other Names: *Yerba del Perro*
Nahuatl: *Piploxóchitl, Pipiloxíhuitl*
Maya: *Ak'ab-yom*

This ornamental native Mexican bush is cultivated in gardens. Its name refers to the slender trumpet-shaped flowers that open at night, exuding a beautiful sweet scent. When the bushes are in bloom, the aroma in the air can be almost overwhelmingly sensuous. The berries that follow are considered poisonous. In traditional medicine an infusion of the leaves, together with other plants, is used to treat epilepsy.

Part Used: Leaf
Property: Antispasmodic

Huizache
Sweet Acacia

Botanical Names: *Acacia farnesiana, Mimosa farnesiana*
Other Names: *Guisache, Palo Huisache, Binorama*, Cassia flower, Cashaw
Nahuatl: *Huaxin*
Maya: *Xkantiriz*
See also: *Acacia, Espino Blanco, Uña de Gato*

This wild Mexican shrub with thorny stems and clumps of fragrant yellow flowers grows plentifully in the Sonoran desert and in tropical and subtropical climates throughout Mexico. It is cultivated ornamentally in gardens both in the Americas and in southern Europe where it is also grown commercially for its flowers, which are used in perfumes.

Huizache has been used since pre-Hispanic times as a food and a dye, and in the manufacture of perfume. Fray Bernardino de Sahagún reported that the Aztecs considered the edible seedpods an aphrodisiac. Today the plant is used medicinally to treat bladder problems and as a topical antiseptic. Like other species of the *Acacia* genus, the herb is soothing to the mucous membranes. The astringent fruit is used to treat dysentery.

Parts Used: Entire plant
Properties: Diuretic, astringent, anti-inflammatory
Used to Treat: Sore throat, wounds, skin and gum problems

Incienso
Brittle Bush

Botanical Name: *Encelia farinosa*
Other Names: *Rama Blanca, Yerba del Vaso, Palo Blanco*

The Spanish dubbed this little shrub *incienso* when they discovered that its resinous stems could be burned as incense. It grows wild in the deserts of Arizona, southern California, and northwestern Mexico, and several species are cultivated for ornamental use. In the spring the bushes are covered with yellow daisylike flowers, but they lose their glamour as the summer progresses and the silvery leaves fall off. In his early eighteenth-century medical text, the Jesuit physician Juan de Esteyneffer included *incienso* in more than fifty remedies, many of which are still in use today.

Parts Used: Young stem, leaf, sap
Properties: Analgesic, expectorant, induces perspiration
Used to Treat: Gum problems, toothache, fever, arthritis

Inmortal
Milkweed

Botanical Names: *Asclepias asperula, Asclepias* spp.
Other Names: *Yerba del Indio, Candelilla, Lichens,* Candlelit, *Yamato, Raíz de Pleurisy,* Antelope Horns, Pleurisy Root
Nahuatl: *Tlalacxoyatl, Tlalayotli, Tlatlacoctic*
See also: *Yerba del Indio*

The *Asclepias* genus is a group of weeds common throughout much of the United States and northern Mexico. Most of them are low to the ground with long, oval leaves. Small flowers bloom in the summer months, followed by seedpods. The various species are called *inmortal* because the plant grows again from the root with seeming immortality. It is also called *raíz de pleurisy* because of its use as a remedy for chest congestion. The Aztec Herbal of 1552 recommended the root as a purgative and used it in a remedy for chest congestion. Fray Bernardino de Sahagún reported that the indigenous Mexicans used it as a laxative. The root of the plant is still used for both these purposes today.

Some elderly people take a little of the root sprinkled in a glass of cool water as a morning tonic. Sniffing the powder causes sneezing, a remedy for stuffy nose.

Parts Used: Root, milky sap
Properties: Expectorant, purgative, tonic
Used to Treat: Colds, chest congestion, kidney problems, delayed menstruation

Not for use during pregnancy or in conjunction with cardiac medications.

Jalapa
Mexican Morning Glory

Botanical Name: *Ipomoea purga*
Other Names: *Raíz de Jalapa, Brionía, Michoacán,* Jalap Root
Nahuatl: *Chichicamolli, Tlanoquiloni*
Maya: *Xtabentum*
See also: *Tumba Vaqueros*

The roots of these tropical morning glories have been used as purgatives since pre-Hispanic times. The seeds are hallucinogenic. Aztec priests used them to induce a trancelike state in which they believed they could contact the spirits of the dead and predict the future.

The Spanish called the herb *mechoacán* since it was first discovered growing plentifully in the state we now call Michoacán, or *jalapa,* after the city of Jalapa in the state of Vera Cruz. In his book *Joyfulle Newes Out of the Newe Founde Worlde,* the sixteenth-century physician Nicolás Monardes tells the story of a Franciscan friar who fell gravely ill in New Spain shortly after the conquest. The local Aztec lord, who had befriended the friar, brought his personal physician to treat the poor man. The friar, thinking that he was at death's door and had nothing to lose, agreed to try the Aztec doctor's remedy, a little powdered *mechoacán* root in pulque liquor. After drinking this remedy, the friar purged so much that he immediately began to feel lighter, and his condition improved with each passing day.

As this joyful news was passed from friar to friar and across the seas to Madrid, the root was embraced as a miracle cure and renamed the Rhubarb of the Indias, replacing the Rhubarb of Barbary as the favorite purge of the day. The root eventually became so popular that it was exported to Europe in great quantities and sold at such a premium that fortunes were made in the purge business.

Jalapa, still considered a useful laxative, is an ingredient in some over-the-counter products sold in pharmacies today.

Part Used: Root
Property: Purgative
Used to Treat: Intestinal parasites

Not to be given to young children or nursing mothers. Not to be used for an extended period of time. A potentially strong purgative.

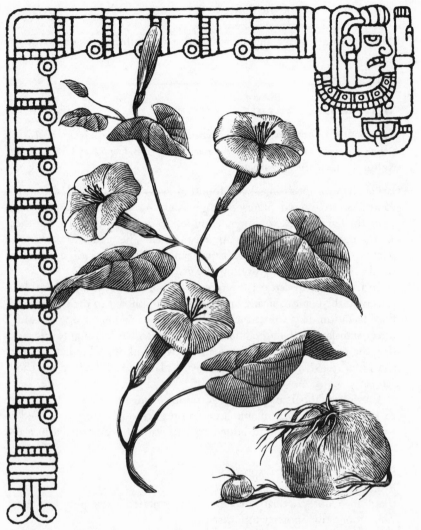

Jalapa / Mexican Morning Glory

Jamaica
Hibiscus

Botanical Name: *Hibiscus sabdariffa*
Other Names: *Flor de Jamaica, Tulipán*

The ornamental hibiscus is a tropical shrub native to the Caribbean (hence its name in Spanish), Central and South America, Florida, and southern Mexico. This species is distinguished by its red stems and pink to purplish red blossoms. Mexican restaurants serve a delicious and refreshingly cool red *jamaica* tea that is also used as a diuretic and is thought to help lower fevers. In Sonora the flowers as well as the roots and bark are used to make a wash for eye infections, sores, and wounds.

Part Used: Calyx of the flower
Properties: Diuretic, emollient
Used to Treat: Fever, digestive disorders, eye infections, sores, wounds

Jarilla
Willow Groundsel

Botanical Names: *Senecio salignus* syn. *Barkleyanthus salicifolius, Senecio flaccidus*
Other Names: *Yerba del Caballo, Veneno de los Perros, Consueldo, Chilca Atzóyatl*
Nahuatl: *Itzcuinpatli, Azumiatl*

Jarilla is a low, spreading shrub found growing along roadsides from the southwestern United States through Mexico and Central America. It bears the familiar yellow flowers common to many wild shrubs, but these are distinguished by a particularly nasty smell. The plant's English name refers to common groundsel, a European species that is such a voracious weed it seems to literally swallow the ground.

In the sixteenth century, Hernández reported that indigenous Mexicans used the plant topically on tumors and applied it to the breast to induce lactation. It is sometimes called *veneno de los perros,* or dog poison, a direct translation of its Nahuatl name, *itzcuinpatli.* According to Hernández, the powdered plant was actually used to kill dogs. He laments that sheep and pigs who grazed on the wild plant were killed by the thousands.

Obviously, this is not a plant you want to ingest. Modern uses relate to *jarilla's* topical anti-inflammatory properties. The infusion is used to wash irritated eyelids and added to bathwater for arthritic aches and pains.

Parts Used: Fresh leaf, sprout
Property: Anti-inflammatory
Used to Treat: Arthritis, rheumatism, irritated eyes, pimples, sores, chest congestion, postpartum distress

For external use only. Toxic if taken internally.

Jarita
(see *Sáuz*)

Jazmín
Mexican Mock Orange

Botanical Name: *Philadelphus mexicanus*
Other Name: *Mosqueta*
Nahuatl: *Acuilotl*

This fragrant evergreen shrub is not related to true Asian jasmine, but its creamy white blossoms have a similarly sweet aroma that is reminiscent of orange blossoms. The Aztecs used the fragrant blossoms in garlands and distilled them to make a cologne. They crushed the leaves in pulque liquor to make a remedy for adult colic and used the leaves as a plaster. In the sixteenth century, Francisco Hernández reported that this remedy was effective "beyond belief" in dissolving tumors. Today an infusion of the flowers is taken to treat nervousness and melancholy.

Part Used: Flower
Properties: Sedative, digestive

Jengibre
Ginger

Botanical Name: *Zingiber officinale*
Other Names: *Ajenjibre, Jenjibre*

A native of Asia, cultivated in tropical countries, *jengibre* has been adopted by Mexicans and Mexican Americans as a flavoring and a remedy. Some people consider it more effective than Dramamine in combating motion sickness, and the spice adds flavor to many herbal infusions. It is also used to combat fever.

Part Used: Root
Properties: Stimulates appetite and circulation; induces perspiration
Used to Treat: Stomachache, gas, indigestion, colds, nausea, fever

Not to be used during pregnancy or in the presence of gallstones.

Jojoba
Jojoba

Botanical Names: *Simmondsia chinensis, Simmondsia californica*
Other Names: *Cohobe,* Goat Nut, Deer Nut, Quinine Plant

A popular ingredient in commercial shampoos, jojoba is also used medicinally. It is a venerable desert plant with a life expectancy of up to one hundred years. An erect shrub with leathery leaves, its flowers give way to the bitter-tasting brown nuts from which jojoba oil is produced.

In his eighteenth-century medical text, Juan de Esteyneffer claimed the oil was a cure for all sorts of cancer, a notion that persisted for some time. In Sonora the oil is still used to treat wounds, as it was in Esteyneffer's day, and in remedies for water retention, eye irritation, and sore throat. In Baja California, where jojoba bushes grow plentifully along the highways, the oil is used as a hairdressing.

Parts Used: Leaf, seed

Properties: Anti-inflammatory, emollient, soothes mucous membranes

Used to Treat: Asthma, emphysema, sore throat, tonsillitis, pharyngitis, vaginitis, hemorrhoids, stomach ulcers, oily skin conditions, dandruff

Lantén
Common Plantain

Botanical Name: *Plantago major*

Other Names: *Llantén, Planten, Pastorcito,* Broad-leafed Plantain

Nahuatl: *Acaxílotl, Totoncapatli*

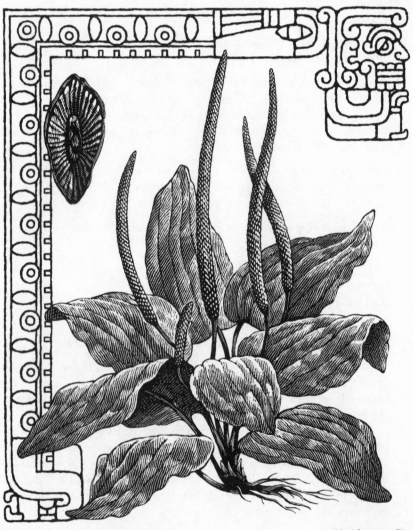

Lantén / Common Plantain

Not to be confused with the banana-like plantain, this is a low shrub with broad, fuzzy oval leaves and tiny brown and white flowers clustered at the ends of long stalks. Of the species growing wild in Mexico and the southwestern United States, several are natives while others are escaped garden plants brought to Mexico from Chile, Argentina, and Peru by the Spanish. One species, *Plantago psyllium*, produces the seeds we call psyllium, a high fiber food that was part of the Aztec diet and is the active ingredient in "colon cleansers" sold in health food stores today.

Parts Used: Leaf, seed
Properties: Anti-inflammatory, emollient, promotes healing, laxative
Used to Treat: Dysentery, wounds, burns, bruises, insect bites, canker sores, eyes and throat, inflammation, headache, vaginal irritation

Laurel
Bay Leaf

Botanical Names: *Laurus nobilis, Litsea glaucescens*

In the sixteenth century when the Spanish began to examine the flora of the New World, they occasionally came across a tree or plant that looked so much like something they knew back home, they gave it the same name. Such is probably the case with this shrub, which would explain why the leaves of the European laurel (*Laurus nobilis*) and a similar North American native (*Listea glaucescens*) are both called laurel and can be used interchangeably in cooking and traditional medicine. Both plants have since been classified as members of the Laurel family, although they do not belong to the same genus.

In some parts of Mexico the leaves of either plant are used as a tea for colic and are added to the bathwater for an invigorating soak.

Part Used: Leaf
Property: Astringent
Used to Treat: Sore throat, colic

Lechuguilla
(see *Maguey, Palmilla*)

Lengua de Buey
(see *Salvia Real*)

Lengua de Vaca
Yellow Dock

Botanical Names: *Rumex crispus, Rumex mexicanus, Rumex pulcher*
Other Names: *Yerba Colorado, Raíz Colorado*, Curly-leaf Dock
Nahuatl: *Atlinan, Axixpatlicóztic*
See also: *Cañaigre*

Lengua de vaca is a common weed found throughout most of the world. It's a low herb with long curly leaves and clusters of flowers giving way to green seeds that turn red as they mature. The shape and reddish color of the root must have reminded somebody of a *lengua de vaca,* a cow's tongue.

The Aztecs called the plant *atlinan,* "its mother is water," because of its proclivity for growing in streambeds. They also called it *axixpatlicóztic,* meaning "yellow urine medicine," which referred to its use as a diuretic. In his Treatise on the Heathen Superstitions That Today Live Among the Indians Native to This New Spain, written in 1629, the cleric Hernándo Ruiz de Alarcón described an Aztec remedy using the herb in an enema to treat stomachache and fever. The roots and leaves were also ground into a powder and sprinkled on wounds and sores. In Europe the herb has been used as a purgative since the time of the ancient Greeks.

Parts Used: Leaf, root
Properties: Astringent, laxative, tonic, liver decongestant
Used to Treat: Sore throat, wounds and abrasions, gum problems, headache, liver problems

Limón
Lemon Tree

Botanical Names: *Citrus aurantifolia, Citrus limonium*
See also: *Azahares*

The lemon tree was exported to Europe from Asia by the Romans and from Europe to the Americas by the Spanish. The trees adapted well to the warm Mexican climate, and the medicinal uses of the fruit and leaves were quickly adopted by the native people. In eighteenth-century New Spain, the Jesuit physician Juan de Esteyneffer prescribed lemon to treat liver problems, intestinal worms, vomiting, and melancholy. Mexican Americans still use lemon to treat all these ailments and numerous others.

Parts Used: Leaf, fruit
Properties: Astringent, disinfectant
Used to Treat: Intestinal inflammations, diarrhea, fever, colds, respiratory problems, cuts, sores, nosebleeds, bee stings, rheumatism, liver problems

Linaza
Flax

Botanical Name: *Linum usitatissimum*
Other Names: *Linasa, Lino,* Linseed

Often used as an ornamental garden border, flax is a delicate blue flower on a slender stalk. Fossilized prehistoric flax was found in Swiss caves, making it arguably the first nonfood plant ever cultivated. It is the source of fiber for linen cloth, the same linen the Egyptians used to wrap their mummies and in which Christ is believed to have been wrapped when he was entombed. Flax was exported from Europe to the New World where it has flourished both as an industrially cultivated plant and as an escaped weed. The seeds are pressed to make linseed oil, used in painting and furniture making, and baked in whole grain breads.

The plant has been used medicinally for centuries. When cooked in water, the seeds exude a mucilage that is an effective emollient and is an ingredient in commercially packaged cough medicines. In traditional medicine, a lubricating infusion of flaxseeds is used to treat mucous membrane inflammations, such as cystitis, and gingivitis. The seeds, which are high in fiber, also have a laxative effect, and the oil, which has a coating action, is a traditional treatment for burns. Flaxseeds are sold at health food stores and some pharmacies.

Part Used: Seed
Properties: Emollient, anti-inflammatory, purgative, laxative
Used to Treat: Burns, abscesses, cough, urinary tract inflammations, boils, swellings, gingivitis

Only mature seeds should be used internally. Seeds that have not fully ripened can be toxic.

Liquidámbar
Storax

Botanical Name: *Liquidambar styraciflua*
Other Names: *Ococote, Ococotzl, Styrax*
Nahuatl: *Xochiocotzotl, Xochiocotzocuahuitl, Xochicuahuitl*

The name *liquidámbar,* liquid amber, originated with the sixteenth-century Spanish physician Nicolás Monardes, who devoted a chapter of his *Joyfulle Newes Out of the Newe Founde Worlde* to this resin. It's a syrupy sap collected from incisions in the bark of a fragrant flowering tree that resembles a maple.

The emperor Motecuhzoma II smoked an after-dinner pipeful of tobacco flavored with *liquidámbar,* a practice soon taken up by the Spaniards. In the sixteenth century, Francisco Hernández raved at length about the virtues of the *liquidámbar*-tobacco combination, which he said would alleviate headaches caused by colds and induce sleep, as well as act as a tonic on the head, stomach, and heart. He attributed a variety of cures to the sap—everything from relieving flatulence to dissolving tumors.

Rancheros once used *liquidámbar* to heal the wounds of horses and cattle. More recently it has been used as an expectorant ingredient in commercial cough syrups.

Parts Used: Resin, refined
Properties: Expectorant, mildly antiseptic
Used to Treat: Cough

Maguey
Century Plant

Botanical Names: *Agave salmiana, Agave americana, Agave lechuguilla, Agave* spp.
Other Names: *Lechuguilla, Mescal*
Nahuatl: *Metl, Tlacametl, Teometl*

According to an Aztec legend, at the beginning of time, demons abducted the beautiful goddess Mayahuel from the celestial level and took her to the Sonoran desert where they chopped her body into pieces. The plumed serpent god Quetzalcóatl, taking pity on her, transformed her bones into the first *maguey* plant. Plentiful in arid areas of Mexico and the southwestern United States, maguey is one of the most useful plants on earth.

For as long as man has traveled the deserts of Mesoamerica, *maguey* has provided food, drink, and medicine. It is most famous and perhaps most prized as the source of tequila, pulque, and mescal. Long fibers from the leaves of some maguey species are the source of sisal hemp that is woven into hammocks, fishing nets, and baskets. The heads, with the leaves trimmed off, are roasted and eaten. The tall stalks are chopped into pieces and chewed like cane sugar. Some species are used to make soap.

Francisco Hernández marveled at the countless uses of *maguey*. In his monumental sixteenth-century catalog of New World flora and fauna, he reported that the indigenous Mexicans used mescal to help ease the pain of childbirth, to promote lactation in nursing mothers, as a diuretic, and to rid the body of lice. The sixteenth-century Franciscan chronicler Fray Bernardino de Sahagún recommended mescal mixed with a yellow chili and gourd seeds as a tonic for one who has suffered a relapse after recovering from an illness. He reported that indigenous Mexicans applied *maguey* juice to cuts and knife wounds, and noted that a cowardly man, who was about to be whipped for some crime, coated his back with *maguey* juice in order to lessen the pain of the lash. Many *maguey* remedies have been in continuous use since pre-Hispanic times. They are still used today for mouth sores, digestive disorders, and bronchial inflammations.

The eighteenth-century Spanish botanist Luis Née was so impressed with *maguey's* usefulness that in his report to the crown he declared that Spain must not be long without it. He realized that maguey could be happily transplanted to Andalusian soil, where it can be found growing today.

Legend has it that *maguey* lives for a hundred years before it flowers and then dies, which is why it is called the century plant. Actually, most of these plants live no more than thirty years, but the fatal flowering can be spectacular. In some species a shoot two stories high is topped by an enormous cluster of white or yellow flowers.

With its rosette of sharply barbed spears, *maguey* resembles the smaller desert plant *sábila* (aloe vera), and the two are often substituted for each other, depending on availability. A beverage made with the juice, called *aguamiel*, literally "water honey," is prepared by roasting one of the spears until it begins to turn brown, then squeezing the liquid from it. This liquid is simmered over a low flame, sometimes with the addition of a cinnamon stick for flavor.

Parts Used: Entire plant
Properties: Antiseptic, diuretic, anti-inflammatory
Used to Treat: Digestive disorders, eye inflammation, liver problems, bronchitis, arthritis, menstrual problems, cuts, wounds, mouth sores

Malabar
Malabar

Botanical Name: *Solanum verbascifolium*
Other Names: *Berenjena, Berenhenilla, Galantea, Yerba Mora*
Nahuatl: *Tzompachtzin*

Malabar is a region in southern India where cardamom is produced, so the name "Malabar" can refer to the plant that produces cardamom seeds or the seeds themselves. But the "Malabar mix" sold in *botánicas* and markets is more often bits of stem and dried leaves of *Solanum verbascifolium*, a small tree or bush with clothlike velvety leaves and round yellowish fruit found throughout most of Mexico. It's a nightshade, a relative of the eggplant and the potato. Many species of *Solanum*, including this one, are also known as *berenjena*, which means eggplant—but they're not really eggplant, which is *Solanum melongena*, a native of Asia.

Parts Used: Leaf, twig
Property: Digestive

Mala Mujer
Treadsoftly

Botanical Name: *Croton ciliato-glandulosus*
Other Names: Scented Croton, *Yerba de la Cruz*

A number of plants are given the name *mala mujer*—"bad woman." In Morelos and Sonora the name refers to a species of *Croton*, a spurge with large, downy, oaklike leaves that inflict a stinging rash on anyone who touches them. It's not really much of a medicine, although some people claim they can remove warts by intentionally stinging themselves with the leaves.

Part Used: Leaf
Used to Treat: Warts

Malva
Mallow

Botanical Names: *Malva rotundifolia, Malva sylvestris, Malva neglecta*
Other Names: *Malva del Campo, Yerba del Negro*
Nahuatl: *Alahuacciopatli*

Mallow grows wild in Europe and North and Central America. It is a common weed, three or four feet high, with downy, tooth-edged leaves and purple flowers that give way to pods containing a single seed. All the mallows are nontoxic and contain a mucilage that is very soothing.

The Aztecs used mallow in easing childbirth and as a remedy for burning urination. In early eighteenth-century northern New Spain, the Jesuit physician Juan de Esteyneffer prescribed it as a remedy for palsy, stomachache, colic, liver obstructions, hemorrhoids and water retention. It is especially useful for relief from inflamed mucous membranes.

Parts Used: Leaf, flower
Properties: Anti-inflammatory, emollient, diuretic, expectorant
Used to Treat: Sore throat, urinary tract inflammation, vaginal inflammation, inflamed gums, fever, boils, abscesses, cough, digestive disorders, hemorrhoids

Manzanilla
German Chamomile

Botanical Names: *Matricaria chamomila* syn. *Matricaria recutita;* also *Anthemis nobilis,* Roman Chamomile
Other Name: *Camamilla*

Manzanilla, a New World émigré, was imported from Europe, but it has been wholeheartedly embraced by generations of Mexicans and Mexican Americans and tops the list of favorite medicinal herbs. It is, after all, a very lovable little plant. An infusion of its tiny flowers tastes sweet and delicious. It's nontoxic, safe even for young children, and useful in a variety of ailments. Most of all, *manzanilla* is soothing; it calms the nerves, settles upset stomachs, and cools burning eyes and skin.

It is also a woman's herb; it is used to ease menstrual cramps and in childbirth. Its botanical name, *Matricaria,* is derived from the Latin word for womb. In rural Mexico an infusion of *manzanilla* is sipped during labor and after delivery to ease the pain. A handful of the herb may also be boiled in a pot which can then be placed below the vagina so that the soothing vapors can reach the cervix. Some midwives massage the mother's swollen belly with an ointment made from *manzanilla* leaves and onions fried in lard to lessen labor pains.

Part Used: Flower
Properties: Digestive, sedative, anti-inflammatory, antispasmodic
Used to Treat: Menstrual cramps, colic, indigestion, inflamed eyes, cold, fever, insomnia, hemorrhoids

Maravilla
Four-O'Clock

Botanical Names: *Mirabilis multiflora, Mirabilis jalapa, Mirabilis longiflora*
Other Names: *Amarilla, Chuyem*
Nahuatl: *Quetzalatzonyatli, Tlaquiln*
Maya: *Tsutsuy-xiu*

A flowering hedge native to the warm climates of the Americas, *maravillas* are cultivated in gardens. They are called "four o'clock" because their trumpet-shaped blossoms open in the late afternoon, and close again at dawn. The roots have been used as a purgative and a remedy for stomachache, and are sometimes chewed to depress the appetite, but the plant can be narcotic and is toxic if taken internally. So its primary use today is in liniments and ointments to relieve aches and pains.

Part Used: Root
Property: Analgesic
Used to Treat: Arthritis, rheumatism, bruises

For topical use only. Toxic if taken internally.

Mariola
Mariola

Botanical Names: *Parthenium incanum, Parthenium stramonium;* also *Solanum hinsianum*
Other Names: *Ocotillo, Yerba Mora*

Mariola #1: In the southwestern United States and parts of Mexico the name *mariola* refers to a desert plant *(Parthenium incanum)* from the same family as *estafiate* and all the other *Artemisias.* It is used in a cold infusion—not heated—to treat fever, stomach disorders, liver problems, and the nausea of morning sickness.

Mariola #2: In Baja California the name *mariola* refers to a completely different plant, a flowering desert bush *(Solanum hinsianum)*, a member of the nightshade family that includes *yerba mora* and *florifundio,* as well as eggplant and tobacco. This *mariola* is brewed in a tea to treat stomach trouble.

Parts Used: *Mariola #1:* Stem, leaf; *mariola #2:* leaf, flower
Properties: *Mariola #1:* Morning sickness, liver problems, fever. *Mariola #1 and # 2:* Stomach problems

Marrubio
White Horehound

Botanical Name: *Marrubium vulgare*
Other Names: *Manrubio, Mastranso*

This aromatic, low, flowering bush arrived in the New World with the Spanish friars and now grows wild throughout the temperate zones of Mexico and the southern United States, having escaped no doubt from many a mission garden.

Marrubio's medicinal use goes back at least as far as ancient Greece. It has been prescribed as a treatment for coughs and colds since the Middle Ages and was a popular ingredient in commercial cough drops until quite recently.

The plant is highly mucilaginous, so it is soothing to the throat and makes a good expectorant. Because of its bitter flavor, it is also used as a tonic to stimulate the appetite.

Parts Used: Leaf, stem, root
Properties: Expectorant, tonic
Used to Treat: Coughs, nausea, digestive problems, menstrual difficulties

Not to be used during pregnancy.

Mastranso
Apple Mint

Botanical Name: *Menta rotundifolia*
See also: *Marrubio*

Mastranso is used in much the same way as more popular mints such as *poleo* (brook mint) and *yerba buena* (spearmint). The leaves are pressed with the back of a spoon in a cup to release the essential oils before boiling water is poured over them. In some parts of the southwestern United States the name *mastranso* is also given to horehound.

Part Used: Leaf
Used to Treat: Sore throat, stomachache, wounds

Mastuerzo
Garden Nasturtium

Botanical Name: *Tropaeolum majus*
Other Names: Indian Cress, *Mexixi*
Nahuatl: *Mexixquílitl, Pelonmexixquíltl*

The Spanish sent Mexican species of this little flower home to Spain and introduced Peruvian varieties into Mexico. Today the nasturtium is commonly cultivated throughout the temperate zones of the world for ornamental use, as a condiment, and as an ingredient in cosmetics. The flowers, which are a good source of vitamin C, were once used to treat scurvy. They are perfectly edible and add color and a spicy flavor to salads. The plant should always be used as a cold maceration, because it loses potency when heated.

Parts Used: Flower, leaf
Properties: Astringent, expectorant, antiseptic, digestive, high in vitamin C
Used to Treat: Anemia, mouth sores, skin problems resulting from vitamin deficiencies

Matarique
Indian Plantain

Botanical Names: *Psacalium decompositum, Cacalia decomposita, Odontotrichum decompositum*
Other Name: Buffalo Root

This pretty aromatic herb can be found on both sides of the border throughout the higher altitudes of the Sonoran desert. Its leaves are a delicate filigree of green lace, from which a tall stalk ascends, topped with white blossoms that turn into feathery seed balls.

Mexican Americans widely regard the plant as a remedy for the early stages of adult-onset diabetes. Animal studies conducted in Mexico have indicated the presence of some hypoglycemic properties, which may explain its apparent effectiveness.

Matarique is also a topical analgesic, considered useful for various aches and pains. In the Mexican states of Sonora and Chihuahua the fresh leaves are applied to wounds to speed healing.

Part Used: Root
Properties: Hypoglycemic, analgesic, antiseptic, purgative
Used to Treat: Adult-onset diabetes, arthritis, rheumatism, wounds, constipation

Strong doses can cause nausea and vomiting. Not to be used internally with insulin medicines, or by those with liver or kidney diseases.

Maté
(see *Mejorana*)

Mejorana
Sweet Marjoram

Botanical Name: *Mejorana hortensis*
Other Names: *Maté, Yerba Maté*
See also: *Salvia*

A culinary herb native to Asia, *mejorana* is often confused with common oregano *(Origanum vulgare)* or Mexican oregano *(Lippia berlandieri)*. Medicinally it is used as a tea to treat digestive problems and menstrual cramps.

Part Used: Leaf
Properties: Digestive, tonic, antispasmodic
Used to Treat: Stomachaches, menstrual cramps

Not to be used in therapeutic doses during pregnancy.

Membrillo
Quince

Botanical Name: *Cydonia oblonga*

The quince tree is an Asian native, transplanted to Europe and the Americas. The fruit, which has an astringent quality, is sometimes used in combination with various herbs as a remedy for digestive problems and diarrhea. The seeds make an emollient remedy for coughs.

Parts Used: Fruit, seed
Properties: Astringent, emollient
Used to Treat: Diarrhea, indigestion, cough

Menta
Peppermint

Botanical Name: *Mentha piperita*

Common peppermint is sometimes used in the same way as the more popular *yerba buena* (spearmint): primarily for digestive problems.

Parts Used: Leaf, flowering top
Properties: Antispasmodic, digestive
Used to Treat: Indigestion, nausea, menstrual cramps

Persons with gallstones should consult a physician before using mint medicinally.

Mercadela
(see *Caléndula*)

Mezquite
Mesquite

Botanical Names: *Prosopis julifera, Prosopis glandulosa, Prosopis pubescens*
Nahuatl: *Mizquitl, Quetzalmizquitl*

A common thorny desert shrub, mesquite became chic when it was discovered that it gave a wonderful flavor to foods if added to the coals in the grill or barbecue. But for centuries before anyone thought of mesquite-grilled chicken salad, indigenous Mexicans were using the plant for food, medicine, and rituals. The sweet pods were used in cooking. The gum, which exudes from incisions made in the trunk, was called the "tears of the moon goddess" and was burned as incense in her honor. Medicinally the gum was used as a remedy for lip sores and eye infections.

Mesquite is still considered a useful remedy for a wide variety of infirmities. Used externally, it soothes burns, sores, and hemorrhoids. Used internally, it works like Mylanta or Pepto Bismol to coat the stomach.

Part Used: Resin
Properties: Soothing, astringent, antiseptic
Used to Treat: Stomach inflammations, diarrhea, cough, laryngitis, wounds, sores, burns, hemorrhoids, eye irritation

Mimbre
Desert Willow

Botanical Name: *Chilopsis linearis*
Other Names: *Jano, Flor de Mimbres*

A willowy bush with heavily aromatic clusters of pink or purple trumpet-shaped flowers that give way to long slender seedpods, *mimbre* is native to the arid regions of northern Mexico and the southeastern United States. In Sonora it is used to treat a weak heart. In other parts of Mexico and the southwestern United States, the infusion is used topically as a wash or compress, or the dried herb is powdered and sprinkled on cuts and scratches.

Parts Used: Leaf, twig, bark, flower
Properties: Antifungal, antiseptic, digestive
Used to Treat: Indigestion, yeast infections, cough, skin infections, cuts, scratches

Mirto
Red Texas Sage

Botanical Name: *Salvia microphylla*
See also: *Salvia, Chía, Té de Monte*

The sage genus encompasses hundreds of species of plants in all shapes and sizes. The leaves are usually grayish green spears with that wonderful sagey aroma. *Mirto*, an ornamental species native to Mexico, has tubular red flowers. It is used medicinally to treat diaper rash and is one of the aromatic herbs sometimes used in the spiritual cleansing rituals called *limpias*. The name *mirto* is also given to several other plants, including *Satureja oaxacana*, *Bouvardia*, and various species of sage and common myrtle.

Parts Used: Leaf, stem, flower
Used to Treat: Deafness, diaper rash

Momo
(see *Hoja Santa*)

Mondarda
(see *Orégano del Campo*)

Muicle
Mexican Honeysuckle

Botanical Name: *Justicia spicigera* syn. *Jacobinia spicigera*
Other Names: *Muitle, Chuparrosa, Trompetilla, Mayotl, Mozote, Yerba de Añil*
Nahuatl: *Mohuitl*
Maya: *Yich-kaan*

Showy orange or red flowers that bloom all summer and attract hummingbirds make this native American bush a garden favorite throughout the southwestern United States. It should not be confused with *chuparrosa* (*Justica californica* syn. *Beloperone californica*), which has similar flowers but very few leaves.

The Aztecs used *muicle* to cure dysentery and scabies, and to reduce excessive menstrual flow. It has been used to make a natural bluing agent for laundry and a blue dye. Its most common use in traditional medicine today is as a tonic to "purify the blood."

Parts Used: Leaf, flower
Used to Treat: Blood impurities, menstrual difficulties

Nance
Nance

Botanical Name: *Byrsonima crassifolia*
Other Names: *Nanche, Nananche, Nan-Chi*
Nahuatl: *Nantazin, Nantzixócotl*

The fruit of this small, crooked tree looks like a yellow cherry and tastes like a lemon. The juice makes a lemonade-like beverage, and the fruit is served as a complement to tamales. *Nance* is cultivated in gardens and

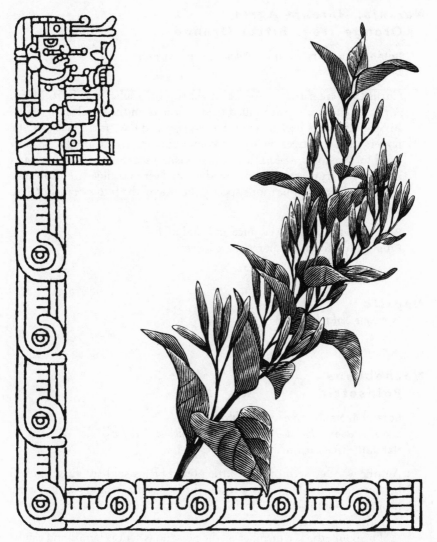

Muicle / Mexican Honeysuckle

grows wild from the central valley of Mexico south to the Yucatán peninsula. The Aztec name means "acid fruit of the mothers," referring to its use as a postpartum purgative. The bark, which has astringent properties, is powdered and sprinkled on skin ulcers and brewed in a tea to remedy diarrhea and indigestion.

Parts Used: Leaf, fruit, flower, bark
Properties: Astringent, digestive, purgative, antifungal
Used to Treat: Diarrhea, *empacho,* poor lactation in nursing mothers, skin and gum problems

Naranja, Naranja Agria
Orange Tree, Bitter Orange

Botanical Names: *Citrus aurantium, Citrus vulgaris*
See also: *Azahares*

Citrus trees are native of Asia, brought from the subcontinent to North Africa by the Arabs, who called them *naranj*, from the Sanskrit *nagaranga*. In Spain the trees became known as *naranjos*, and their fruits *naranjas*. The flowers of citrus trees, which are commonly referred to by the Spanish word for blossoms, *azahares*, are used to make a sedative tea. The juice and rind of the fruit are used in remedies for liver and digestive problems. Many medicinal applications specify the use of the bitter orange *(Citrus aurantium)*.

Parts Used: Leaf, flower, juice and rind of fruit
Properties: Sedative, diuretic, astringent

Negrito
(see *Sáuz, Yerba del Negro*)

Nochebuena
Poinsettia

Botanical Name: *Euphorbia pulcherrima*
Other Names: *Flor de Pascua del Monte, Catalina, Tabachín*
Nahuatl: *Cuitlaxóchitl*

Anyone who has seen only the little potted plants sold at Christmas will be amazed at the huge proportions the poinsettia achieves in its native habitat. In southwestern Mexico it is a large bush or small tree covered with the bright red flowers.

The poinsettia is a member of the poisonous spurge family and can be dangerous if taken internally. Nevertheless, nursing mothers in rural Mexico sometimes drink an infusion of the flower petals to increase the flow of milk, a holdover from the ancient Aztecs who believed that the plant might increase lactation because of the milklike sap it exudes when the stems are broken. Some people remove body hair by allowing the milky sap to dry on the skin and then pulling it off. Poultices of the leaves are applied to skin inflammations.

Parts Used: Petal, sap, leaf
Used to Treat: Skin inflammation

For external use only. Toxic if taken internally.

Nogal
Walnut Tree

Botanical Names: *Juglans regia, Juglans mexicana, Juglans major*
Nahuatl: *Quauhcacáoatli*

The walnut tree is native to Asia and the Mediterranean as well as North and South America. It is a very common tree in Mexico where the leaves and bark are used in traditional medicine. This is one of those confusing plants that seems to be at cross purposes. The bark is used as a mild laxative, while the leaves are used for the opposite problem—as a remedy for dysentery.

Parts Used: Leaf, bark, green nut
Properties: Astringent, detoxifier
Used to Treat: Constipation, dysentery

Nopal
Prickly Pear Cactus

Botanical Name: *Opuntia* spp.
Other Names: *Tuna, Duraznilla*
Nahuatl: *Tlatocnochtli, Tzapotlnochtli*
Maya: *Pak'an*

According to Aztec history this is the cactus on which an eagle perched, flapping its wings wildly, a sign from the great god Huitzilopochtli that the wandering Mexica tribe had at last come upon the place where they could found their city. The name of the ancient Aztec capital, Tenochtitlán, can be roughly translated "place of the prickly pear cactus."

The Aztecs used *nopal* as both food and medicine. In the sixteenth century, Fray Bernardino de Sahagún reported that women who were having difficulty in childbirth were given a beverage made with the peeled ground paddles, in the belief that the slippery juice would help the baby slide out. *Nopales* were among the first plants sent back to Europe by the Spanish expeditions. By the year 1576, when Francisco Hernández completed his monumental *Historia natural de la Nueva España*, he was able to write that *nopal* "had been known for many years in our Old World." Hernández also explained that the term "tuna" was a Haitian word for the plants. The Aztecs called the cactus *nochtl* and distinguished the many species by their fruits or flowers.

The edible fruits of the *nopal* are popularly known as prickly pears or *higos de las Indias*, figs of the Indias. The cactus paddles are sold in the produce section of many supermarkets. Peeled and eaten as a salad or side dish, or added to stews, they are a natural diuretic and a good source of vitamins.

Parts Used: Paddle, root, fruit
Properties: Diuretic, hypoglycemic, anti-inflammatory
Used to Treat: Toothache, canker sores, kidney stones (roots), adult-onset diabetes, abscesses, wounds, burns, urinary tract inflammation

Nuez Moscada
Nutmeg

Botanical Names: *Myristica fragans, Myristica officinalis*

The spice we call nutmeg is an acorn of sorts from a cultivated tree native to Asia. Medieval Arab physicians prescribed it as an aphrodisiac, but Mexican Americans just use it for indigestion, especially when an excess of stomach gas is involved.

Part Used: Seed
Properties: Digestive
Used to Treat: Stomachache, intestinal gas

May be toxic if large quantities are taken or if used for a prolonged period of time.

Ocote
Pine

Botanical Names: *Pinus teocote, Pinus edulis, Pinus* spp.
Other Names: *Trementina de Piñon, Aguarrás*
Nahuatl: *Ocotl, Oxitl, Ocotzotl, Ocoxóchitl*

The ancient Mexicans used the resin of the pine tree to make an ointment which they believed was invented by the goddess of medicine, Tzapotlatenan. In his Aztec Herbal of 1552, Martín de la Cruz included pine needles and flowers in a recipe for a liquor to be anointed on the armpits of sick people in order to remove the evil smell. He also mentions the bark in a recipe for an enema to alleviate dysentery.

In traditional medicine today this resin, which is called *trementina* or *aguarrás,* is used to make a liniment for arthritis. It is taken internally in small doses for dry mouth, dry and sore throat, and bronchitis. Pine needles are also brewed to make an expectorant tea.

Parts Used: Resin, bark, needle
Properties: Expectorant, antiseptic, anti-inflammatory
Used to Treat: Rheumatism, arthritis, chest congestion, excess mucus

Not to be used internally by persons suffering from bronchial asthma or whooping cough.

Ocotillo
Candlewood

Botanical Name: *Fouquieria splendens*
Other Name: *Mariola*

These tall desert plants look like a bunch of green sticks spreading out from a center base, similar to the spokes of an umbrella. They are covered with nasty spikes and, after the rainy season, small leaves. In early spring when the desert is in bloom, each stick is topped with a flower that resembles a long crimson feather. Hillsides in New Mexico and Arizona are covered with *ocotillo*. If you drive through eastern Arizona at that time of year, you'll notice that they add a festive red accent to the center divider of Interstate 8.

In Sonora another plant, *Parthenium stramonium*, is also called *ocotillo*.

Parts Used: Root, bark
Properties: Anti-inflammatory, lymph drainage stimulant
Used to Treat: Varicose veins, hemorrhoids, fatigue, swelling

Not to be used during pregnancy.

Orégano
Mexican Oregano

Botanical Names: *Lippia berlandieri, Lippia origanoides, Lippia dulcis;* also *Origanum vulgaris*
Other names: *Yerba Dulce*, Wild Marjoram, *Salvia Real*
Nahuatl: *Ahuiyaxíhuitl*
See also: *Orégano del Campo*

The name "oregano" is used to refer to three different plants. European oregano *(Origanum vulgaris)* is common everyday cooking oregano. Mexican oregano is one of several species of the *Lippia* genus, which smells and tastes a lot like the European oregano. To make matters even more confusing, still another plant, one or another species of the *Monarda* genus, is also called oregano, although many people just call it by its Latin name to save themselves the headache. Herb shops in the Southwest sometimes simply label the herb *Monarda*.

Mexican Americans use all three plants medicinally. European oregano has been used as a remedy at least since the time of the ancient Greeks. Mexican oregano was used medicinally by the Aztecs. The sixteenth-century physician Francisco Hernández identified the herb called *coapatli* as a relative of European oregano, similar in smell, taste, and form to European oregano, which the indigenous Mexicans used to treat flatulence. The two oreganos are used somewhat interchangeably for a wide range of ailments.

Parts Used: Entire plant
Property: Antiseptic
Used to Treat: Colic, indigestion, intestinal parasites, seasickness, swellings, menstrual cramps, cough, earache, toothache, snakebite, itchy skin

Not to be used during pregnancy.

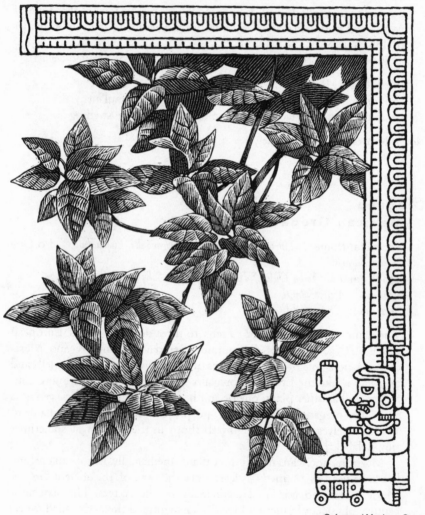

Orégano / Mexican Oregano

Orégano del Campo
Monarda

Botanical Names: *Monarda menthafolia, Monarda pectinata*
Other Names: *Orégano de la Sierra, Monarda*
See also: *Orégano*

This plant is really not oregano at all but a look-alike. Both herbs have purple flower heads and fragrant leaves. They are used for similar purposes: in cooking as a flavoring, and medicinally for cough, fever, sore throat, and indigestion. Monarda is an attractive garden plant, and the tea has a nice spicy flavor.

Parts Used: Leaf, stem
Property: Induces perspiration
Used to Treat: Stomachache, fever, respiratory ailments

Orozús
Licorice

Botanical Name: *Glycrrhiza glabra*
Other Names: *Regaliz, Yerba Dulce, Palo Cuate, Coahtli*

Botánicas and supermarkets in Mexican-American neighborhoods sell packets of a little black stick called *orozús.* Although there is a wild licorice native to the Americas, these packets probably contain the roots of the cultivated plant native to Asia.

Licorice has been used for centuries throughout the world as a remedy for colds, stuffy nose, coughs, and chest congestion of all sorts. The ancient Greeks, the Chinese, and the Ayurvedics in India all prescribed licorice for respiratory ailments.

In early eighteenth-century northern New Spain, the Jesuit Juan de Esteyneffer prescribed a juice made with licorice for sore throats, asthma, and burning urination. In rural Mexico today a cough syrup is made by boiling the roots in water.

Ounce for ounce, licorice root is fifty times sweeter than sugar, so the powdered root is used pharmaceutically to disguise nasty-tasting medicines and to coat pills. In traditional medicine a little powdered licorice root is sometimes used to mask the flavor of bitter herbs.

Licorice has been studied extensively. Modern scientists have discovered that it may help the body utilize other hard-to-absorb herbs, giving credence to the Chinese practice of adding it to herbal formulas for "balance." Its expectorant and anti-inflammatory properties have been documented by chemical analysis, and it has been studied as a potential remedy for duodenal ulcers. It is still used in commercially sold cough syrups and cough drops, but most of the licorice candies sold in the United States today are flavored with anise oil and contain little or no real licorice.

Part Used: Root

Properties: Expectorant, antiviral, anti-inflammatory, antibacterial, estrogenic, light laxative, tonic

Used to Treat: Cough, sore throat, wounds, gastrointestinal ulcers, menstrual problems

May be toxic if large quantities are taken over a prolonged period of time. Should be avoided by pregnant women, nursing mothers, and persons suffering from diabetes, cardiac problems, or hypertension.

Ortiga
Stinging Nettle

Botanical Names: *Urtica dioica, Urtica urens*
Nahuatl: *Tlaltzitzicaztli, Atzixicaztli, Tzitzicazquilitl, Chichicazatli*
Maya: *La'al*

Nettle is a mean little plant covered with stinging hairs. It looks enough like mint to be its evil twin, but it lacks the minty aroma. Its formidable defense system has failed to protect it from becoming a food source. In medieval Europe the tops of young plants were cooked as a vegetable (it has the same amounts of vitamins A and C as the more mild-mannered spinach). The ancient Greeks used nettle juice as an antidote for the infamous poison hemlock as well as for snakebites and scorpion stings.

The Aztecs made medicinal use of the several species of nettle native to Mexico. The Aztec Herbal of 1552 recommends sniffing a mixture of crushed nettles in milk to stop a nosebleed. (Modern chemical analysis has shown that nettle has hemostatic qualities that would stop bleeding.) The Aztec Herbal also prescribed a combination of nettles crushed in water and boiled as a poultice for arthritis.

Nettle continues to be used today for arthritis pain. In Germany it is used to treat high blood pressure because of its diuretic action. And in the United States it has recently become a popular and effective remedy for the symptoms of hayfever.

The herbal antidote for nettle stings is yellow dock (*lengua de vaca*). Rub a good leaf over the spot where the bad leaf got you.

Parts Used: Leaf, seed
Properties: Astringent, diuretic, hemostatic
Used to Treat: Rheumatism, kidney problems, water retention

Oshá
Porter's Lovage

Botanical Names: *Ligusticum porteri, Levisticum porteri*
Other Names: *Chuchupate,* Indian Parsley, Bear Medicine, Colorado Cough Root
Nahuatl: *Chuchupatli, Acocotli*

Oshá is one of the most treasured of herbs, a remedy for all sorts of ailments. It is most commonly used in northwestern Mexico and the southwestern United States where it grows wild in the pine forests of the upper elevations.

Other species of the genus found further south in Mexico were used medicinally by the Aztecs. The sixteenth-century royal physician Francisco Hernández found what he considered a "foreign species of *ligústico* with the same properties as the *ligústico* of our land."

In the Middle Ages a European species (*Ligusticum officinale*) was eaten in salads, fermented to make a sweet wine, and used to treat stomachache, fever, and delayed menstruation. In China a similar plant of the same genus (*Chuan Xiong, Ligusticum wallichii*), has a revered place in the materia medica, where it is used to lower blood pressure and as an aid in childbirth. In the past few years, species of the plant have been under scientific investigation for their antibiotic properties, their potential ability to stimulate interferon production, and possible uses in the treatment of cancer. Like the more famous echinacea, *oshá* is considered to have properties that are antimicrobial and enhance the immune system. The herb is considered particularly valuable in fighting viral infections.

Oshá is a relative of curly parsley, with big, lacy leaves and flat-topped heads of tiny white flowers that give way to edible seeds. It has a fresh aroma and makes a tasty tea. The root is carried as a talisman to ward off snakes.

The herb is wildcrafted, picked in the wild rather than cultivated, but harvesting it is a tricky business because of its strong resemblance to the poisonous hemlock plant. Be sure you are buying it from a reliable supplier. Some of its constituents are only partly soluble in water, so it is often prepared as a tincture, steeped in alcohol or simply chewed raw. Some health food stores sell *oshá* in capsules.

Parts Used: Root, stem
Properties: Anti-inflammatory, fungicide, disinfectant, promotes healing, diuretic, expectorant, induces perspiration
Used to Treat: Colds, respiratory tract problems, sore throat, stomachache, intestinal gas, cuts, wounds

Not to be used during pregnancy or by nursing mothers.

Palmilla
Yucca

Botanical Names: *Yucca schidigera, Yucca valida, Yucca* sp.
Other Names: *Amole, Datilla, Lechuguilla,* Spanish Dagger
Maya: *Sak-tuk, X-tuck*

The yucca is a spear-leafed desert bush similar to agave and aloe vera, with which it is sometimes confused. Like maguey, it is a plant with many uses. The fibers of the leaves are woven into sandals, baskets, and cloth.

According to legend, the cloth that bore the image of Our Lady of Guadalupe was woven of yucca fiber. Both the flower stalks and the fruits that follow are eaten. A laxative is made from the roots, but it is considered too strong to be safe.

A larger species, *Yucca valida*, grows at lower elevations. These trees are beautiful in gardens; their graceful palmlike branches arch toward the sky then explode in huge bursts of white blossoms. Paper is made from the trunks and leaves. The flower buds, called "*datile*," are eaten raw or cooked and brewed to treat arthritis. The roots are used to make a soap or shampoo called "amole."

Part Used: Root
Properties: Anti-inflammatory, purgative
Used to Treat: Arthritis, rheumatism, constipation

Palo Azul
Kidneywood

Botanical Name: *Eysenhardtia polystachya;* also *Caesalpinia bonducella*
Other Names: *Palo Dulce, Palo Cuate, Cualaldulce, Varadulce, Taray*
Nahuatl: *Cohuatli, Tlapalezpatli*

A small tree or shrub native to northwestern Mexico with aromatic leaves, white flowers, and long red or orange seedpods, *palo azul* has been used since the time of the Aztec empire to treat kidney ailments. All the early colonial sources mention this herb. In the Aztec Herbal of 1552, Martín de la Cruz listed the tree in a cure for hiccups. Fray Bernardino de Sahagún noted its use as a diuretic and a treatment for fever. Francisco Hernández reported that the indigenous Mexicans used the herb to treat kidney problems and that it diminished acid in the urine. In his *Joyfull Newes Out of the Newe Founde Worlde,* Dr. Nicolás Monardes prescribed it for "infirmities of the Urine" for "them that doeth not pisse liberally" and for those who pissed with pain. His instructions on the preparation of the herb, written in 1574, are still followed today. Small bits of the wood are soaked in clear, clean water. After half an hour the water will turn a yellowish orange color, but if it is held up to the light, it will appear blue. The strained infusion, which is tasteless, is drunk in place of water throughout the day.

Parts Used: Wood chips
Properties: Hypoglycemic, diuretic, anti-inflammatory
Used to Treat: Kidney disorders, urinary tract disorders, toothache, stomachache, fever

Palo Blanco
(see *Palo del Muerto*)

Palo Brasil
(see *Brasil, Tabachín*)

Palo Colorado
(see *Tabachín*)

Palo Cuate
(see *Palo Azul*)

Palo Dulce
(see *Palo Azul, Orozús*)

Palo del Muerto
Palo del Muerto

Botanical Names: *Ipomoea arborescens, Ipomeoa muricoides*
Other Names: *Palo Santo, Cazahuate Prieto, Arbol del Muerto, Palo Blanco*
Nahuatl: *Cuahazahuatl, Micacuahuitl*
See also: *Guayacán*

Palo del muerto is a member of the Ipomoea genus, which includes the many species of flowering vines we call "morning glories" in English. This one, though, is not a vine at all but a native Mexican tree with smooth white bark and big white morning glory–like flowers. When in bloom, it has almost no leaves. Since it appears to survive without water, the Aztecs believed it was a divine plant from the heavenly garden ruled by Tláloc, the water god.

In Morelos it is believed that the tree can cause imbecility and that it is poisonous to livestock and horses—which accounts for its foreboding name, meaning "death stick." In Sinaloa, pieces of the bark, which exude a gummy sap, are sold in the market to be used in a bath for paralysis and snakebites. Mexican Americans use the bark to make a purgative tea.

Parts Used: Wood chips
Property: Purgative

Palo Mulato
(see *Copal*)

Palo Santo
(see *Guayacán, Palo del Muerto*)

Palo Verde
Jerusalem Thorn

Botanical Name: *Parkinsonia aculeata*
Other Names: *Retama,* Horsebean

This little shrub is almost leafless, which may explain why the Spanish named it *palo verde,* green stick. Lots of very tiny little leaves appear and then disappear from its slender branches. The pretty yellow blossoms seem to have one mutant red-spotted leaf. After the blooming season, rows of beanlike seedpods hang from the branches.

The name of this plant is very confusing. Similar plants also called *palo azul* (blue stick) are species of the *Cercidium* genus, and there are at least two other plants called *retama.*

Parts Used: Twig, leaf, flower
Properties: Diuretic
Used to Treat: Fever, indigestion

Pañete
(see *Alacrán*)

Papaya
Mexican Papaya

Botanical Name: *Carica papaya*
Other Names: *Melón Zapote, Papaya Real, Papaw,* Melon Tree
Nahuatl: *Chichihualxóchitl*
Maya: *Chi'ich'put*

The active ingredient in *papaya,* papain, is used as a meat tenderizer, so imagine what it can do in your stomach to help you digest a steak dinner. The most potent form of papain is in the sap collected by making incisions in the unripe fruit. It's an enzyme that breaks down protein, virtually predigesting meats.

The Aztecs called *papaya* "flower of the chest," and it is still used in some parts of Mexico to treat chest-related infirmities such as bronchitis and asthma. In the sixteenth century, Francisco Hernández reported that the sap from the unripe fruit was used to cure prickly heat and ringworm, and the juice of the mature fruit was used for bellyaches. In some parts of the tropical Americas the leaves are still used to make a soap for washing clothes.

The sap is used to remove warts and lighten freckles, and the dried seeds are eaten as a digestive aid. Meats are cooked wrapped in the leaves, which contain smaller amounts of the tenderizing properties.

Parts Used: Fruit, seed, leaf, sap
Properties: Anti-inflammatory, digestive
Used to Treat: Indigestion, intestinal parasites, freckles

Passiflora
Passion Flower

Botanical Names: *Passiflora edulis, Passiflora mexicana, Passiflora* spp.
Other Names: *Passionaria, Granadita, Granadilla*
Nahuatl: *Coanenepilli*
Maya: *Poochil, Kansel-ak*

This American vine is grown in gardens for its beautiful flowers and sweet fruit. The Aztecs called the plant "snake tongue" and used it in remedies for snakebite, fevers, and other ailments. The Spanish missionaries called the plant *passionaria* after the Passion of Christ because the circle of little hairs that emerge from the corona of the flower reminded them of the crown of thorns and the three stalks of the pistil reminded them of the stigmata. In his *Joyfulle Newes Out of the Newe Founde Worlde*, Dr. Nicholás Monardes called the fruit *granadilla* because of its resemblance to *granadas,* pomegranates. He reported that both the Spanish and the native Mexicans enjoyed sipping the juice, which he said relieved them of stomach pains. In the Mexican-American community, *passiflora* tea is a much loved sedative, taken at bedtime to remedy sleeplessness.

Parts Used: Stem, leaf
Properties: Sedative, antispasmodic, anti-inflammatory
Used to Treat: Nervousness, insomnia, stomach cramps, symptoms of menopause, headache

Pazotillo
(see *Simonillo*)

Pegapega
(see *Yerba del Buey*)

Perejil
Curly Parsley

Botanical Name: *Petroselinum crispum* syn. *Carum petroselinum*

The common grocery store parsley that adorns many a platter has a history of medicinal use as well. Medieval doctors thought parsley was a remedy for pleurisy and dropsy, and even prescribed it as a cure for the plague. The herb is well known for its diuretic properties. The essential oil called apiol, which is extracted from the seeds, is sold in capsule form in health food stores as a remedy for water retention. Drinking fresh parsley juice has a similar effect. In traditional medicine a boiled tea made from the roots is used as a laxative and as a treatment for premenstrual symptoms.

Parts Used: Root, seed, leaf, stem
Properties: Diuretic, laxative, astringent, blood purifier
Used to Treat: Water retention, premenstrual syndrome, insect bites

Not to be used medicinally during pregnancy or in the presence of inflammatory kidney conditions. Parsley seed can be toxic in large doses.

Pericón
Mexican Tarragon

Botanical Names: *Tagetes lucida, Tagetes filifolía, Tagetes micrantha*
Other Names: *Anís, Yerba de Anís, Anisella, Santa María, Periquillo, Curucumín, Flor de Veinte, Yerba del Venado, Cinco Llagas,* Mexican Marigold, African Marigold, Sweet Mace
Nahuatl: *Yauhtli, Cuauhiyauhtli, Iyauhtli, Tepepapaloquilitl*
See also: *Cempasúchil*

These wildflowers are relatives of the common garden marigold, but the flowers are sparse—small yellow blooms with only five petals. Mexicans sometimes call the plants *anís* or *yerba de anís* because of their rich aniselike aroma and flavor. For the same reason the plants are called Mexican tarragon in English.

The Aztecs grew *pericón* for culinary, medicinal, and ritual uses. It added a spicy flavor to the royal *chocólatl,* a drink made with cocoa from which we get the English word "chocolate." In the Aztec Herbal of 1552, Martín de la Cruz describes the use of the plant as a talisman, rubbed on the chest to ensure safety when crossing a river. The Aztecs burned *pericón* as incense, and the flowers were used decoratively in many religious ceremonies. In parts of rural Mexico today *pericón* is laid in each corner of the cornfield before the harvest, and nailed in the shape of a cross to the doors of houses to ward off evil spirits. The flowers are one of the herbs used during rituals to cleanse the spirit.

Pericón was also an important medicine in ancient Mexico. It was named for the water goddess Ayauh. As the plant fell under the provenance of the water gods, it was used medicinally to treat the illnesses those gods controlled. Many of the remedies for which the plant is used today are survivors of Aztec medicine, echoes from the pages of the sixteenth-century chronicles. Infusions of the flower petals are used to treat the common cold, intestinal gas, and diarrhea.

Parts Used: Entire plant
Properties: Diuretic, induces perspiration
Used to Treat: Colic, common cold, fever

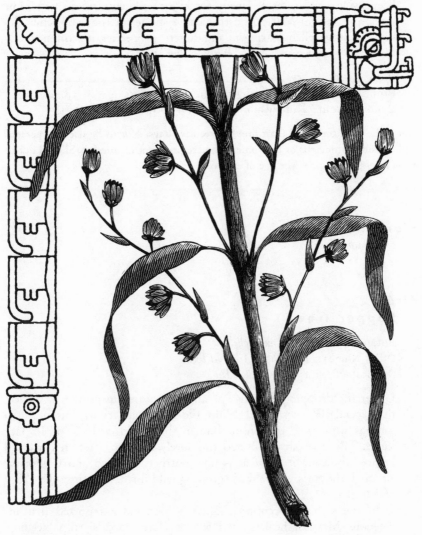

Pericón / Mexican Tarragon

Pingüica
Uva Ursi

Botanical Names: *Arctostaphylos uva-ursi, Arctostaphylos manzanita, Arctostaphylos pungens*
Other Names: *Manzana, Manzanita, Corallino, Coralillo,* Bearberry
Nahuatl: *Tomazquitl, Tepeizquitl, Tepesquisúchil*

Found throughout most of the Northern Hemisphere, these trailing shrubs form ground-covering mats with clusters of waxy pink or white urn-shaped flowers giving way to red berries. European herbalists have been using *Uva ursi* as a remedy for kidney ailments since the Middle Ages, and ancient Mexicans used a native species of the same genus. Because of its excellent astringent and diuretic properties, it is often among the herbs included in blended herbal "diet" teas.

Parts Used: Berry, leaf
Properties: Diuretic, astringent, antiseptic
Used to Treat: Kidney ailments, bladder problems, bronchitis

Not to be used for more than four consecutive days. Not to be used by persons with sensitive stomachs or by women who are pregnant or nursing. Should not be given to children under the age of twelve.

Pionillo

(see *Barbasco*)

Pirú
Pepper Tree

Botanical Name: *Schinus molle*
Other Names: *Perú, Pirul, Arbol del Peru*
Nahuatl: *Pelonquáhuitl, Copalquáhuitl*

Under the drooping branches of an old *pirú* tree in northern Mexico, the legendary *curandero* El Niño Fidencio held court, meeting the throngs who came to consult him in the speckled shade of its lacy leaves. The Spanish discovered this lovely flowering tree in Peru and began cultivating it in what is now northern Mexico and California, although the trees were already growing wild further south in the Valley of Mexico.

In the sixteenth century Francisco Hernández reported that indigenous Mexican healers used *pirú* to close wounds, stop bleeding, heal hemorrhoids, ease the pain of arthritis, and make cataracts disappear, and that the sap of the tree was dissolved in water to make a purgative.

Today the leaves and fruits are still used to treat wounds, toothache, and constipation. The branches are used in the traditional spiritual cleansings called *limpias*.

Parts Used: Fruit, sap, bark
Properties: Emollient, expectorant, diuretic, antiseptic
Used to Treat: Bronchitis, backache, wounds, tooth and gum problems, urinary tract disorders

Plumajillo
Yarrow

Botanical Names: *Achillea lanulosa, Achillea millefolium*
Other Names: *Plumbajillo, Milenrama, Real de Oro, Alcanfor, Yerba de los Carpinteros*
Nahuatl: *Tlalquequetzal*

Species of the genus *Achillea* are native to Europe, Asia, and the Americas. The Latin name is derived from the legend that Achilles used it to treat his soldiers who were wounded in battle. Yarrow has been used for centuries to stop bleeding and speed the healing of wounds. Medieval physicians mixed the herb with grease to make a poultice for wounds that had been "made with iron" —for example, running into a spear. The herb has been called "soldier's wound wart" in English and the "carpenter's herb" in both French and Spanish. It was among the herbs used to dress wounds during the American Civil War. It contains alkaloids, which may help stop bleeding, and the essential oil azulene, which is an anti-inflammatory.

Yarrow has also been used to treat a wide variety of ailments including toothache, hiccups, headaches, and indigestion. The Aztecs used it as a poultice on sores and drank it to cure coughs, diarrhea, and other digestive problems. It was one of the herbs used to increase contractions during childbirth, and taken in large doses, it was used as a purge after overeating. The Aztec name for the plant, *tlalquequetzal*, includes the suffix for earth, "tla," and plumes, "quetzal," referring to its feathery leaves. The plants are aromatic and have flat-topped heads of tiny white daisylike flowers.

Parts Used: Flower, leaf, root
Properties: Anti-inflammatory, astringent, antibacterial, tonic, diuretic, induces perspiration
Used to Treat: Fever, wounds, skin and digestive problems, cough, colds

Not to be used during pregnancy.

Poleo
Brook Mint

Botanical Names: *Mentha arvensis, Mentha pulegium*
Other Name: *Poleo Casero*
Nahuatl: *Chichilticxíhoitl, Tlalatóchietl*

Poleo is a native American mint that was used medicinally by the Aztecs. In the sixteenth century Francisco Hernández reported that the indigenous Mexicans used it in much the same way it is used today: in an infusion to treat flatulence, stomach pain, and colic, and to induce perspiration. The Aztecs bundled the herb and kept it for use during the course of the year, just as we dry and store herbs.

Poleo grows wild along the banks of streams and brooks, and is cultivated in gardens. The leaves look like mint, but the small, round purple flowers look like pennyroyal *(poleo chino)*, for which it is often mistaken. In Sonora an infusion of the leaves is used to treat insomnia. Mexican Americans use this mint as a remedy for colic.

Part Used: Leaf
Property: Sedative
Used to Treat: Stomach irritations, nausea, diarrhea, insomnia

Not to be used during pregnancy.

Poleo Chino
Pennyroyal

Botanical Names: *Hedeoma oblongifolia, Hedeoma pulegioides*
Other Names: Dwarf Pennyroyal, American Pennyroyal

Although pennyroyal is only a distant cousin of *poleo,* Mexican Americans sometimes use the two plants interchangeably. The difference is in the stem, which in *poleo chino* (pennyroyal) is branching, while *poleo* (brook mint) has only one stem.

Parts Used: Entire plant
Used to Treat: Fevers, menstrual cramps, indigestion

Not for use during pregnancy.

Poleo de Monte
Poleo de Monte

Botanical Names: *Cunila lythrifolia, Cunila longiflora*
Other Names: *Poleo de Campo*
Nahuatl: *Atochietl*

This *poleo* grows wild in the temperate zones of the Valley of Mexico. It has slender stalks with small, widely spaced, spear-shaped leaves and tiny blue or purple flowers. It looks a lot like brook mint, but it belongs to a different genus. The Aztec Herbal of 1552 lists a plant that can be identified as *poleo de monte* in remedies for cough, runny nose, and excess phlegm. The herb is still used in teas, compresses, and rubdowns to treat those symptoms. A liniment made with this *poleo* is also applied in a warm compress for headaches.

Part Used: Leaf
Property: Expectorant
Used to Treat: Bronchitis, cough, runny nose, headaches

Popotillo
Mormon Tea

Botanical Names: *Ephedra torreyana, Ephedra viridis*
Other Names: *Cañutillo del Campo, Cañutillo del Llano, Tepopote, Té Mormona, Itamo Real, Retamo Real,* Torrey's Ephedra, Desert Tea

Ephedra is one of the oldest medicinal herbs in continuous use. Fossilized evidence of the plant has been found in a Neanderthal cave in Iraq. The herb is native to Europe, Asia, and the Americas. Asian ephedra contains a vasoconstrictor called ephedrine which is used to treat asthma. Synthesized ephedrine, pseudoephedrine, is the most widely used ingredient in over-the-counter decongestants.

Popotillo, which is American ephedra, lacks this property, but it's a useful

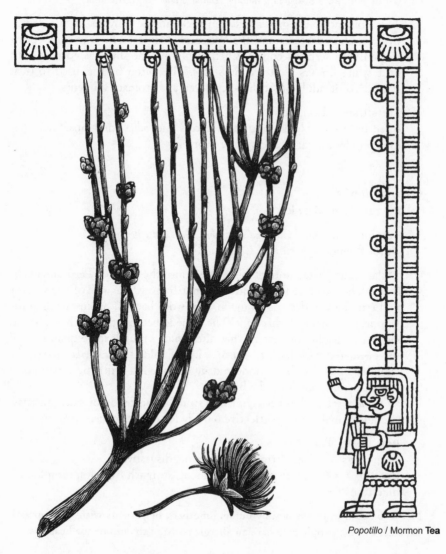

Popotillo / Mormon **Tea**

diuretic and astringent. Because it can be effective in treating burning urination, it was once considered a remedy for venereal disease. The small leafless desert shrub has hollow stems, like the reedy *cola de caballo*. Both plants are sometimes referred to as *cañutillo* in Spanish, which means little reed.

Part Used: Stem
Properties: Diuretic, astringent, tonic
Used to Treat: Kidney and bladder problems, stomach disorders, diarrhea

Prodigiosa
Bricklebush

Botanical Names: *Brickellia cavanillesii, Brickellia grandiflora, Brickellia californica*
Other Names: *Rodigiosa, Hamula, Amula, Mala Mujer, Atanasia*

This compact bush grows between rocks in the canyons of the southwestern United States and the Valley of Mexico. The leaves are spearshaped with serrated edges. When in bloom, the shrub is covered with little white flowers scattered on stalks. This bitter herb is used to treat symptoms of adult-onset diabetes, fever, and stomach ailments.

Parts Used: Leaf, flower
Used to Treat: High blood sugar, excess bile *(bilis)*, adult-onset diabetes, liver problems, diarrhea, digestive problems

Quina Roja
Peruvian Bark

Botanical Names: *Cinchona succirubra, Cinchona officinalis*
Other Names: *Quina Rojo, Chincona*

Malaria was a fatal, untreatable disease until the Incas of Peru taught the Spanish how to cure fevers with *quina roja*. In 1640 the wife of the Viceroy of Peru, the Condesa de Chincón, sent word back to Spain extolling the wondrous powers of this bark. The remedy became popularly known as *chincona* in her honor. Later, when the Jesuits brought large quantities of the powdered bark back to Europe, it was sold as *polvos de la condessa*, the countess's powders. The modern drug quinine is a synthetic version of a chemical component of the bark.

   Quina roja bark has been shown to stimulate secretion of saliva and gastric juices, making it an effective remedy for digestive disorders.

Part Used: Bark
Properties: Tonic, astringent, antiseptic, disgestive
Used to Treat: Chills, fever, sore throat, stomach troubles, pimples, indigestion

Not to be used in pregnancy, by nursing mothers, or patients with gastrointestinal ulcers. Some people may have an allergic reaction to quinine medications.

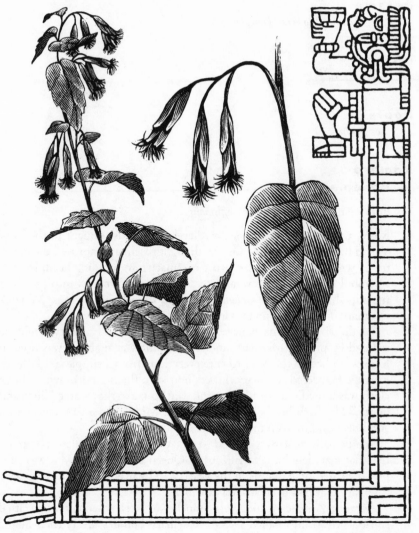

Prodigiosa / Bricklebush

Raíz del Indio
  (see *Yerba del Pasmo*)

Raíz de Jalapa
  (see *Jalapa*)

Raíz de Pleurisy
  (see *Inmortal*)

Regaliz
  (see *Orozús*)

Retama

(see *Hojasen, Palo Verde, Tronadora*)

Ricino

(see *Higuerilla*)

Roble

(see *Encino*)

Romero
Rosemary

Botanical Name: *Rosmarinus officinalis*

Rosemary is one of the classic medieval medicinals brought to the New World by the Spanish. The Greeks thought rosemary improved the memory if worn in the hair. They wove rosemary into wedding headpieces as a symbol of loyalty in love and tossed rosemary wreaths into graves at funerals. In Shakespeare's *Hamlet*, the mad Ophelia wryly says, "There's rosemary. That's for remembrance."

Medieval physicians believed that nightmares and anxiety could be avoided by placing rosemary under one's pillow at night. It was used in lotions applied to the head to cure everything from a simple headache to insanity. Powdered rosemary flowers bound to the right arm with a linen cloth was a medieval antidepressant, said to make the wearer "light and merry." The herb has been used since the Middle Ages to scent clothes and linens and to keep moths away.

Medicinally, rosemary is used to ease the pain of rheumatism, a practice that may date back to Elizabeth, Queen of Hungary, who was supposedly cured of paralysis in the year 1235 by massaging her joints with rosemary that had been soaked in wine.

Mexican Americans today use branches of fresh rosemary in the ritual spiritual cleansings called *limpias*. Rosemary bundles are burned in the corners of a room to cleanse it spiritually, possibly a survival of the medieval practice of burning rosemary to keep away the plague. The herb is also used as a disinfectant to wash floors.

Parts Used: Leaf, flower, stem
Properties: Antibacterial, tonic, astringent, disinfectant
Used to Treat: Digestive disorders, rheumatism, delayed menstruation

Not to be used in therapeutic doses during pregnancy.

Rosa de Castilla
French Rose, Red Rose, etc.

Botanical Names: *Rosa gallica, Rosa chinensis, Rosa* spp.

The roses brought to Mexico by the Spanish were probably species of *Rosa gallica,* the Adam and Eve of endless varieties of garden roses and the only species known to have been cultivated in Europe in the fifteenth century. Some varieties grew wild in western Europe, while others were introduced to France from North Africa during the Crusades. Many of the roses cultivated today are hybrids of an Asian species, *Rosa chinensis,* which was not introduced into Europe from China until the eighteenth century.

Medieval physicians made a syrup by steeping rose petals with sugar in hot water and then straining the mixture. They used it as a remedy for feebleness, melancholy, even cholera. In his medical text of 1719, Juan de Esteyneffer described more than one hundred ways in which roses were used medicinally in New Spain.

Mexican Americans use soothing infusions of rose petals to treat inflammations and diarrhea.

Part Used: Petal
Properties: Astringent, soothing to mucous membranes
Used to Treat: Infantile diarrhea, inflamed gums, sore eyes, sore throat, fever

Ruda
Rue

Botanical Names: *Ruta graveolens, Ruta chalepensis*
Other Names: *Ruta, Lota, Lula, Luta, Lura*

Rue is one of the most ancient of the herbs still in current use. Its name is derived from the Greek word *rua,* which means to set free, since rue was believed to free people of disease. Pliny reported that in ancient Rome rue was used by painters and engravers to sharpen and preserve their eyesight. It has been considered an antidote since at least the first century. According to legend, King Mithradates of Asia Minor survived his enemies' attempts to poison him by eating rue. In the Middle Ages rue was one of the herbs used to ward off witches. Judges kept bunches of strong-smelling rue at the bench to protect themselves from the foul odors and infectious diseases brought into court from the jails by wretched prisoners. In Shakespeare's *Hamlet* when Ophelia, in her delirium, intones, "There's rue for you and here's some for me; we may call it herb of grace o' Sundays," she is referring to the use of brushes made from rue for sprinkling holy water at a ceremony before Sunday mass.

Rue was brought to Mexico by the Spanish. It's one of the aromatic herbs sometimes used in *limpias,* spiritual cleansings. Long considered a "woman's plant," it was one of the herbs midwives used to speed uterine contractions during labor.

A small perennial shrub with straight, branched stems it has small, blue-green or ash-green leaves and clusters of tiny yellow-green flowers in summer. The shape of rue leaves was used as a model for the spade suit in playing cards.

Parts Used: Leaf, stem, flower
Properties: Antispasmodic, stimulant
Used to Treat: Menstrual cramps, earache, headache, nosebleed, insect repellent

Rue can be toxic if taken in large doses. It can cause increased photosensitivity, and exposure to the fresh plant can cause a poison ivy–like reaction in some people. It should never be used internally by pregnant or nursing women.

Sábila
Aloe Vera

Botanical Names: *Aloe barbadensis, Aloe vulgaris, Aloe mexicana*
Other Names: *Zábila*

One of the most highly regarded medicinal plants of all time, the aloe is a native of Africa. Legend has it that Cleopatra used aloe to maintain her gorgeous complexion, and according to the apostle John, the body of Christ was embalmed in aloe. By the early fifteenth century, aloe had been naturalized on the European side of the Mediterranean. The Spanish called the plant *sábila* after the Arabic word for it, *saber*, which means "patience." Aloe had long been valued for its ability to help heal battle wounds, and it was among the first plants to arrive in the New World from Europe. Even before the conquest of Mexico, aloe was heavily cultivated on the island of Barbados. For this reason a botanical synonym for *Aloe vera* is *Aloe barbadensis.*

Aloe is a low plant with barbed, spear-shaped leaves similar to *maguey*, with which it is often confused. Columbus himself assumed that the *maguey* he discovered in the New World was a species of the aloe he knew in Spain, and he brought a sample back with him.

The plant is a favorite remedy of Mexicans and Mexican Americans who grow it in gardens and on windowsills. It grows wild throughout Mexico and the southwestern United States, and can even be found on hillsides and empty lots in the urban sprawl of Los Angeles.

Studies have confirmed its healing properties and the presence of a substance that encourages cell growth, which explains why it is often used to treat burns. Modern herbalists also consider aloe juice useful in eliminating toxins from the body.

Parts Used: Leaf, juice
Properties: Emollient, promotes healing, anti-inflammatory, antibacterial, laxative
Used to Treat: Burns, skin irritations, wounds, rheumatism, gastric ulcers, heartburn, constipation, indigestion

Ingestion of the juice may irritate the mucus membranes of the intestines if overused. Not to be used by persons suffering from inflamed hemorrhoids, stomach, or intestinal inflammations. Not to be used by pregnant women or those with liver disease. Not to be taken internally by children under the age of twelve.

Sabino
(see *Ahuehuete*)

Salvia
Common Sage

Botanical Names: *Salvia officinalis, Salvia lavanduloides*
Other Names: *Alhucema de la Costa, Té de Mar, Yerba de Santa María*
See also: *Chía, Mejorana, Mirto, Salvia Real*

True sage, which is a species of the genus *Salvia*, is often confused with native Mexican plants of the *Buddleia* genus, which are commonly called *salvia real*, meaning royal sage. The two plants are used interchangeably for many of the same remedies. To add to the confusion, true sage has lots of other names in the lexicon of Mexican herbal remedies. It is variously known as *alhucema de la costa* (lavender of the coast), *té de mar* (tea of the sea), and *yerba de Santa María*, a name it shares with other plants. Species of yet another genus, *Leucophyllum*, are known as purple sage.

In their *Handbook of Mexican Roadside Flora*, Charles and Patricia Mason counted some 280 species of *Salvia*. Most sage sold as a medicinal herb is probably either some variety of *Salvia officinalis*, which is common garden sage, or *Salvia lavanduloides*, which is Mexican bush sage, although many species of the genus are considered to have medicinal properties. When in bloom the plants can be quite attractive, with showy tube-shaped red or blue flowers. Nurseries in the southwestern United States sell them for ornamental use in gardens.

Medieval physicians extolled the antiseptic virtues of sage. Its name comes from the Latin word *salvus*, meaning health. Maude Grieve, in her *Modern Herbal* of 1931, quotes a medieval Latin proverb: *Cur moriatur homo cui Salvia crescit in horto?* Why should a man die while sage grows in his garden? Medieval physicians pounded the leaves to make poultices for infected wounds, boiled them to make a wash for itching skin problems, and prescribed sage tea with honey to soothe a cold. All these old remedies are still used by Mexican Americans today.

Parts Used: Leaf, stem
Properties: Digestive, astringent, antiseptic
Used to Treat: Stomach gas, sore throat, sore gums

Salvia de Bolita

(see *Salvia Real*)

Salvia Real
Butterfly Bush

Botanical Names: *Buddleia americana, Buddleia wrightii, Buddleia cordata, Buddleia perfoliata, Buddleia* spp.
Other Names: *Salverial, Cantue, Cantuesa, Lengua de Buey, Salvia de Bolita, Tepozan*
Nahuatl: *Topozán, Tlatlanili, Mispatli, Zayolitzcan*

These small trees and bushes are grown ornamentally in gardens to attract butterflies. Most of the cultivated species originated in China, but some tropical and subtropical species are Mexican natives. Most of the genus is distinguished by spiky flower heads densely covered with bright yellow, pink, or purple blossoms and woolly, aromatic leaves that can smell a lot like true sage.

Parts Used: Entire plant
Properties: Diminishes bodily secretions such as perspiration, saliva, mucus
Used to Treat: Stomach disorders, pimples, cough, colds

Sangre de Drago
Limberbush

Botanical Names: *Jatropha dioica, Jatropha macrorhiza, Jatropha* spp.
Other Names: *Sangregado, Palo Sangriento, Sangre de Cristo, Telondilla*
Nahuatl: *Tzontecapatli, Chicioaquáhuatl, Quauhayohuachtli*

The Spanish called this desert plant *sangre de drago*, blood of the dragon, because its yellowish stems are blood red inside and exude a sticky sap. It is called limberbush in English because the stems are so pliable they bend easily without breaking and are used to weave baskets. The Aztecs called it *tzontecapatli*, wound medicine. They used the sticky sap to close wounds and made a purgative drink with the toasted nuts. Today an infusion of the leaves is used as a mouthwash, eyewash, and a wash for infected wounds. When taken as a tea, it's considered a tonic.

A cousin of the poinsettia, *sangre de drago* grows wild throughout the Sonoran desert on both sides of the border in lower elevations. Tiny white flowers are nestled among the spear-shaped, deeply toothed leaves.

Parts Used: Branch, root, sap
Properties: Anti-inflammatory, astringent, tonic
Used to Treat: Mouth sores, inflamed gums, surface wounds

Santa María
(see *Altamisa Mexicana, Pericón, Salvia*)

Santa Rita
Indian Paintbrush

Botanical Names: *Castilleja arvensis, Castilleja* spp.
Other Names: *Flor de Santa Rita, Garañona, Enchiladas, Yerba del Cancér, Cola de Borrego*

These tall, deep green stalks topped by brush-shaped blossoms with red-tipped petals splash color through the high chaparral. In their *Selección de Plantas Medicinales de México*, Edelmira Linares, Beatriz Flores Peñafiel, and Robert Bye reported that in Mexico City's great marketplace, the Mercado Sonora, the herb is recommended for kidney problems, as a wash for wounds, to treat measles and coughs, and as a bath *"de señoras"* to treat "women's problems."

Part Used: Leaf
Property: Diuretic

Sapote
(see *Zapote Blanco*)

Saúco
Elder flower

Botanical Names: *Sambucus mexicana, Sambucus nigra, Sambucus racemosa*
Other Names: *Flor Saúco, Azumiate, Guarico, Negrito, Tápiro*
Nahuatl: *Xúmetl*
Maya: *Tlsolos-ché*

Elder trees and bushes are native to all the temperate regions of the globe. Their medicinal use dates back to the Egyptians. One legend has it that the cross on which Christ was crucified was made from elder wood. Medieval European herbalists considered the elder a cure-all. Elder sticks were even used to drive away evil spirits.

The Aztecs used the leaves in a poultice for headaches, nosebleeds, wounds, and skin ulcers. At the turn of the century the dried flowers were used in a lotion to clear the complexion of freckles. The berries were baked into pies and fermented to make the famous elderberry wine.

Today an infusion of the flowers is used to treat fever in childhood diseases and to relieve stomach gas. A simmered tea made with the bark is used as a purgative.

Part Used: Flower
Properties: Anti-inflammatory, antifungal, induces perspiration

Used to Treat: Fevers in children, childhood diseases, colic, intestinal gas, colds, pimples, bruises

Sáuz
White Willow

Botanical Names: *Salix bonplandiana, Salix goodingii, Salix taxifolia, Salix* spp.
Other Names: *Sáuce, Jarita, Taray, Ahuejote, Negrito*
Nahuatl: *Quetzalahuexoltl*

Searching for an inexpensive substitute for that natural miracle cure, the Peruvian quinine bark, nineteenth-century scientists decided to have a look at the willow, which had been used medicinally at least since the time of Greek physician Dioscorides, primarily as an astringent. Meanwhile, back in Tenochtitlán, the Aztecs had been treating fever with their own *quetzalahuexotl*, royal-plume-water-willow, for centuries. Fray Bernardino de Sahagún reported that Mexican willow bark, administered to young children and old people alike, "removes the fever."

But willow's fever-fighting prowess was not apparent to the rest of the world until the late 1890s when, after some tweaking by a chemist working for the Friedrich Bayer company, a synthetic version of its active ingredient finally hit the drugstores. Acetylsalicylic acid, renamed aspirin, has been reducing fever big time ever since, but some people still continue to prefer good old willow bark. *Sáuz*, is sold in barrio markets. The infusion is used as a fever-reducing tea, a gargle for sore throats, and a compress for arthritic pain, sores, and burns.

Parts Used: Leaf, bark
Properties: Anti-inflammatory, analgesic, fever reducer

Siempreviva
Stonecrop

Botanical Names: *Sedum dendroideum, Sedum* spp.
Other Names: *Cola de Borrego, Doradilla*
Nahuatl: *Texiotl, Tetzmitl, Tezmitic*

There are some four hundred species of *Sedum*, most of them low, ground-covering succulents with flat, fleshy, spade-shaped leaves that form little flowerlike clusters. The Aztec Herbal of 1552 lists plants identified as *Sedum* in remedies for mouth inflammations, and Fray Bernardino de Sahagún reported its use in the sixteenth century as a remedy for irritations of the eye. The plant is used today in much the same way for the anti-inflammatory properties recognized by the Aztecs. In Morelos the juice is applied to eye irritations and burns. The leaves are chewed to alleviate the discomfort of sore gums and toothache, and a warmed leaf is just the right size to place carefully inside an aching ear.

Parts Used: Leaf, sap
Properties: Anti-inflammatory, astringent
Used to Treat: Backache, earache, inflamed gums

Simonillo
Horseweed

Botanical Names: *Conyza confussa, Conyza filaginoides, Conyza canadensis*
Other Names: *Pazotillo, Texiote,* Canadian Fleabane
Nahuatl: *Zacachichic, Tlalyetl*

Depending on the species, *simonillo* can be a small or a big weed topped with insignificant white flowers. It grows from the central Valley of Mexico north to the dry climates of the southwestern United States, from the canyons of New Mexico to the vacant lots of East L.A. It can also be found neatly packaged in cellophane in markets and *botánicas.*

Its use for digestive disturbances has been validated by at least one study, conducted in Mexico City at the Instituto Médico Nacional, which showed that the plant was effective in relieving gastric inflammation and vomiting. In the sixteenth century, Fray Bernardino de Sahagún described a plant that may have been *simonillo* which the Aztecs used topically to treat hemorrhoids and venereal ailments. Herbalists still recommend the plant to relieve hemorrhoids.

Parts Used: Leaf, stem, flower
Used to Treat: Gastric disturbances, *bilis,* diarrhea, colitis, hemorrhoids

Can be toxic if taken in large doses or for an extended period of time. Not recommended for persons of advanced age or in frail health.

Sinvergüenza
(see *Yerba del Pollo*)

Solano Negro
(see *Yerba Mora*)

Sueldo
Common Comfrey

Botanical Name: *Symphytum officinale*
Other Names: *Consueldo,* Knitbone
See also: *Cardo Santo*

Comfrey is one of the medieval herbs brought to Mexico by the Spanish. The gluey substance in its roots made people think it might be good for setting broken bones, and the greens were used in stews and salads. In early eighteenth-century New Spain, the Jesuit physician Juan de Esteyneffer used it as a poultice for toothache and bruises.

It contains allantoin, which is also present in mother's milk, a substance that speeds healing by increasing the production of new cells, so it makes a good poultice for sores and wounds. The herb also has a long history of internal use for urinary and pulmonary inflammations, kidney and gallbladder distress, and stomach ulcers. But in 1978 a study showed that rats ingesting the herb developed cancerous liver tumors. Although those findings are now much disputed, comfrey's reputation was ruined, and it's now recommended for external use only. It is an ingredient in some commercial salves and ointments.

Parts Used: Root, leaf
Properties: Anti-inflammatory, astringent, promotes healing
Used to Treat: Skin infections, insect bites, ulcers, wounds, burns, bruises

Should not be used topically on broken skin. Not to be used during pregnancy without first consulting a physician.

Tabachín
Mexican Bird of Paradise

Botanical Name: *Caesalpinia pulcherrima* syn. *Poinciana pulcherrima*
Other Names: *Palo Colorado, Brazíl, Noche Buena, Camarón, Barbona, Cabellitos de Angel, Guacamaya,* Dwarf Poinciana, Peacock Flower, Barbados Flower
Nahuatl: *Chacaloxóchitl, Chamolxóchitl, Xiloxóchitl*
Maya: *Chink-in, Kan-zink-in*

This beautiful flowering bush is native to the tropical Americas. It is sold in nurseries in the southwestern United States as an ornamental plant and is cultivated in gardens throughout Mexico for its fernlike foliage and sprays of fragrant delicate red-and-yellow flowers that bloom from spring through early fall.

The Aztecs called the plant "shrimp flower" and used it as a purgative for intestinal parasites and in a remedy for fever. Mexican Americans use it to treat coughs, colds, and a variety of other ailments, sometimes substituting it for *boldo* (bold) as a laxative.

Parts Used: Leaf, flower, root, bark
Properties: Purgative, antifungal, astringent
Used to Treat: Respiratory problems, liver ailments, mouth sores, sore throat, eye inflammation, skin problems

Tabaquillo
Rancher's Tea

Botanical Names: *Hedeoma piperita*
Other Names: *Santo Domingo, Té de Rancheros, Té del Monte, Yerba del Borracho*
See also: *Poleo Chino*

A relative of American pennyroyal, this herb has many stems with opposing leaves and tiny white flowers. It is known to have a high menthol content. In Mexico, it is used as a tea, sometimes combined with a little bicarbonate of soda, to treat nausea, particularly the vomiting associated with heavy drinking. Topically, it's used as a poultice on abscesses.

Parts Used: Entire plant
Properties: Nausea, abscesses

Tamarindo
Tamarind

Botanical Name: *Tamarindus indica*

The tamarind tree, a native of Asia and Africa, was imported to the Americas by the Spanish and is now cultivated widely in tropical climates throughout the world. The fruit, which is rich in potassium, is available in some U.S. supermarkets. Tamarind syrup is used in cold beverages. Mexican Americans eat the stewed fruit as a laxative and a digestive aid, and take an infusion of the leaves to expel intestinal parasites.

Parts Used: Fruit, leaf
Properties: Digestive, laxative, diuretic, antiparasitic

Tanceto
Tansy

Botanical Name: *Chrysanthemum vulgare* syn. *Tanacetum vulgare*
Other Names: *Tanse, Ponso*

Tansy is another of the medieval medicinal herbs exported to the New World from Europe. An aromatic creeper with ferny leaves and clusters of yellow-orange flowers, it has a camphorlike aroma. In the sixteenth century, cakes made with tansy leaves were eaten at Easter to represent the bitter herbs of Christ's last supper.

An infusion of the leaves was used to dress wounds. The tea was once prescribed for delayed menstruation, chills, and fever, and taken as a tonic. But recent studies suggest that the herb may be dangerous if taken in significant doses. It contains an essential oil called thujone that is toxic to the nervous system.

Its use as an insect repellent, though, is harmless and worth a try. Some people hang bunches of the herb in kitchen windows or rub the flowers on tabletops and windowsills to repel flies and ants.

Part Used: Leaf
Properties: Antispasmodic, soothing, insect repellent
Used to Treat: Delayed menstruation, fever

Can be toxic if taken internally.

Taray
(see *Palo Dulce*)

Té de Coral
(see *Aceitilla*)

Té de Milpa
(see *Aceitilla*)

Té de Monte
Savory

Botanical Names: *Satureja macrostema, Satureja laevigatum*
Other Names: *Té de Borracho, Tochil, Tabaquillo Grande, Yerba Buena*
Nahuatl: *Cuencuentzpatli*
See also: *Mirto, Tabaquillo*

There are thirty species of *Satureja*, all small, aromatic shrubs native to the Northern Hemisphere. The Mediterranean species we call summer savory *(Satureja hortensis)* has been used as a culinary herb since the time of the ancient Greeks and once enjoyed a reputation as an aphrodisiac. Both summer and winter savory *(Satureja montana)* flavor salami and sausage.

The city of San Francisco was originally named Yerba Buena after the species *Satureja douglasii*, which is native to the Pacific Coast. The Mexican species *Satureja macrostema* is used in an infusion to treat stomachache and flatulence, to induce perspiration and to bring on delayed menstruation. Because it is a popular hangover remedy, the herb is also sometimes called *yerba del borracho*, drunk man's herb. In Oaxaca, wedding wreaths are made from the flowering branches.

Part Used: Leaf
Properties: Antiseptic, astringent
Used to Treat: Hangover, menstrual problems, stomach gas, fever

Té Limón
Lemongrass

Botanical Names: *Cymbopogon citratus* syn. *Andropogon citratus*
Other Names: *Zacate Limón, Ocozacatl*

This aromatic grass with a pleasant citrusy flavor is a native of Asia and is used in Thai cuisine. Mexican Americans often combine the herb with *yerba buena* (spearmint) or one of the other mints to brew a calming tea. *Té limón's* pretty blue-green hue and fresh scent make it a favorite in kitchen gardens.

Part Used: Leaf
Properties: Digestive, sedative

Not to be used during pregnancy.

Té Mormona
(see *Popotillo*)

Té de Sena
(see *Hojasen*)

Tejocote
Mexican Hawthorn

Botanical Names: *Crataegus pubescens, Crataegus mexicanus*
Other Names: *Chisté, Manzanilla, Manzanita*
Nahuatl: *Texócotl*

Tejocote is the Mexican cousin of the European hawthorn berry (*Crataegus mongyna* Jacq., *Crataegus laevigata*) which has recently attracted attention for its ability to lower blood pressure by dilating the blood vessels.

This native American species is a big-leafed, thorny shrub or small tree. The white blossoms, which have an unpleasant scent, give way to yellow-orange berries. It grows wild in mountainous regions and is cultivated in gardens. Mexican Americans treat coughs and colds with the berries, eaten raw or in jams or marmalades. An infusion of the leaves is also used as a cold remedy. The roots are believed to have diuretic properties. In Michoacán a diuretic tea made from the leaves, roots, or bark is used to treat symptoms of adult-onset diabetes.

Parts Used: Leaf, fruit, root, bark
Properties: Diuretic, tonic
Used to Treat: Cough, colds, kidney inflammation

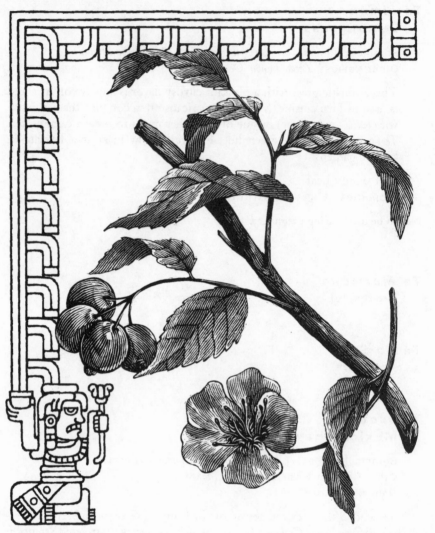

Tejocote / Mexican Hawthorn

Telondilla
(see *Sangre de Drago*)

Tepopote
(see *Popotillo*)

Tepozan
(see *Salvia Real*)

Tila
Linden

Botanical Names: *Tilia mexicana, Tilia americana, Tilia vulgaris, Tilia* spp.
Other Names: *Flor de Tila, Tilia*

Linden trees grow in the temperate zones of Europe, Asia, and the Americas. The American species are native to mountainous regions of the United States, Canada, and Mexico. Since pre-Hispanic times, *tila* has been used when an antispasmodic or sedative was needed. In Europe, linden leaves and flowers were used similarly, to treat hysteria and indigestion.

The linden tree is tall and majestic, with heart-shaped leaves. It's so intensely fragrant when in bloom that it has inspired passionate lines of poetry for centuries. Honey from bees fed on the nectar of linden flowers is considered a great delicacy.

Parts Used: Leaf, flower
Properties: Mild sedative, antispasmodic, induces perspiration
Used to Treat: Fevers, nerves, insomnia, muscle spasms, coughs, colic, nervous indigestion, menstrual cramps

Tlachichinola

Botanical Name: *Kohleria deppeana,* also *Tourneforta capitata, Plumbago pulchella*
Other Names: *Tlachichinoa, Tlachinola, Tochimitllo, Tochomitl, Yerba Rasposa*
Nahuatl: *Tlachichinolxóchitl, Tlepatli*

Fray Bernardino de Sahagún reported in the sixteenth century that the Aztecs used "the *tlachichinoa xiutil*" to treat fever in the mouth or abdomen, festering sores, and itching. Francisco Hernández cataloged eleven different herbs whose names incorporated the Nahuatl word *tlachichinol*, which can be roughly translated as "over the fire remedy." In Sonora the name refers to a species of *Plumbago*, and in other parts of Mexico it could refer to some species of *Tournefortia, Stevia,* or *Helitotropium.*

Most often, though, the name *tlachichinola* or some variation of it refers to *Kohleria deppeana*, a small bush native to Mexico that has bright red flowers and bitter-tasting leaves. The infusion is used as a douche for vaginitis and a tea for gastroenteritis and kidney congestion. A packet of *tlachichinola* sold by a south Texas-based distributor was recommended for stomach problems. In parts of Mexico, nursing mothers drink the tea to increase the flow of milk.

Parts Used: Leaf, stem
Properties: Astringent, disinfectant
Used to Treat: Vaginitis, digestive disorders

Toloache
(see *Florifundio*)

Tomate
Mexican Ground Cherry

Botanical Names: *Physalis subulata, Physalis angulata, Physalis ixocarpa*
Other Names: Husk Tomato, *Tomatillo*
Nahuatl: *Xaltomatl*
Maya: *P'akmuul, P'ak-kanil*

This is not your basic supermarket tomato but a smaller fruit that comes enclosed in a papery husk. It is an ingredient found in chile sauces. The Aztecs used the juice to treat fevers. Today the fruit is used topically as a cure for earache, sore throat, and tonsillitis. The little tomatoes are cooked and mashed with salt and then, while still hot, plastered on the throat or ear of the afflicted party.

Parts Used: Fruit
Used to Treat: Earache, sore throat, tonsillitis

Tomillo
Garden Thyme

Botanical Name: *Thymus vulgaris*
Nahuatl: *Tohmiyoxihutil*

The ancient Greeks and Romans burned thyme to fumigate their homes. Its name may have been derived from the Greek word *tumus*, meaning courage. Medieval ladies presented their knights with scarves embroidered with images of bees hovering over sprigs of thyme, a symbol of bravery.

In the Aztec Herbal of 1552 a plant identified as thyme was included in an elaborate remedy for nursing mothers whose breasts failed to produce the necessary supply of milk. Today the herb is used primarily to calm coughs and as a digestive aid. Thyme oil on a cotton ball is applied to a toothache. Because of its antiseptic qualities, thyme is sometimes an ingredient in herbal toothpaste.

Parts Used: Leaf, flower
Properties: Antispasmodic, expectorant, antibacterial
Used to Treat: Cough, indigestion, toothache

Excessive use of thyme can be irritating to the stomach. Not to be used in therapeutic doses during pregnancy.

Toronjil
Giant Hyssop

Botanical Names: *Agastache mexicanum* syn. *Cedronella mexicana;* also *Melissa* spp.
Other Names: *Toronjil Morado, Toronjil Rojo, Toronjil Blanco, Té de Menta*
Nahuatl: *Tlalhaueuetl, Tlalámatl, Tzompilihuitzpatli, Tzompilihuitzxíhuitl*

A member of the mint family, *Toronjil* is distinguished by long spikes of deep red flowers. The Aztecs used the plant ornamentally and in the treatment of wounds. In Mexico it is still used as a salve made with lard. Mexican Americans use it primarily in remedies for nervous disorders, insomnia, headache, and the gas and cramping associated with nervous indigestion. Lemon balm (*Melissa* spp.) and various species of mint are also sometimes called *toronjil.*

Another member of the mint family, called dragon's head in English (*Dracocephalum moldavica*), is known as *toronjil chino* or *toronjil azul,* Chinese or blue *toronjil,* referring to its Asian origins and its stalk of purply-blue flowers. These two plants are often combined in remedies.

Properties: Antispasmodic, anti-inflammatory
Used to Treat: Nerves, insomnia, digestive disorders, menstrual cramps

Torote
(see *Copal*)

Trébol Morado
Red Clover

Botanical Name: *Trifolium pratense, Trifloium repens*

Red clover is the familiar rampant weed that covers meadows, backyards, and vacant lots all over the Northern Hemisphere. When it is in bloom, the reddish stems and three-lobed leaves are accented by little white, rose, or purple flower balls. It's easy enough to pick your own free supply, and dried *trébol morado* is an herbal staple often found at markets and *botánicas* in Mexican-American neighborhoods.

Part Used: Flowering top
Properties: Mildly sedative, antispasmodic, expectorant
Used to Treat: Cough, colds

Trementina de Piñon
(see *Ocote*)

Tripa de Judas

Botanical Name: *Cissus sicyoides*
Other Names: *Tlayapaloni, Tripa de Vaca, Bejuco, Yerba del Buey*
Nahuatl: *Temecatl, Tepemecatl*
Maya: *Ya'ax-tabakanil*

These climbing vines are members of the Mexican branch of the grape family. The fruits they produce are not edible and can actually be toxic if taken internally, but the stems have been used topically since pre-Hispanic times to treat rheumatism, pimples, and boils. The colorful Spanish name translates literally as "intestines of Judas," or "cow intestines."

Part Used: Stem
Property: Anti-inflammatory
Used to Treat: Rheumatism, aches, pains

For external use only. Can be toxic if taken internally.

Trombita

(see *Florifundio*)

Trompetilla
Bouvardia

Botanical Name: *Bouvardia ternifolia* syn. *Bouvardia triphylla*
Other Names: *Cantaris, Cerillito, Contrayerba, Yerba del Indio, Yerba del Pasmo, Mirto*
Nahuatl: *Tlacoxóchitl, Tlacoxihuitl*

These small flowering shrubs, native to Mexico, Central America, and the southern United States, are sold in nurseries as ornamental garden plants. They are prized for their sprays of bright red, trumpet-shaped flowers.

In sixteenth-century New Spain, Fray Bernardino de Sahagún described the plant in a remedy for fever with copious perspiration. Francisco Hernández reported that the plant was useful in cases of fatigue and that the powdered roots were used to treat old sores. Today, handfuls of the plant are boiled to make a wash for snakebite and insect stings. In parts of Mexico *trompetilla* is still used to treat fatigue and dysentery.

Parts Used: Entire plant
Used to Treat: Snakebite, scorpion bite, other insect stings, dysentery, fatigue

Trompillo

(see *Anacahuite*)

Tronadora
Trumpet Bush

Botanical Name: *Tecoma stans* syn. *Stenolobium stans*
Other Names: *Retama, Flor de San Pedro, Flor Amarillo, Palo de Arco,* Yellow Elder
Nahuatl: *Tecomaxóchitl, Nextamalxóchitl*
Maya: *K'anlol, Xk'anol*

A popular ornamental bush, *tronadora* is cultivated in warm climates for its fragrant trumpet-shaped flowers, which bloom all summer and attract hummingbirds. Its Nahuatl name can be roughly translated as "flower in the form of a vase." The Aztecs used the plants both medicinally and ornamentally.

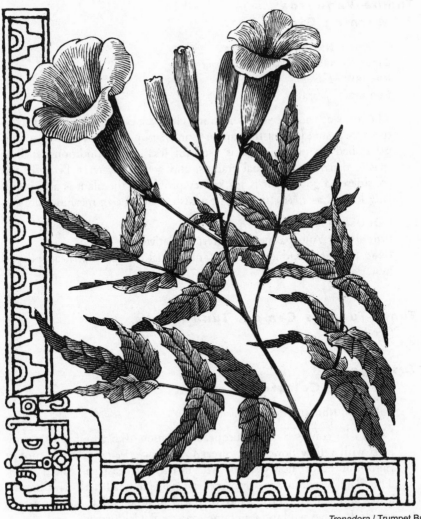

Tronadora / Trumpet Bush

Mexicans and Mexican Americans treat adult-onset, insulin-resistant diabetes with an infusion of *tronadora*. A study reported in the *Journal of Ethnopharmacology* in 1985 indicated that the chemical constituents of the plant had hypoglycemic properties. In 1991 a subsequent study of plants used in Mexico to treat diabetes confirmed these findings. Some people also take an infusion of the stems of *tronadora* to remedy the symptoms of a hangover. A tea made with the roots is considered an effective diuretic.

Parts Used: Flower, leaf, branch, bark, root
Properties: Hypoglycemic, antibiotic, anti-inflammatory, diuretic
Used to Treat: Symptoms of adult-onset diabetes, gastric disturbances associated with a hangover

Tumba Vaqueros
Morning Glory

Botanical Name: *Ipomoea Stans.*
Other Names: *Riñona, Espanta Vaqueros*
Nahuatl: *Tlaxapán*
See also: *Jalapa*

The roots of this species of morning glory are considered such an effective antispasmodic that they are used in a syrup to treat epilepsy. A simple boiled tea of the roots is used for less severe conditions, such as spastic diarrhea, menstrual cramps, and general hysteria. Because it is considered a good remedy for kidney problems, the plant is also popularly known as *riñona*, from the Spanish word *riñones*, meaning kidneys.

Part Used: Root
Properties: Antispasmodic, diuretic, sedative
Used to Treat: Kidney problems, menstrual cramps, diarrhea, epilepsy, hysteria

Tuna, Tuna de Campo, Tuna Mansa
(see *Nopal*)

Tusilago
Western Coltsfoot

Botanical Name: *Petasites palmatus*

Not to be confused with European coltsfoot (*Tusilago palmatum*), a low herb with yellow flowers, or Sweet Coltsfoot (*Petasites hybrides*), another European import now growing wild in the northeastern United States. The plant Mexican Americans call *tusilago* is a small herb with big flat leaves and stalks of little white or purplish flowers that bloom in early spring. It grows wild in mountainous areas of California.

Part Used: Leaf
Properties: Antispasmodic, sedative
Used to Treat: Cough

Uña del Gato
Cat Claw

Botanical Name: *Acacia gregii*
Other Names: *Acacia*
See also: *Acacia, Huizache, Espino Blanco*

This is not the famous Brazilian rain forest plant *(Unicaria tomentosa)* but a tall desert bush with flowers that look like pussywillow. Common from Colorado to Baja California and in Texas, Chihuahua and Sonora, these bushes are covered with nasty curved thorns that give them their Spanish name meaning "cat's claw." A powder made with the dried seedpods and leaves is sprinkled over inflamed irritated skin. A compress made with an infusion of the leaves is applied to sore muscles. The ground pods are also brewed like coffee.

Parts Used: Pod, leaf
Properties: Anti-inflammatory, antimicrobial, astringent
Used to Treat: Muscle pain, diaper rash, superficial wounds

Uvalama
(see *Aceitunillo*)

Valeriana
Garden Helioptrope

Botanical Names: *Valeriana ceratophylla, Valeriana officinalis, Valeriana mexicana*
Other Names: *Yerba del Gato*
Nahuatl: *Cuitapatli*

Valeriana was so highly regarded by physicians in medieval Europe that it was given the name "all heal." Long before the Spanish arrived, the Aztecs made medicines with Mexican species of the plant. The Aztec name is a compound of the Nahuatl words for smelly, *cuitla*, and medicine, *patli*, referring to the nasty odor of the roots. Both the European and Mexican species contain an acid that has antispasmodic and sedative properties.

Part Used: Root
Properties: Sedative, antispasmodic
Used to Treat: Insomnia, nervousness

Can be toxic in large doses.

Varadulce
(see *Palo Azul*)

Varbulilla
(see *Contrayerba*)

Veneno del Perros
(see *Jarilla*)

Verbena
Vervain

Botanical Names: *Verbena canadensis, Verbena carolina, Verbena officinalis, Verbena* spp.
Other Names: *Dormilón, Moradilla*
Nahuatl: *Axixipatli*

Verbena is one of the oldest medicines known to civilization. According to Egyptian mythology, the plant represents the tears shed by the goddess Isis when she was grieving over her beloved Osiris. Legend has it that *verbena*, found growing at the base of the cross where Christ was crucified, was used to stop the bleeding of his wounds. In medieval Europe, physicians hung *verbena* around a patient's neck at night to prevent disturbing dreams.

Although some species of the plant, such as the medicinal *Verbena officinalis*, originated in Europe, others, like the creeping *Verbena canadensis*, are native to the southwestern United States and Mexico. The Aztecs called it "medicine for urinating" and used the mashed roots as a diuretic. In early eighteenth-century New Spain, the Jesuit Juan de Esteyneffer prescribed the herb as a remedy for headache, jaundice, and other ailments. Mexican Americans today use *verbena* tea to treat bad colds and flu.

American *verbena* is a low plant with white flowers topping tall spikes. The species originally imported from Europe now grow wild. Ornamental hybrids are cultivated in gardens. This plant should not be confused with lemon verbena, a totally different genus (*Lippia citriodora* syn. *Aloysia citriodora*) that looks similar.

Parts Used: Leaf, flower
Properties: Sedative, diuretic, induces perspiration
Used to Treat: Colds, flu, stomach problems, *bilis*

Yerba Buena
Spearmint

Botanical Name: *Mentha spicata*

Yerba buena, the good herb, is perhaps the best loved and most used of all the Mexican-American medicinal herbs; it is rivaled for the number one spot only by *manzanilla* (German chamomile). The name can be given to a number of mints, but most often it refers to the strongly flavorful spearmint. A native of the countries bordering the Mediterranean, *yerba buena* came to the Americas with the Spanish friars. Its medicinal use goes back at least to ancient Egypt, where the Greeks and Romans learned of it. It contains essential oils that increase the flow of digestive juices, stimulate perspiration, and diminish catarrh. Used topically, it is slightly antiseptic.

The herb is, above all, gentle, comforting, and delicious. It can be used to mask the nasty taste of some of the other herbs without diminishing their effectiveness. For example, a tea of bitter rue, taken for menstrual cramps, is perfectly palatable if a sprig of *yerba buena* is added to the cup.

Parts Used: Leaf, stem
Properties: Digestive, antiseptic, anti-inflammatory, antispasmodic, external analgesic, induces perspiration
Used to Treat: Colic, flatulence, headache, indigestion, respiratory ailments, diarrhea, nausea

Yerba de la Cruz
(see *Mala Mujer*)

Yerba del Alacrán
(see *Alacrán*)

Yerba de la Víbora
Snakeweed

Botanical Name: *Zornia diphylla*
Other Names: *Viborina, Raíz del Víbora*
See also: *Escoba de la Víbora*

This small yellow-flowered herb grows throughout Mexico and parts of the southwestern United States. It is primarily used to reduce fevers and to treat coughs and colds. It should not be confused with *escoba de la víbora*, or snake broom. In Mexico at least half a dozen plants are also given the name *yerba de la víbora*.

Part Used: Leaf
Property: Induces perspiration
Used to Treat: Fever, stomachache, colds

Yerba del Borracho
(see *Tabaquillo, Té de Monte*)

Yerba del Buey
Gum Weed

Botanical Name: *Grindelia aphanactis*
Other Names: *Pegapega, Tripa de Judas*

Yerba del buey, herb of the ox, is a weedy bush found in dry climates of California, Arizona, and New Mexico. Its English name refers to the gooey stuff that exudes from the yellow flowers.

Parts Used: Flower, leaf
Traditional Uses: Expectorant, antispasmodic, tonic

Used to Treat: Colds, cough, sore throat, kidney disorders

Not to be used in high doses.

Yerba del Burro
Burrobush

Botanical Names: *Hymenoclea* sp.; also *Spigelia longiflora*
Other Names: *Romerillo, Sangre de Toro*

At least ten different plants are known as *yerba del burro,* donkey herb, in various parts of Mexico. In northern Mexico and the southwestern United States the name is likely to refer to some species of *Hymenoclea.*

Another plant commonly called *yerba del burro, Spigelia longiflora,* is a native of the Mexican state of Hidalgo. The roots of this plant are boiled to make a purgative tea, but it **should be used with extreme caution because it is known to be toxic.**

Part Used: Root *(Spigelia)*
Used to Treat: Arthritis, rheumatism *(Hymenoclea);* purgative for intestinal worms *(Spigelia)*

Spigelia longiflora **can be toxic.**

Yerba del Caballo
(see *Jarilla*)

Yerba del Cancer
(see *Cancerina*)

Yerba del Carbonero
(see *Yerba del Pasmo*)

Yerba del Gato
(see *Valeriana*)

Yerba del Golpe
Evening Primrose

Botanical Names: *Oenothera kunthiana, Oenothera pallida, Oenothera rosea*
Other Names: *Flor de San Juan,* Rose of Mexico
Maya: *Chan-xmuk*

Yerba del golpe means "herb for bruises," a name given to many bruise-healing plants. Most often it refers to some species of the primrose. These little shrubs are native to both North and South America. Widely cultivated and hybridized, their four-petaled yellow, pink, red, or white flowers make a familiar garden border.

They exude a lovely aroma in the evenings, attracting not so lovely nocturnal bugs. Evening primrose oil, which is extracted from the seeds, is sold in health food stores for the treatment of premenstrual syndrome.

Mexican Americans make a poultice of the leaves to treat burns, bruises, sore throat, and chest congestion. They take an infusion of the flowers to treat kidney problems and menstrual cramps.

Parts Used: Leaf, flower
Properties: Anti-inflammatory, astringent, antispasmodic, expectorant
Used to Treat: Wounds, bruises, burns, chest congestion, kidney spasms, urinary tract inflammation, menstrual cramps.

Not to be used during pregnancy.

Yerba del Indio
Indian Root

Botanical Names: *Aristolochia mexicana, Aristolochia watsonii, Aristolochia wrightii*
Other Names: *Raíz del India, Inmortal, Comino, Guaco, Yerba del Pasmo,* Birthroot, Snakeroot, Dutchman's Pipe
Nahuatl: *Tlacopatli*

In the Middle Ages, physicians subscribed to a theory called the Doctrine of Signatures, which held that nature gave us a sign to let us know what purpose a plant might have in the service of mankind. *Yerba del indio,* the *Aristolochia* vine, offers an excellent illustration of that theory. Its huge, bent, tubular flowers reminded someone of the human womb, so it was decided that the plant must be useful in childbirth. The Latin botanical name, *Aristo-lochia,* uses the Greek words for best and birth, while in England the plant became known as birthwort, wort being an old English word for herb. Medieval midwives administered doses of the herb in an attempt to speed the birth process.

In the sixteenth century, when Francisco Hernández was laboring at the monumental task of cataloging the flora of New Spain, he came across a plant that he thought looked much the same as the herb he knew back in Europe (although the tropical Mexican species can have enormous flowers). He reported that the native Mexicans used it to treat abscesses, dysentery, deafness, and various other ailments.

Today the herb is under scientific scrutiny, particularly in Germany and China. It has been found to have antibiotic properties and may also be an effective anti-inflammatory and analgesic. Other studies have shown, however, that some species can be toxic to mammals in large doses.

In the markets of Mexico it is recommended as a treatment for snakebite. Interestingly, in a study conducted half a world away in Taiwan in 1974, another species of the same genus appeared to effectively inactivate snake venom.

Parts Used: Root, flower, stem
Properties: Antiseptic, antibiotic
Used to Treat: Snakebite, scorpion bite, vaginal infections, flu, fever, arthritis, toothache

Not to be used by nursing mothers. Can be toxic if taken internally in large doses. Should not be used for an extended period of time.

Yerba del Negro
Desert Hollyhock

Botanical Names: *Sphaeralcea angustifolia, Sphaeralcea* spp.
Other Names: *Yerba de la Negrita, Mal de Ojo, Negrito, Plantas Muy Malas,* Globemallow
Nahuatl: *Tlaltzacutli, Tlalaala, Tlixíhuitl*
See also: *Malva*

These desert herbs can be found throughout the dry regions of the western United States and Mexico. Bright pink- to peach-colored five-petaled flowers bloom along the branches, hollyhock-style. The sticky hairs that cover the foliage are irritating to the skin and eyes, which is why the plant is sometimes known by the Spanish names *mal de ojo* and *plantas muy malas* (evil eye or very bad plants). The Aztec name means "wild sticky plant."

They can be annoying little creatures, but they're not all bad. Cousins of *malva*, they have similar emollient properties and are useful in making soothing washes or poultices. In the sixteenth century, Francisco Hernández reported that native Mexicans used the powdered leaves alone or with sage in a remedy for diarrhea and to cure hives.

Parts Used: Leaf, stem, flower
Property: Emollient
Used to Treat: Eye irritations, sore throat, hemorrhoids, bruises, insect bites, skin irritations

Yerba del Pasmo
Desert Broom

Botanical Names: *Baccharis multiflora, Baccharis* spp.; also *Haplopappus sonorensis*
Other Names: *Escoba Ancha, Romerillo, Yerba del Carbonero, Escobilla, Tepopote, Raíz del Indio*
Nahuatl: *Quauhizquiztl, Tepopotli, Huitzpatli*

Pasmo is Spanish for spasm, but Mexican Americans sometimes use the word to mean a swelling or infection caused by a chill. For instance, one could be afflicted with *pasmo* from drinking a very cold beverage on a hot day, from standing in a cold draft, or from getting caught in the rain. Some *pasmo*-related illnesses might include bronchitis, menstrual problems related to *fría de matríz* (cold womb), aching bones, and sore muscles.

Plants from the species *Baccharis* are commonly used to remedy these symptoms. The branches of these woody shrubs are leafless at the bottom but get very bushy at the top, giving them a decidedly broomlike appearance. The plant is called "desert broom" in English and is sometimes called *escoba ancha,* meaning "broad broom," in Spanish. The plants are still bundled to make brooms in Mexico today.

Species of *Baccharis* are native to both Europe and the Americas. They have been used medicinally since the time of the ancient Greeks, as a diuretic and to provoke menstruation. In Mexico the plant has been used for centuries to bathe women after childbirth. In the sixteenth century, Francisco Hernández listed the herb as a remedy for venomous stings, earache, and toothache, and reported that the mashed leaves applied as a poultice to the head could help with hair loss. In Sonora *yerba del pasmo* is recommended as a contraceptive, a tea for digestive orders, chest congestion, and fever. In Baja California the stems are still chewed to relieve toothache. *Yerba del pasmo* is one of the plants sometimes used in the spiritual cleansings called *limpias.*

Plants of the genus *Haplopappus* are also called *yerba del pasmo. Haplopappus* and *Baccharis,* both members of the Astor family, are used to treat similar infirmities.

Part Used: Leaf
Properties: Astringent, expectorant
Used to Treat: Stuffy nose, sinus headache, insect bites, delayed menstruation

Yerba del Pescado
(see *Alacrán*)

Yerba del Pollo
Mexican Dayflower

Botanical Names: *Commelina coelestis, Commelina pallida, Commelina* spp.
Other Names: *Sinvergüenza*
Nahuatl: *Matlalxihuitl, Coapatli, Matlaliztic*

The Aztecs, who were constantly at war, became quite expert in the art of dressing battle wounds. The herb they called *coapatli* or *matlalxihuitl* was effectively used as a compress to stop bleeding. Modern chemical analysis shows that the plant has properties that can provoke the constriction of the capillaries.

Species of the plant are sometimes used as garden ornaments for the sky blue "day flowers" that close in the afternoon.

Parts Used: Entire plant
Properties: Hemostatic (stops bleeding)
Used to Treat: Wounds, nosebleeds, postpartum bleeding, bleeding after tooth extraction

Yerba del Sapo
Button Snakeroot

Botanical Name: *Eryngium* sp.
Other Names: Sea Holly
Nahuatl: *Huitzcolohtili*
See also: *Chicuría*

Species of this blue thistle are native to both Europe and the Americas. The Aztecs used the root as a restorative tonic after an illness. In Europe it was considered an effective antiflatulent. A seventeenth-century London confectioner sold the candied root as a remedy for liver ailments and a tonic for the aged. Today the herb is sold in Mexican-American neighborhoods as a remedy for kidney problems and a aid for weight loss. The mashed leaves are sometimes used as a poultice for sore eyes. The plant also has reputedly been used to induce abortion.

Parts Used: Leaf, flower, and stem
Properties: Diuretic, anti-inflammatory, antiflatulent, aphrodisiac, stimulates uterus
Used to Treat: Delayed menstruation, kidney problems, cough, rheumatism

Not to be used during pregnancy.

Yerba del Venado
Deerweed

Botanical Names: *Porophyllum* spp.
Other Names: *Odora, Maravilla*
Nahuatl: *Papaloquilitl, Tepepapaloquilitl*
Maya: *Pech'uk-il*

Yerba del venado is a small plant with yellow or purplish flower heads and a strong aroma. The Aztecs ate the roots as a vegetable and used them in remedies for hiccups.

Part Used: Leaf
Used to Treat: Indigestion, colic

Yerba Dulce
(see *Orégano*)

Yerba Luisa
(see *Cedrón*)

Yerba Mansa
Swamp Root

Botanical Name: *Anemopsis californica*
Other Names: *Yerba del Manzo, Bavisa, Raíz del Manso,* Lizard Tail

Despite the unappealing name, "swamp root," *yerba mansa* is really a lovely aromatic creeper, with spikes of fragrant white flowers and flat, oval leaves. It just happens to like swamps and other wet places. Mexican Americans call it *yerba mansa,* "gentle herb," because of its mild flavor and soothing properties. An effective anti-inflammatory, it is used to treat the discomfort of arthritis in a variety of ways: as a tea, a liniment, and a bath. It's easy to find growing wild in the southwestern United States or northern Mexico, and is sold in *botánicas* and markets.

Parts Used: Leaf, root
Traditional Uses: Anti-inflammatory, antibacterial, antifungal, diuretic
Used to Treat: Urinary tract infections, wounds, bruises, skin inflammation, inflamed gums, vaginal inflammation, arthritis, aches, pains

Yerba Mora
Black Nightshade

Botanical Names: *Solanum nigrescens, Solanum nigrum*
Other Names: *Malabar, Solano Negro, Buena Mujer, Mariola, Chichiquelite,* Garden Nightshade, Petty Morel

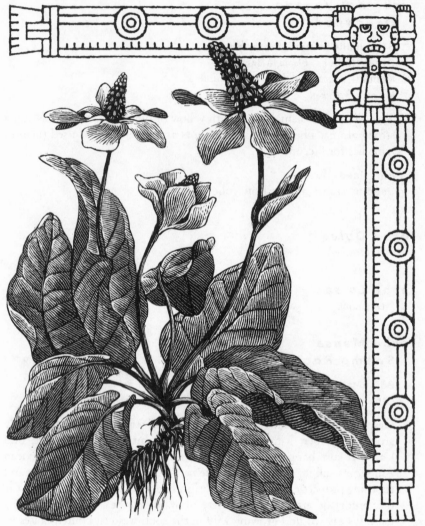

Yerba Mansa / Swamp Root

Nahuatl: *Chichiquilitl, Huitztomatzin, Tzopilotlacuatl*
Maya: *Bahalkan, Ich-kan, Pak'al-kan*

Like all nightshades, *yerba mora* is a relative of the eggplant and the potato, as well as a number of poisonous plants such as ominously named deadly nightshade *(Solanum dulcamara).* The species called *yerba mora,* or black nightshade, has white or bluish flowers and black berries. Nightshade berries can be toxic, particularly if they are eaten before they are ripe. The young leaves are considered to be edible, however, and are used as a culinary herb.

Parts Used: Leaf
Properties: Anti-inflammatory, antifungal
Used to Treat: Wounds, skin irritation, diaper rash, vaginal infection, skin softener

Berries can be toxic.

Yerba Santa
(see *Hoja Santa*)

Yoyote
(see *Ayoyote*)

Yucca
(see *Palmilla*)

Zábila
(see *Sábila*)

Zacate Limón
(see *Té Limón*)

Zapote Blanco
White Sapote

Botanical Name: *Casimiroa edulis*
Other Names: *Matasano Sapote, Sapotilla, Chapote, Zapote Dormilón*
Nahuatl: *Cochizápotl, Cochizxihuitl, Itzaczápotl*
Maya: *Yuy*

Many of the fruits common in the New World today—all the citrus fruits, apples, and pears—were imported after the Spanish conquest, so most of the fruit in the diet of pre-Hispanic Mexico was some variety of *zapote.* It's a sweet pulpy fruit, roughly the size of an orange and the shape of a quince, with a thin skin like an apple. It most closely resembles an Asian pear.

Its Nahuatl name means "sleep fruit," a compound of the words for sleep, *chochi,* and sweet fruit, *zápotl.* The leaves of the *zapote blanco* have been used for centuries as a sedative, and Mexican Americans use it to lower blood pressure. Recent animal studies conducted at the National University of Mexico have supported the possible effectiveness of the plant for both these purposes. The seeds are said to have hypnotic properties.

Part Used: Leaf
Properties: Sedative, analgesic
Used to Treat: Insomnia, nervous disorders, high blood pressure, *empacho*

Zarsaparilla
Sasparilla Root

Botanical Names: *Smilax medica, Smilax aristolochiaefolia, Smilax mexicana, Smilax* spp.
Other Names: Red China Root, *Cocolmeca*, Greenbrier
Nahuatl: *Mecapatli, Cozumecatl*
Maya: *Koh-keh*

The sixteenth-century physician Nicholás Monardes devoted two chapters of his *Joyfulle Newes Out of the Newe Founde Worlde* to *zarsaparilla*, a compound Spanish word meaning "little bramble vine." An enthusiastic proponent of the root, Monardes was something of a *zarsaparilla* gourmet, extolling the virtues of the Honduran variety over the one brought in from Mexico and comparing the roots imported from Peru and Ecuador. Monardes followed the theory, generally held at the time, that an illness was something that had invaded the body, and the cure therefore involved some means of getting it out, either through bleeding, diuretics, laxatives, or, in the case of *zarsaparilla*, through profuse perspiration. He describes an arduous cure in which a thick juice is made by soaking and then boiling the chopped root or root bark. The afflicted person was made to drink this juice three times a day, forsaking all other nourishment with the exception of a little chicken. Wrapped in warm clothing, the patient would then proceed to "sweat it out." The treatment was a prolonged one, lasting more than two weeks, but according to Monardes it was highly effective against a variety of ills.

Not the least of these was syphilis. Although the true origin of the disease is arguable, Columbus's sailors were blamed for discovering it along with the New World and bringing it home with them. Following another medical theory which held that you'll find the cure where you found the ailment, the New World plant *zarsaparilla* became the standard treatment for venereal disease.

By the mid-nineteenth century the root had become wildly popular. In 1831, 176,854 pounds were imported into England alone. In the United States it was the principal ingredient of many patent medicines, such as Ayer's Sarsaparilla. Cowboys in the wild west might have ordered a bottle of sarsaparilla instead of beer at the saloon, particularly if they had recently visited the local brothel.

Today it is still used to flavor soft drinks. Look for it listed under "natural and artificial flavors" next time you open a bottle or can of root beer. Mexican Americans use a strong tea made with the roots as a laxative and tonic.

Parts Used: Root, leaf
Properties: Astringent, analgesic, hemostatic (stops bleeding), tonic for pregnant women
Used to Treat: Diarrhea, adult-onset diabetes, menstrual cramps, excessive menstrual bleeding, premenstrual syndrome

Zempazúchil

(see *Cempasúchil*)

Zoapatle

Botanical Name: *Montanoa tomentosa*
Nahuatl: *Cihuapatli*

This herb has been used since the time of the Aztecs and for untold eons before as an aid in childbirth. *Zoapatle* is a relative of the sunflower, a tropical shrub with triangular leaves and clusters of small white, daisylike flower heads. It is a wild herb, native to Mexico, and it is also cultivated in kitchen gardens.

The plant has been studied both in the United States and in Mexico for its possible usefulness in modern medicine. A tea of the leaves apparently induces uterine contractions and dilation of the cervix. Because women used the tea to prevent pregnancy, the plant has also been studied as a potential oral contraceptive. In addition to its use by midwives, the infusion is sometimes taken for menstrual pain and excessive menstrual bleeding, but it can be a dangerous herb if used incorrectly. In Mexico, where *zoapatle* is used to induce abortion, its sale has been banned by the Secretary of Health.

Part Used: Leaf
Property: Increases the intensity of contractions during childbirth
Used to Treat: Women in childbirth

Can be toxic.

PROFILES: PROFESSIONAL HEALERS

Lee Cantu's Healing Center (Austin, Texas)

Mrs. Cantu had been very kind on the telephone, but it was clear that an interview with her husband, the healer, would have to be carefully arranged. She spoke in the reverential tone the papal secretary must assume when booking an appointment with His Holiness. Two days and several phone calls later, the healer agreed to meet with me for a few minutes.

The Cantu's shop is open at the owner's discretion. The business hours posted on the door are only times when the store *might* be open. When the healer is in, piñatas suspended from the awning dance in the breeze. At the appointed hour I drive around the quiet streets, circling back, waiting for the festive signal that the Cantus have decided to open.

Cantu's Mexican Hierberia Imports & Lee's Healing Center is in a gradually gentrifying, barrio-adjacent neighborhood across the river from the bright lights and wide boulevards of downtown Austin. Their advertising slogans are "where you find experts in every item that is recommended & fully explained instructions" and "a little bit of Mexico in every corner." Display cases offer a colorful assortment of serapes, tortilla warmers, candles, plastic statuettes of the saints, amulets, and magical sprays to protect your home or your car. Along one wall the Virgin of Guadalupe, draped in ropes of Christmas lights, presides over her altar. Another wall is covered with hundreds of cellophane packets of dried herbs, carefully arranged in alphabetical order. A sign behind the cash register reads: PRICES ARE CHEAPER IN MEXICO, BUT THIS IS THE UNITED STATES. THANKS!

Waiting for my moment with the healer, I have plenty of time for a cozy chat with his wife, who quickly warms up to me in her south Texas Spanglish. Mary Lou Cantu is a small, sweet-faced, middle-aged woman who is sincerely in awe of her husband. Before Lee Cantu was called to the practice of healing, she tells me, they were teachers at a community college. Her field was business occupations. His was welding. She proudly informs me that her husband has an associate minister certificate. He is a nondenominational minister at St. Paul's Church of Religious Science and the founder of the First Church of El Niño Fidencio, which venerates the legendary Mexican *curandero*. She is sure they are doing God's work in their *botánica*: helping people. Their steady clients call them Mom and Dad.

"My mother, my daughter, just down the line, we've done herbal healing," she confides. "And then my husband's mother was Aztec, blood Aztec, so she had a lot of knowledge about the herbs. It just comes natural. You don't have to study it or learn it from books, *m'ija*, because you just know."

At five o'clock business in the store picks up as clients drop in on their way home from work. Some have appointments with the healer, others are merely shopping. A man asks for *flor de tila*. "*Ah, sí*," Mrs. Cantu says, "*para dormir, para nervios*." For sleep, for nerves. Take it four times a day.

She counsels a woman who has a court appearance the next day, telling her to buy two lucky candles—one for herself, the other for the judge. "If it works, you'll see me tomorrow," the woman tells her. "If not, they're gonna put me away."

Finally, the healer finishes with a client and comes out of his private office behind the store to meet me. A tall, pale, heavyset man with thinning gray hair, Lee Cantu is not sure he wants to be interviewed. He tells me he has been burned by writers who came in to steal his remedies without buying so much as a candle. I explain that I already know a lot of remedies, that what I am interested in learning about is him. But maybe he doesn't want to be in my book. I can certainly understand. Hearing this, he begins to thaw a little and launches into his story.

"My mother claims that I cried in the womb and she never told nobody, and that's how you're supposed to do it. If you don't tell nobody, the child who is born of the person is very gifted. From the time I was two years old my mother encouraged me to touch people. If there was a little sore or something like that, she let me touch it with my saliva. If a baby was coming breach, she let me touch the stomach of the lady and the baby would turn. There was a lot of reactions that took place. And, of course, it was very uncomfortable for me because I wanted to go and play. I didn't want to be touching people with sores or ringworm or stuff like that. Even though I was born with a gift and my mother told me to do things, I never took it serious. I would not do it. It was not until I had an encounter that I started to do this work.

"When I was working for the refiners in Corpus, I had a fall and I messed up my back, and I had two, three vertebrae that had to be fused. I was in a wheelchair for nineteen months. While I was in the wheelchair, I had an encounter that lasted two days where I spoke with something that was higher than my own realm here. It told me that the reason I was in a wheelchair was because I wasn't using the gift and the mission that I was supposed to be doing. It told me to work with people on a one-on-one basis. I was already doing healing with the Church, but that wasn't enough. It wanted me to be more involved with the people.

"So after that I agreed to help people out. And I had a chance to get my back operated on. I only had a forty percent chance that I would be able to walk again, and I took that chance and, sure enough, I did get well. And that's what triggered the idea of doing the healing part. So I started going to different towns in a van full of teas and herbs and powders and started counseling. I went to Victoria; I went to Houston. I would go here, to Austin, and then I would go back south to Alice."

The Cantus eventually settled in Austin, where they have been in business for fifteen years.

The room where Lee Cantu meets his private clients is furnished with a massage table, a desk, and chairs. It is decorated with candles and altars to the Virgin Mary and to El Niño Fidencio. He has posted his menu of services on the door: *limpias,* chakra cleanings, spiritual alignments, color definitions, card readings, aura cleansings, water readings, psychic acupuncture, past life regressions, and dream interpretation. The fee for half an hour of any one of these treatments is $35. "He even does exorcisms," his wife whispers furtively. "Oh, it scares me to death, but it just has to be done." Lee Cantu pretends not to hear but doesn't hesitate to mention that he has also effectively managed spiritual cleansings of prized horses and dogs.

And who am I to say his treatments don't work? Maybe he really does have psychic powers or, at the very least, a particularly empathetic nature. He must be doing something to make his clients feel better. Why else would they keep coming back?

Socorro Vázquez, *Componedora* (Pico Rivera, California)

Beyond the old barrio of East L.A., the Mexican-American community sprawls eastward, following the Pomona Freeway through the smoggy suburbs of Rosemead, Whittier, and Pico Rivera. Take any off-ramp east of the L.A. river, and everyone on the street speaks Spanish. We drive slowly along Rosemead Boulevard, not sure where we're going, chasing the dim memory of a *curandera* visited years before. My friend, crippled by an attack of sciatica, shifts miserably in the driver's seat, an ice pack tied against the small of her back.

Mid-morning on a weekday, the streets of Pico Rivera are deserted. The light is white and shadowless. The only soul in sight is an elderly man watering his parched lawn, apparently in vain. *¿Por favor señor, la conoce Usted . . . ? Ah, sí, claro.* For sure, he knows where the *curandera* lives. Anyone in the neighborhood could have told us it was the corner house with the glass ornaments hanging from the porch roof. But she is seeing clients at her daughter's shop today.

Tucked into a neighborhood strip mall, the Botánica Vázquez offers herbal teas, soaps, ointments, religious items, talismans—nearly all of it imported from Mexico. We inquire discreetly. There is a reason to be careful. Sometimes *curanderas* are accused of practicing medicine without a license. We are ushered into a long and windowless waiting room hidden behind a curtain in back of the shop and take our places on metal folding chairs lined up against a wall.

Socorro Vázquez has a large and faithful clientele. They come in family groups—grown children with an elderly father, young parents with a baby. The old man tells us he was paralyzed by a stroke and the doctors couldn't help him, but *la señora* has given him back the use of his arm. The young parents tell us they had been unable to conceive a child until Señora Vázquez helped them. *¡Y mira!* The proof is right here in the stroller.

When her turn comes, my friend limps, bent over, into the treatment room. A few minutes later she emerges smiling, standing upright, no more ice pack, no more pain—at least for now.

Socorro Vázquez does not call herself a *curandera;* instead, she has chosen the title *componedora*, fixer. She mends her patients. But in her flowered smock and clear plastic gloves, she looks more like a beauty parlor operator about to give her next client a permanent wave. She is happy to talk with me. After all, God has given her this gift, and she ought to share it with the world. Removing her gloves, she takes my hand and tells me that I have so much energy, too much. You see, *m'ija*, she says solemnly, I can tell everything about a person just from touching them. Maybe she can.

She was born in the state of Jalisco sixty-nine years ago. Her mother, too, was a *componedora*, and her mother's father, and her father's mother, and one of her great-grandmothers, and one of that great-grandmother's sisters. She had sixteen brothers and sisters, but only Socorro and one of her brothers have inherited the ability to heal.

When she was fourteen, she discovered that she had gifted hands. A *muchacha* was suffering terribly in childbirth. Soccoro took her turn at trying to help. Massaging the girl's belly, she was able to reposition the baby, and in just a few minutes, *"ya estaba el chiquillo afuera,"* that baby came out. *"Allí mismo supe que podía componer."* Right then she knew that she could fix people, that she could heal.

After she was married, she worked in a mechanic's shop. Each time somebody got hurt, they would say, "Go get the wife of Margarito Chinchín," and she would fix them. In 1954 she came to the United States. "In the factory where we began working, my daughter and I, we saw such injustice because the majority were undocumented workers. If one would hit himself with a brush, I would heal his jaw and then go back to my work. An arm I would heal, a leg, a back—right there I would heal it. Even the owner, who was a gringo. I fixed his hand, and he tells me, 'I went with the same pain five times to the chiropractor and he didn't do anything, and you, with the one fix that you gave me, you healed it. Why don't you go to work as a healer?'

"But I didn't believe I could do such a thing here because it's a much different country than ours." She retired from the factory after nine years when her eight children began to grow up and leave home. She had become ill. She believes that so many years working in front of an industrial oven had overheated her bladder.

At last she was able to fix people full-time. "In this fixing, there is much satisfaction. *Con eso ya te sientes felíz,"* she says. "When I go to mass, my patients see me and they hug me tightly. . . . There are many gifts in the hands, more gifts than I can begin to mention."

She claims to have particular success in treating infertility. She says she repositions the womb by externally massaging the woman's abdomen. Then she wraps a tight bandage around the belly that must be kept in place for three days to keep the womb from slipping back to the wrong spot. During this time there must be no relations with the husband, no mopping, no sweeping. After the woman's next menstrual period ends, Señora Vázquez prescribes an herbal douche made with *romero, altamisa mexicana, artemisia, gobernadora,* and a little pine twig. "You put some water on to boil, then you add a little pinch of each herb. You let it cool a little. . . . It should be lukewarm." This is to warm up the womb *"después de la descompostura,"* she says, using a Spanish expression that implies the womb has been left in a state of disarray after menstruation. "Being *descompuesto* will make it cold, and sometimes the fixing doesn't want to work because its cold. This is done every month. Although, sometimes with the douche, after one period they're already expecting before the next one.

"I have a family that couldn't have kids, and now they have fourteen kids, all male. I ask them when are they going to quit, but they tell me, 'No, señora, we were crying for a child, and if God has given us this harvest, He has done it for a reason.'"

Señora Vázquez has eight children, three in the States and five back in Mexico. Her daughter Victoria, who owns the *botánica*, is also a *componedora*, continuing the family legacy of healing. Perhaps the legacy will end with her. She thinks perhaps the youngest of her three children may have the gift. "But they are not interested. They are *más incrédulos*, skeptical. Still, when something happens to them—'mommy this hurts, mommy that hurts'—then they come to me."

Bonnie Ochoa, *Yerbera* (Las Cruces, New Mexico)

Driving south from Las Cruces on the old highway that leads toward El Paso, the strip malls and traffic lights quickly disappear in my rearview mirror. On one side of the road, the Organ Mountains seem to form a continuous monumental backyard fence behind miles of comfortable old houses. On the other, the flat expanse of the Mesilla valley rolls eastward from the Rio Grande. At high noon on a late spring Sunday, the piñon and birch cast flat shadows on the sandy white ground in brave defiance of the sun's brutality. And the fine dust that powders my windshield is heading into town on a hot wind blowing up from the Chihuahua desert.

Three miles south of Mesilla I find Bonnie Ochoa in her garden pulling up a tangled mass of coriander plants turned dry and rust-colored by the heat. Sixtyish, feisty, with a quick but cautious smile for the curious gringa, she refuses my help with a load of herbs almost the size of her tiny frame and hauls her harvest onto one of the tables on a shaded patio.

Her garden is well tended and well decorated, with fountains, weather vanes, and bells. An assortment of little birds chirps so vehemently, I have to strain to hear her. "Look at the swallows! They're here because we let 'em build a nest over there. They're making a mess," she complains.

Mrs. Ochoa grows and dries most of the herbs she sells in the tiny shop at the side of the house and at the Las Cruces farmer's market. "You don't need very much," she explains. "You can just have a little bit of everything." She starts her chamomile crop very early, in the winter, then harvests it and uses the space to plant something else. Basil will soon take the place of the coriander she has just pulled up. Every other year she plants *toronjil morado*, purple hyssop.

"The rue is right here," she says, showing me. "It stinks. I have pennyroyal over there. This is the [*yerba*] *mansa*; it smells so pretty. And I have aloe vera there." Bright purple echinacea flowers dominate a corner of the front yard. Patches of *epazote* and *estafiate* flourish in the shade behind the house; huge rosemary bushes flank the side door.

What she can't grow, she collects, wildcrafting in the desert and the forest. "I go clear up to Taos to get the *oshá*. I don't collect an herb if I don't know very well about it." *Cenizo*, she instructs me, is a sage bush that blooms lavender. "It's right there by the road, by my sister's place." And *yerba anís*, "is very delicate, that thing. The flower is tiny, tiny, yellow. Well, you get to the desert, everything's yellow." She gets her eucalyptus leaves from a tree belonging to a friend of her husband. Every year a nephew ships her a box of orange blossoms from his orchard in Escondido, California.

Bonnie Ochoa's mother was a *yerbera* who took her along when she visited patients, teaching her about the herbs. "When everybody was dying of influenza, my mother was curing people right and left. So much that you can learn about herbs, so much.

"But you never learn unless you grow up in a family that knows and you hear about them from when you're little until you get old. This is the best. And then you have to stay in the business a long time to know them. When you prescribe to people and they take the herbs, then you really find out. There are a lot of herbs that my mother said, 'Don't do this with them. Don't do that.' Like that wormwood. You can't drink that more than a week because it thins your guts. You have to come to an herbalist like me. You have to learn what all the herbs do."

Bonnie Ochoa's Hot Weather Remedy

"This is very important in the summer," Bonnie Ochoa tells me, "because we eat so many vegetables and fruits that have acid. *Azafrán* is for the acid in the stomach that can eat up your guts and make your face break out. In the summer when it's very hot out and you're going outside, be careful with the sun and the acid in your stomach. It just eats up your skin. You drink this, right away you feel good."

One heaping teaspoon of *azafrán* (safflower petals)
One quart of water

Add the *azafrán* to the water and shake well. Strain and drink.

Bonnie Ochoa's *Té Coral* Recipe

Té Coral is a blend of herbs sometimes sold prepackaged in markets and *botánicas*. Bonnie Ochoa has her own formula. "It's good for the heart, it's good for blood pressure, migraine headaches, colitis. Doctors don't cure colitis," she says. "This cures it."

Use equal parts of the following herbs:

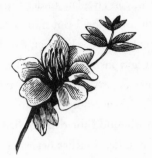

toronjil morada (purple giant hyssop)
azahares (orange blossoms)
flor de tila (linden flowers)
tumba vaqueros (morning glory)
brasil (Brazilwood)
valeriana (garden heliotrope)
poleo (brook mint)
albahaca (basil)
yerba mansa (swamp root leaves)
retama

Mix well. Add one teaspoon of the herb mixture to a teacup. Cover with boiling water and infuse for ten or fifteen minutes. Strain. Drink three or four cups a day.

Drying and Storing Herbs:
Bonnie Ochoa's Advice

If, like Bonnie Ochoa, you grow some of your own herbs, you may want to dry part of the harvest for later use. As a general rule, the best time to pick herbs is in the late morning, just after the dew is gone and before they've started to wilt from the heat. Pick flowering herbs while they are in bud, before the blooms have opened.

Drying herbs is a very uncomplicated business. "Keep them in the shade, never in the sun!" Mrs. Ochoa admonished me. "The sun discolors them and they lose flavor. It does make a difference." And you will need to be sure air

211

can circulate around the plants so that all surfaces dry evenly. Herbs are dried either hanging upside down in bundles or laid out on screens.

Mrs. Ochoa dries some of her herbs suspended from the ceiling of a shaded side porch. "We used to have *vigas*. How do you call them?" *Vigas* are the ceiling beams of southwestern- or hacienda-style houses, the classic place to hang bundles of herbs for drying. "But now I dry the herbs on boards. "

Screen Method

Mrs. Ochoa balances ordinary window screens over a couple of boards so that the air can circulate under them. "I put tissue paper on the screens, and then I put my herbs. I put more tissue paper on top, and I tie it," she told me. By drying the herbs between two layers of tissue paper, she keeps them clean of dust and insects. She stores the screens under a bed for a couple of weeks. "They dry so green and pretty!" And they do. The herbs she sells have all retained their color and aroma beautifully. This screen-drying method is particularly good for delicate herbs with lots of volatile oils, such as mint and chamomile. Sturdier herbs, especially those with woody stalks, such as rosemary, can more easily be dried using the hanging method.

Hanging Method

I don't have *vigas* in my house, either, but I do have a pantry closet with louver doors. The closet is fitted with the inexpensive wire shelving sold in many home supply or hardware stores. I bundle each herb separately and wrap the stems with wide rubber bands a couple of inches from the cut edge. Then I just tie them upside down to the underside of a shelf, close the door, and forget about them for a week or two. Drying times depend on climate. Mrs. Ochoa has an advantage living in southern New Mexico where the humidity is usually very low.

Oven Method

Mrs. Ochoa was horrified when I suggested it to her, but I have also had good results oven-drying some of the fleshier herbs such as borage. You may lose a bit of the volatile oil this way, but it's very fast and the dried leaves stay green and flavorful. I remove the leaves and flowers from the stems, place them in a single layer on a cookie sheet, and bake them in the oven on the very lowest setting—under 150 degrees Fahrenheit—with the door slightly ajar so that the air can circulate. It can take half an hour or more for the leaves to dry fully, and it is important to keep checking. You don't want them to start to brown. If you are drying leaves and flowers on the same sheet, the flowers may dry first. The minute they are ready, remove the herbs from the oven and allow the leaves to cool before handling them.

Some people are desperate to try this in their microwaves, but it can be tricky. The microwave is really airtight, so as the moisture evaporates from the leaves, it can get reabsorbed. And it is more difficult to control. A few seconds can make a big difference, so overdrying is always a danger. That lovely aroma that wafts up from the microwave as you dry the herbs probably means you're losing a lot of the volatile oils, so this method works better with sturdier herbs.

If you'd like to experiment, place your leaves in a single layer on a paper towel, cover with another paper towel, nuke the herbs on a high setting for one minute, then check to see if they need a little more drying time. Power and time settings will vary depending on the type of microwave you are using and the type of leaf you are drying.

Roots and Seeds

When I found Mrs. Ochoa pulling up her coriander plants by the roots, they had already gone to seed. She just removed the seeds from the plants, sifted them clean of bits of leaves and dirt, and stored them.

Roots require some drying time. Place clean roots in a single layer in a shallow cardboard box or basket, and store them in a dark place.

Storing Dried Herbs

Mrs. Ochoa keeps her dried herbs for a year or two. The shelves of her shop are lined with neatly labeled glass jars, and more herbs are kept behind the counter in tightly sealed tins. Herbs should be kept in dark, airtight containers. A big glass or plastic jar with a good lid is perfect. Dark glass is great if you can find it, but you can also wrap a clear glass jar with paper to keep the light out. Smaller quantities of herbs, especially if you're planning to use them up within a few months, can be stored in airtight plastic bags and kept in a dark closet.

Before storing, you may want to pull the leaves off the stems or chop the herbs into one-inch pieces, discarding the woody twigs if you won't be using them. Herbs that you plan to use in powdered form, such as roots and seedpods, should be stored whole and ground later as needed.

PART III

PREPARATIONS FOR HERBS

HERBAL TEAS

Hot teas can be prepared as either infusions or decoctions. Both methods are designed to get the active ingredients out of the plant parts and into the water. Always prepare herbal teas in ceramic, glass, or enameled cups or pots. Never use aluminum because components of the metal can leak into the tea.

STEEPED TEAS: INFUSIONS

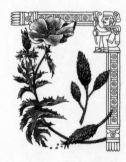

Infusing is the method of choice for herbs that are likely to lose potency through prolonged exposure to heat. Whenever you pour hot water over a tea bag, you're preparing an infusion. Flowers, leaves, and ground roots or bark are usually prepared by infusing. Infusions can also be prepared with seeds if they are first lightly pounded in the pot or cup to release the essential oils.

Some medicinal herbs are now available packaged as tea bags, but most are sold as loose herbs, so you'll need to pour your infusion through a little strainer before drinking.

Examples of herbs usually prepared as infusions are *cola de caballo, epazote, estafiate, malva, manzanilla, romero,* and *yerba buena.*

SIMMERED TEAS: DECOCTIONS

Decoctions are simmered teas, made by adding the herb to cool water, bringing the mixture to a boil, lowering the heat, and simmering, covered, usually for ten to fifteen minutes. The herbs and water are allowed to cool slightly before straining so that they can spend a little more time together. Since some of the water will have evaporated, additional hot water should be added to bring the liquid back to its original measure.

This method is used for herbs that require prodding to get the essence of the plant into the water. Teas made with roots, twigs, bark, or particularly fleshy or woody leaves are often prepared using this method.

Examples of herbs usually prepared as simmered teas are *cardo santo, cáscara sagrada, culantrillo, palo azul,* and *yerba del indio.*

COLD INFUSIONS: MACERATIONS

Some herbs shouldn't be heated at all because they'll lose their potency. These plants are prepared as cold infusions or macerations. The herb is simply placed in a glass jar or enameled pot, covered with cold water, and allowed to steep for several hours or overnight. The liquid is then strained and can be kept, covered, in the refrigerator for a day or two.

Examples of herbs usually prepared as cold infusions are *chaparro amargoso, cuasia, mastuerzo, matarique,* and *oshá.*

TINCTURES

Many modern herbalists have adapted the traditional teas by soaking the herbs in alcohol to make tinctures. There are advantages to this method. Some plant properties are dissolved more easily in alcohol than water, and the alcohol serves as a preservative. It is easier to control dosage with tinctures, too. Ideally, tinctures are made with pure cane alcohol, which is illegal in some states, but gin or vodka can be substituted.

The herbs are chopped very fine, placed in an immaculately clean jar, and amply covered with the alcohol. A general rule of thumb is about four ounces of herbs to a pint of alcohol. The jar is closed with a good lid, and the mixture is allowed to steep for two weeks in a cool, dark place. The jar must be shaken daily.

On the last day, the liquid is poured through a cheesecloth-lined strainer into another jar, then the remaining herbs are squeezed in the cheesecloth, into the strained liquid, to get the last drops of the tincture out.

You can use the tincture directly from the bottle, but you will actually be sipping herb-flavored gin or vodka. You may prefer instead to evaporate the alcohol by adding half a spoonful of tincture to half a cup of boiling water and drinking it as a tea.

MEASURING AND DOSAGE

As the major pharmaceutical companies move into the business of manufacturing herbal remedies, there is a lot of talk about the need for "standardization." But standardization of an organic product is difficult. Two oranges picked on the same day from the same tree will not be equally sweet or contain equal amounts of vitamin C. The sprig of mint you pick tomorrow may not be precisely as potent as the one you pick the day after. Herbal medicine is intrinsically an art as much as a science. It requires the instincts of a cook as well as those of a chemist.

Traditional herbal remedies call for measures of *un manojo, un puñado, tres dedos*—a handful, a fistful, three fingers full. When I asked Concha Talavera how she measured her teas, she tried patiently to explain to me that she used a spoonful of herb in a cup of hot water. When I pressed her for more precise information on exactly how she measured, the look on her face made me fear she must be thinking, "If this gringa is too stupid to make a simple cup of tea, how will she ever manage to write a book?" But she graciously went into her kitchen and retrieved an old teacup and a common teaspoon. She plopped them before me by way of illustration. *"¡Con estos!"* (with these!).

Most teas are made with just those proportions, a rounded teaspoon of the herb to a teacup of water. If the herb is fresh, not dried, you'll need to use two to three spoonfuls instead of one. How long do you steep it? *"¡Cuando está lista!"* (Until it's done!) How can you tell when it's done? You'll know! This usually means about ten or fifteen minutes of steeping time, which is longer than you might think. Most of us are used to dunking a tea bag in a cup for just a minute or two. Steeping times vary with the individual herbs. For example, anyone who has brewed a cup of chamomile tea knows that it requires longer steeping than black tea. Use your instincts and your common sense, and you'll quickly learn how long to steep each tea.

When a *yerbera* recommends a "cup" of tea, she is referring to an old-fashioned teacup-sized dose, not a mugful, and nothing as precise as a measuring cup. Her spoonful is an ordinary teaspoon, not a measuring spoon.

As a general rule, teas are taken three or four times a day for a period of several days. Bonnie Ochoa always recommends that her clients continue taking the teas for a couple of days after they have begun to feel better. Some teas, especially those used to cleanse the kidneys or the blood, are to be taken *"como agua de uso."* You just drink them like water throughout the day, as much as you like. These teas are usually prepared with a handful of herbs in a liter of water.

Other teas should be used in moderation, and most teas shouldn't be used for more than several consecutive days without taking a break. If you notice any problems, stop taking the herb right away. If, on the other hand, the herb doesn't seem to be doing anything at all, it's okay to try taking a little more.

When giving teas to very old people or children, the doses are reduced. Young children are given teas made with only half a spoonful of herb per cup, and babies are always given very diluted infusions.

BASIC BREWING

Not all parts of a plant contain the same properties. We eat the root of the carrot plant, the leaves of the lettuce plant. So, too, with medicinal plants. The roots of the *angélica* plant are used to make a digestive tea, the leaves of the *cédron* plant are used to brew a sedative. The various parts of a medicinal plant require different preparations.

Before brewing teas with dried flowers and leaves, lightly crush them between your fingers to help release the essential oils.

Fresh leaves can be torn into smaller pieces to release the oils and make them easier to measure. Or place a sprig or two of fresh *yerba buena, manzanilla, estafiate,* or *altamisa mexicana* directly into your teacup or pot, and gently bruise the leaves a little by pressing them with the back of a spoon.

Roots, bark, or twigs need to be crushed or ground. If you think of them in cooking terms, garlic is a root prepared by chopping or crushing. Cinnamon is a bark prepared by powdering. These herb parts can be finely chopped, grated, or whirred around in a coffee grinder before brewing. (Most electric blenders are not designed to grind solids.)

Traditionally, the teas mentioned in these remedies are brewed without precise measuring, the way a cook makes a familiar dish, through instinct and experience. But the following basic rules may be helpful. Unless noted otherwise, you can use these proportions as general guidelines for brewing medicinal teas.

To Brew by Infusing

Use
about 1 round teaspoonful of dried herbs in a cup of boiling water
OR
about 2 round teaspoonfuls of fresh herb in a cup of boiling water
then
steep for 5 to 10 minutes before straining.

To Brew by Decoction

Add
about I tablespoonful of crushed seeds to a pint of boiling water;
simmer, covered, for about 10 to 15 minutes before straining.
OR
about 1/2 ounce of crushed, finely chopped dried roots, twigs, or
bark to a pint of boiling water; simmer for about 20 minutes
before straining.

To Brew by Maceration

Place herbs in a clean jar. Add cool water to cover. Seal the jar and
allow to stand for 4 to 6 hours or overnight before straining.

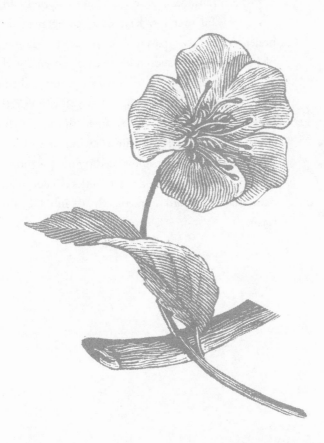

INFUSED OILS

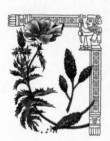

The traditional method is to warm dried herbs in olive oil over low heat in a saucepan or double boiler. At least two parts of oil are used with one part of herbs. The herb should be very well covered with oil. The mixture is heated until it barely simmers, then covered and allowed to simmer slowly for about thirty minutes. The cooled oil is strained through a cheesecloth, then strained again into an immaculately clean dark glass bottle or jar, and sealed tightly for future use. The oil should keep for a few months if kept in a cool, dark place. Discard immediately if mold begins to form.

SALVES AND OINTMENTS

Herbal salves and ointments are traditionally made by cooking the herb in lard over very low heat for a long time, using about three parts of lard to one part herb. It is easier to do this in a double boiler and even easier if you use an electric slow cooker such as a Crock-Pot. Leaves and flowers are usually cooked for at least an hour, roots and bark for at least two hours. The lard is cooled slightly and strained into a jar.

The problem is that lard goes rancid rather quickly. A more modern approach is to substitute olive oil, which has a long shelf life. To make a salve, use three parts oil to one part herb. To make an ointment with a creamy consistency, the infused olive oil is strained, then reheated gently with the addition of a little melted beeswax.

A very simple method uses a commercial petroleum jelly, such as Vaseline. Heat three parts petroleum jelly with one part dried herb very slowly over low heat, just as you would if you were using lard. Cool and strain back into the jar.

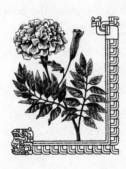

Some herbs, such as powdered chiles, don't need to be simmered at all but can be simply mixed with petroleum jelly, cold cream, or VapoRub.

LINIMENTS

A liniment is just alcohol in which herbs have soaked. To make one, place chopped herbs in a clean glass jar, add enough alcohol so that the herbs are covered plus two inches to allow for evaporation of the liquid and expansion of the herbs as they soak it up. Cover tightly and store in a cool dark place. The recommended soaking time for the various herbs can be as short as a few hours or as long as a couple of weeks.

Fidela Gutiérrez makes a liniment to relieve her arthritic pains by putting a big handful of *florifundio* into a clean jar, filling the jar with enough rubbing alcohol to cover, sealing it, and leaving it in a dark kitchen cabinet for about a week.

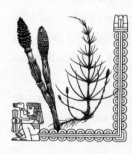

Traditionally, liniments and other remedies were left outside at night, uncovered, to absorb *el sereno,* the cool dew, which some people believed would increase their potency. This belief probably has roots in both medieval Spanish superstitions and ancient Aztec practices.

Many remedies recommend that the herb and alcohol be steeped for nine days, referring to the Aztec magic number. There are nine levels of heaven and nine levels of the underworld, according to Aztec mythology.

COMPRESSES

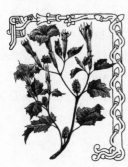

Compresses are made by soaking a clean rag or towel in a warm herbal tea, wringing it out, and placing it on the affected area. More towels can be wrapped over the compress to keep it warm. As the compress begins to cool, it should be replaced with a warm one. Some people keep a hot water bottle on the compress.

Socorro Vázquez told me that in rural Mexico people keep a compress warm with a brick that has been heated in the fire.

POULTICES

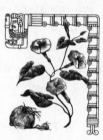

A poultice is made by placing the plant directly on the afflicted area. There are several methods for making a poultice. Fresh leaves are warmed and mashed, and sometimes vinegar and salt are added. Or a paste is made with ground or powdered dried herbs mixed with warm water. The paste is placed between two pieces of gauze or spread on a cloth that is applied to the skin paste side down.

PART IV

LOS REMEDIOS:
TRADITIONAL TREATMENTS
FOR COMMON AILMENTS

HERBS FOR
THE DIGESTIVE SYSTEM

TO AID DIGESTION

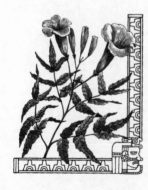

alhucema (lavender)
altamisa mexicana (feverfew)
anís (anise)
azahares (orange blossom)
boldo (bold)
canela (cinnamon)
chía (sage)
clavo (clove)
cola de zorrillo (hop tree)
cuasia (quassia)
diente de león (dandelion)
epazote (American wormseed)
estafiate (mugwort)
hinojo (fennel)
malva (mallow)
manzanilla (German chamomile)
marrubio (white horehound)
mastuerzo (garden nasturtium)
nuez moscada (nutmeg)

orégano (Mexican oregano)

oshá (Porter's lovage)

papaya (Mexican papaya)

pericón (Mexican tarragon)

plumajillo (yarrow)

poleo (brook mint)

popotillo (Mormon tea)

romero (rosemary)

sábila (aloe vera)

salvia real (butterfly bush)

salvia (common sage)

té limón (lemongrass)

tomillo (garden thyme)

yerba buena (spearmint)

Mexican Americans have lots of remedies for indigestion, which is one of the most common disorders to afflict the human body. Most of these herbs make a pleasant bedtime tea.

Herbs to Stimulate Gastric Juices After a Big Meal

Cuasia, like many other bitter-tasting herbs, is used to stimulate the flow of gastric juices. It loses its potency when heated, so it should be prepared as a cold infusion. The herb is used in the form of little wood chips. Soak a level teaspoonful in a cup of water for twelve hours and strain. Drink two cups—one before going to bed at night, and the other first thing in the morning on an empty stomach.

Diente de león combined with **yerba buena** helps the digestive process in two ways: the bitter *diente de león* leaves increase the flow of digestive juices, and the essential oil of the *yerba buena* is a carminative, helping the body to absorb excess gas. Combine equal parts of the dried leaves and pour a cup of boiling water over a heaping spoonful of herbs. Steep for ten or fifteen minutes, strain, and sip.

Mastuerzo, the common garden nasturtium, is believed to have properties that can improve the digestion by increasing the flow of gastric juices. It should always be prepared as a cold infusion. Just add a pinch of the leaves, stems, or seeds to a cup of cool water and steep overnight before straining. This cold tea can be kept in the refrigerator for a day or two.

Tomillo, common thyme, contains an essential oil called thymol, which is considered useful in increasing the secretion of gastric juices. Make an infusion by steeping a rounded spoonful of the leaves in a cup of boiling water for ten or fifteen minutes before straining.

Herbs for Acid Indigestion

Alhucema is recommended for the double whammy of acid indigestion and excess gas. Steep a heaping spoonful of lavender blossoms and leaves in a cup of boiling water for fifteen or twenty minutes before straining.

Cola de zorrillo is used as a remedy for acid indigestion, especially after a big meal. Simmer a rounded spoonful of the clean bark in a cupful of water. The essential oil is alkaloid, which may help to balance excess acid in the digestive system.

Manzanilla is calming to the digestive system. The tea is sometimes combined with a little *yerba buena,* which is good for stomach gas and adds flavor.

Sábila is used for heartburn and stomach ulcers. An aloe vera leaf is peeled and boiled in water to cover, and the resulting liquid can be taken as needed.

Té limón soothes the stomach and aids digestion. This tea can also be effectively combined with an equal part of *yerba buena.*

Yerba buena is one of the oldest and most popular remedies. Spearmint tea helps stimulate the flow of gastric juices. For acid indigestion or heartburn, steep the fresh or dried leaves in hot water and allow the tea to cool to room temperature before adding a little lemon juice and baking soda.

Herbs for Indigestion with Stomach Cramps and Excess Gas

Altamisa is considered to have antispasmodic and anti-inflammatory properties and is taken as a cool tea to settle an upset stomach. Make an infusion by steeping a rounded spoonful in a cup of boiling water for ten or fifteen minutes. Strain and cool to room temperature before drinking.

Azahares, anís, and *hinojo* make a pleasant tea for indigestion accompanied by gas. Combine a spoonful of dried orange blossoms with a pinch of crushed anise seeds and a pinch of crushed fennel seeds. The fennel has anti-spasmodic properties to help with the cramps, and the orange blossoms and anise have a calming effect. Steep in a cupful of hot water for ten or fifteen minutes; strain and sweeten with honey if you like.

Boldo An infusion of *boldo* leaves is taken to alleviate stomach gas. Compresses made with towels or rags soaked in the warm tea are also applied topically to a crampy belly.

Estafiate is considered useful in increasing the flow of gastric juices, and *epazote* is believed to relieve stomach gas. Tea is made by steeping equal parts of the two leaves in a cupful of boiling water for ten or fifteen minutes, straining, and flavoring with cinnamon and sugar.

Marrubio, canela, and *hinojo* make a tasty recipe. Combine a handful of horehound (*marrubio*) leaves and stems with a stick of cinnamon (*canela*) and a stem of fennel (*hinojo*)—the fennel to calm stomach cramps, the horehound to increase the flow of gastric juices, and the cinnamon to help eliminate gas. Add the herbs to a liter of water, bring to the boil, lower the heat, cover and simmer slowly for fifteen minutes. Cool slightly before straining.

Nuez moscada is a remedy for excess stomach gas. A generous pinch of the ground spice added to a cupful of hot water can be taken on its own, or a dash of ground nutmeg can be sprinkled into one of the other digestive teas.

Oshá roots or stems are chewed to relieve a gassy stomach.

Popotillo leaves and stems, flavored with lemon or orange juice, make a tasty and soothing tea.

Romero and *orégano* can be used for a gassy stomach. Try simmering a sprig of rosemary or common oregano in a cup of water. The two herbs can also be combined in a single tea.

Salvia real is considered useful in diminishing the production of excess saliva associated with indigestion. A rounded teaspoonful of the leaves is simmered in a cup of boiling water for ten or fifteen minutes and allowed to cool slightly before straining. The tea can be flavored with honey and lemon.

Salvia, common sage, in an infusion flavored with lemon and honey is a pleasant remedy for stomach gas. Some people like to end a big meal by chewing a few seeds of a sage called **chía** (*Salvia hispanica*) as a digestive aid.

COLIC AND STOMACH CRAMPS

albahaca (basil)

anís (anise)

boldo (bold)

cedrón (lemon-scented verbena)

cempasúchil (Aztec marigold)

eneldo (dill)

hinojo (fennel)

hojasen (senna)

limón (lemon)

malva (mallow)

manzanilla (German chamomile)

papaya (Mexican papaya)

pericón (Mexican marigold)

plumajillo (yarrow)

poleo (brook mint)

rosa de castilla (rose)

yerba buena (spearmint)

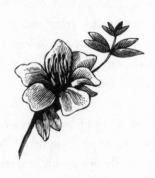

The Spanish word *cólico* refers to a painful, crampy stomach afflicting a person of any age. When applied to an adult infirmity, *cólico* can mean any sort of stomach pain, from simple gas to appendicitis. The remedies listed here are suggested only for the discomfort of indigestion.

Baby colic is treated with many of the same herbs, infused to make a very weak tea and fed lukewarm, not hot. (See Herbs for Babies, page 309.)

Herbs for *Cólico*

Albahaca, cempasúchil, eneldo, hinojo, hojasen, yerba buena, poleo, and *rosa de castilla* are combined in equal parts. The recipe calls for "three fingers full" (a good-sized pinch) of the mixed herbs to be steeped in a liter of water and taken by the cupful on an empty stomach as needed. Basil is thought to have anti-inflammatory properties; both basil and dill are thought to be useful in eliminating stomach gas. The senna increases the flow of gastric juices and will be mildly laxative. The rose petals, *cempasúchil,* and *yerba buena* are soothing.

Boldo is calming to a crampy stomach. The remedy calls for a mild infusion of the leaves taken three times a day.

Cedrón—An infusion of the leaves is soothing and mildly sedative.

Limón and *anís* can be simmered together in a cup of water (a pinch of lemon peel with a few anise seeds). Anise has long been considered a digestive aid and is thought to have antispasmodic properties to relieve stomach cramps.

Malva is soothing to the digestive tract. A spoonful of *malva* leaves can be steeped in a cup of boiling water and taken three times a day.

Manzanilla—An infusion of chamomile flowers is perhaps the best known tea for stomach cramps. Studies have affirmed its antispasmodic properties.

Papaya is a well-respected digestive aid. It contains an enzyme that breaks down protein. The traditional remedy calls for simply eating some of the fruit or drinking papaya juice. Tablets and capsules of papaya derivatives are sold at health food stores and pharmacies.

Pericón, in a tea taken throughout the day in place of water, is believed to stimulate gastric juices and relieve stomach cramps. A small handful of leaves and flowers is brought to a boil in a quart of water, simmered for ten or fifteen minutes, and then allowed to cool before straining

Plumajillo was used by the Aztecs to treat the painful effects of overeating. An infusion of the leaves and flowers is used for the same purpose today. The herb has antispasmodic properties that help calm a crampy stomach.

Fidela Gutiérrez uses a tea made with equal parts of *manzanilla* flowers and *yerba buena* leaves *"para limpiar,"* to cleanse the digestive system. She also uses a tea made from *epazote* leaves for this purpose. For acid indigestion, she uses a tea made with the leaves of a *laurel* tree that grows near her house. She likes to take an infusion of *cedrón* leaves for gas pains.

CONSTIPATION

cáscara sagrada (bearberry)
fresno (evergreen ash)
hojasen (senna)
lantén (common plaintain)
lengua de vaca (yellow dock)
linaza (flax)
nogal (walnut tree, leaves)
sábila (aloe vera)
tabachín (Mexican bird of paradise)

Herbs to Be Taken at Bedtime for a
Laxative Effect in the Morning

Cáscara sagrada and **hojasen** are leading herbal laxatives, the active ingredients in many over-the-counter products. To use them as teas, steep a spoonful of *hojasen* leaves in a cup of boiling water and flavor with a dash of ground ginger. Or bring a spoonful of crushed *cáscara sagrada* bark to a boil in a cup of water. Add a pinch of fennel or a sprinkle of ground ginger to prevent nausea, and simmer for about ten minutes. Add enough hot water to bring the mixture back to a full cup. Flavor with sugar or honey to taste.

Other Herbs Used as Laxatives

Lantén roots and flowers are simmered to make a laxative tea. The seeds are eaten for the same purpose.

Lengua de vaca is used to make a laxative tea. About a teaspoonful of chopped roots are simmered in a cup of water.

Linaza—A tablespoon or two of the seeds is washed down with a big glass of water.

Nogal is prepared by simmering a heaping teaspoonful of the crushed inner bark or root bark in three-quarters of a cup of water.

Sábila juice is heated in a pan over low heat until it produces a dark brown gel, which is taken by the spoonful as a laxative. It should be used in moderation because it can cause cramping and irritation of the intestinal lining. Take no more than one dose of the gel a day, at bedtime. The dosage may be repeated nightly, for no more than a week.

Tabachín leaves or flowers are used to make a laxative tea.

EMPACHO

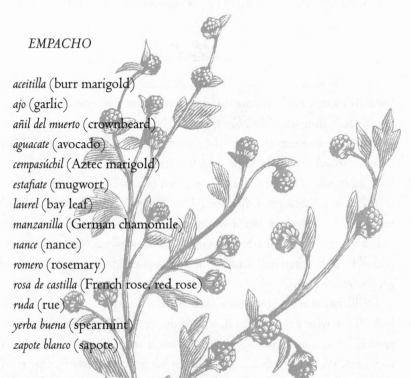

aceitilla (burr marigold)
ajo (garlic)
añil del muerto (crownbeard)
aguacate (avocado)
cempasúchil (Aztec marigold)
estafiate (mugwort)
laurel (bay leaf)
manzanilla (German chamomile)
nance (nance)
romero (rosemary)
rosa de castilla (French rose, red rose)
ruda (rue)
yerba buena (spearmint)
zapote blanco (sapote)

Empacho is the name given to a problem that goes beyond simple constipation. It refers to something more like an intestinal blockage. Some people believe that *empacho* is caused by food that remains stuck to the stomach lining. Eating too much starchy food, eating the wrong foods, or eating too much in general are believed to be causes of the problem. Children who have bad eating habits sometimes come down with a case of *empacho*.

The symptoms can include a bloated stomach, stomach pain, nausea, lack of appetite, and fever. The remedy often calls for a massage of the area. An experienced healer will find the blockage by massaging the stomach and then attempt to break it up with external pressure. The skin on the patient's back, directly behind the stomach, is sometimes pulled between two fingers. When the skin snaps back, the blockage is thought to be loosened.

The massage is followed by an herbal tea to soothe the stomach. A cathartic is also used to eliminate the blockage. Some of the plants traditionally used to treat *empacho* are *aceitillo,* crushed avocado pit, garlic suppositories, a tea of *rosa de castillo* or *cempasúchíl* flowers, *añil del muerto, estafiate, nance, romero* or *yerba del indio* leaves, *copalchí* bark, *contrayerba* root *(Dorstenia contrayerba), zapote blanco,* castor oil, and onion.

Appendicitis is sometimes misdiagnosed as *empacho.* Severe stomach pains and vomiting are always a sign that you should see a doctor right away.

Socorro Vázquez asks clients suffering from *empacho* to come to her *en ayunas,* on a fasting stomach. She gives them a light massage to loosen the blockage, and then she instructs them to take a concoction made with two Alka-Seltzer tablets cooked with *yerba buena, estafiate,* a stem of *ruda,* a leaf of laurel, and a little *manzanilla.* The drink should be taken first thing in the morning on an empty stomach. She gives children 7-Up. "Don't ask me what 7-Up has," she told me. "I don't know, but it works." For babies with *empacho* she prescribes only a quarter of an Alka-Seltzer tablet. She says babies who are more than a year old can be given half an Alka-Seltzer, and children over the age of three get one entire tablet.

Ofelia Esparza told me that when she was a little girl she nearly died of *empacho.* "I got what I think must have been dysentery. My mother said it was *empacho.* She did a little massage on my stomach and found a hard knot on my intestines. We went to the doctor, but I didn't get better. My mother tried her own remedy, half a glass of cool *yerba buena* tea with a little lemon and just a fingernailful of baking soda. Usually that would help me, but not this time. So she consulted an old lady who lived down the street. Following the lady's recipe, my mother picked a *granada* [pomegranate] from a tree in our yard, peeled it, and made a tea with the peels, a few marigold petals, and a little *estafiate.* It was bitter and ugly but I had no more stomach cramps, and after about two days of drinking that tea every few hours, I got well. After that, my mother just gave me a little *poleo* tea with a drop of lemon to keep my stomach soothed. Slowly, I started eating bread and then some of the broth left from cooking beans. My mother and my aunts always said that the doctors here don't know how to cure *empacho.* From then on, whenever my mother had a *granada,* she would dry the peels and save them in a jar for tea."

INTESTINAL INFLAMMATIONS

cancerina (Mexican heather)
cardo santo (Mexican thistle)
jojoba (jojoba)
mezquite (mesquite)
yerba buena (spearmint)

Cancerina and **cardo santo** are used for their soothing properties. The stems, leaves, and flowers of *cancerina* or the chopped roots of *cardo santo* are brought to a boil and simmered for ten or fifteen minutes. The mixture is allowed to cool slightly before straining.

Jojoba is widely considered soothing and emollient. A tea made by steeping a few jojoba leaves in a cup of boiling water is taken to soothe intestinal inflammations and stomach ulcers. The recommended dosage is three cups a day.

Mezquite is used to coat the intestinal tract. A tea is made by pouring half a cup of boiling water over about one and a half teaspoons of clean mesquite bark or seeds. The infusion is allowed to steep for only a minute or two before straining. This tea is taken several times a day as needed.

Yerba buena is soothing. An infusion is made by steeping the leaves or powdered root.

DIARRHEA

aguacate (avocado)
capulín (wild cherry)
cardo santo (Mexican thistle)
crameria (rhatany)
encino (oak bark)
epazote (American wormseed)
estafiate (mugwort)
geranio (geranium)
gordolobo (cudweed)
granada (pomegranate)

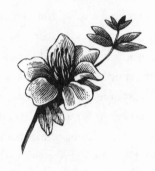

guázima (pricklenut)

manzanilla (German chamomile)

mezquite (mesquite)

nogal (walnut, leaves)

poleo (brook mint)

popotillo (Mormon tea)

prodigiosa (bricklebush)

simonillo (horseweed)

tumba vaqueros (morning glory)

yerba buena (spearmint)

Herbs Used to Make Teas to Treat Diarrhea

As a general rule these teas are taken every three to four hours as needed and are more effective if taken on an empty stomach.

Gordolobo was used medicinally by the Aztecs. Fray Bernardino de Sahagún reported that they treated patients who were on the verge of dying from diarrhea with a remedy made from the herb, so it's probably worth a try if you have a simple case of the runs. The herb is considered to have anti-inflammatory, antispasmodic, and astringent properties, all of which would make it a useful remedy. Steep a teaspoonful of the dried flowers in a cup of boiling water for about fifteen minutes, strain, and drink as necessary.

Guázima, which has antibacterial properties, is a widely regarded remedy for diarrhea. One remedy calls for an infusion made with a spoonful of dried leaves steeped in a cup of boiling water. This tea is taken first thing in the morning on an empty stomach, and again during the day as needed.

Another remedy calls for a tea made by simmering a spoonful of chopped twigs and bark in a cup of hot water for ten or fifteen minutes. This tea is taken cool, three times a day, after meals for three days.

Mezquite works like an herbal Pepto-Bismal, forming a protective coating in the stomach lining. A mild infusion is made with the leaves or bark, using one and a half teaspoons of herb to half a cup of water, and steeping for only a minute or two before straining. Several cups a day can be taken as needed.

Prodigiosa is recommended for treating diarrhea. In his book *Plantas Curativas de México,* Dr. Luis Cabrera writes that the herb slightly paralyzes the peristaltic movements of the intestines.

Herbs Useful Because of Their Astringent Properties

Aguacate is used in a variety of ways to treat diarrhea. One very appealing remedy calls for simmering an avocado pit in half a liter of water for fifteen minutes. During the last few minutes, add a handful of *yerba buena* leaves. Strain the liquid and add a little of it to a cup of hot chocolate.

Another remedy calls for crushing the pit of a ripe avocado, boiling it in water, straining, and drinking the tea on an empty stomach.

The simplest method is to make a tea by simmering a few avocado leaves in a cup or two of water for ten minutes, then straining the liquid.

Cardo santo roots are considered both astringent and anti-inflammatory. Use a big pinch of the chopped roots in a liter of water. Bring the mixture to a boil, simmer for ten or fifteen minutes, and cool slightly before straining.

Crameria can be brewed as a tea by pouring three-quarters of a cup of boiling water over a heaping teaspoonful of the crushed root. Let the infusion steep for fifteen minutes before straining. Drink three times a day before meals.

Encino is prepared by covering clean fresh or dry oak bark with cold water. The mixture is brought to a boil, then removed from the heat and allowed to steep overnight before straining. Half-cup doses are taken four times a day, beginning with a cup first thing in the morning.

Granada's fruit, juice, and rind have astringent properties. One remedy calls for boiling a handful of the rind in about a liter of water, simmering for ten minutes, then cooling and straining. Three glasses are taken throughout the day. A tastier version adds cinnamon, a few hibiscus flowers, and some fresh quince. For children with diarrhea, *granada* juice is boiled together with sugar to make a syrup that can be administered by the spoonful several times a day as needed.

Geranio was used during the nineteenth century to make an astringent tea to remedy diarrhea. A recommended dose is a rounded spoonful of the ground root boiled in half a cup of water. Take a spoonful of the resulting liquid every hour. The tea is considered more effective if a bit of *manzanilla* flowers and *yerba buena* leaves are added.

Nogal—A tea made with walnut leaves is simmered in water and used to treat colitis and chronic bowel irritation.

Herbs Useful Because of Their Soothing Properties

Capulín is thought to have sedative and antispasmodic properties. The remedy calls for a weak infusion of the fresh leaves, taken a couple of spoonfuls at a time, every few hours as needed.

Manzanilla is known to be an effective antispasmodic and anti-inflammatory. An infusion of the flowers is soothing.

Epazote is considered to be soothing to a crampy stomach. An infusion of *epazote* leaves and stems is a classic remedy for diarrhea.

Poleo—An infusion made with its leaves and stems may soothe an intestinal tract irritated by a bout of diarrhea.

Popotillo leaf in an infusion is widely considered a soothing remedy.

Simonillo is considered to be useful for soothing the intestinal inflammation of irritable bowels, diarrhea, and colitis. A strong infusion is made by pouring about a half cup of boiling water onto a couple of spoonfuls of the dried leaves and stems or flowers and steeping for about fifteen minutes. The tea is taken on an empty stomach once a day.

Tumba vaqueros is used to make an antispasmodic and sedative tea for diarrhea that is accompanied by stomach cramps. A spoonful of the chopped root is simmered in a cupful of water.

Yerba buena has properties that help relieve the gas and cramps associated with diarrhea. An infusion is made by steeping the leaves in boiling water.

LACK OF APPETITE

damiana (damiana)
estafiate (mugwort)
jengibre (gingerroot)

Teas for Those Who Are Suffering from a Debilitating Illness or Recovering from One

Damiana has been used at least since the time of the Aztecs as an appetite stimulant. Three cups a day of an infusion of the leaves are recommended, taken first thing in the morning and between meals.

Estafiate in an infusion is used to stimulate the appetite and improve digestion.

Jengibre adds flavor to infusions of soothing herbs such as *yerba buena, manzanilla,* or *poleo,* and has properties that help to combat nausea. A pinch of the powdered root can be sprinkled into a cup of tea.

NAUSEA

anís (anise)
canela (cinnamon)
jengibre (gingerroot)
marrubio (white horehound)
orégano (Mexican oregano)
poleo (brook mint)
yerba buena (spearmint)

Jengibre is widely considered an effective remedy for nausea *but is not considered safe for the morning sickness of pregnancy.*

Yerba buena laced with *canela* or *marrubio* leaves and flowers is used to make a very mild tea for expectant mothers.

Anís seeds or *orégano* flowers can be used in an infusion for nausea and seasickness.

INTESTINAL PARASITES AND AMEBIC DYSENTERY

aguacate (avocado)
albahaca (basil)
anís (anise)
calabaza (squash)
cáscara sagrada (bearberry)
chaparro amargoso (crucifixion thorn)
cuasia (quassia)
durazno (peach tree, leaves)
epazote (American wormseed)

estafiate (mugwort)
granada (pomegranate)
hojasen (senna)
jalapa (jalapa)
limón (lemon)
marrubio (white horehound)
orégano (Mexican oregano)
papaya (Mexican papaya)

The Aztecs had a long list of remedies for intestinal parasites, a problem that has plagued mankind for centuries. In traditional medicine today, herbal teas are used to kill the invaders or drive them out of the body. This treatment is usually followed by purging the bowels with a super-strength dose of a laxative tea such as *cáscara sagrada* or *hojasen*. Getting rid of intestinal worms is a tricky business. Although there are many traditional remedies for the condition, it's a good idea to check with a doctor.

Albahaca and **anís** can be combined effectively. *Albahaca* (basil) contains an essential oil that fights the organisms that cause dysentery and one study showed that anise oil inhibited some microbes that were not affected by the basil oil. A tea made by simmering fresh basil leaves in water for fifteen minutes and then straining and adding a drop or two of anise oil will cover lots of bases, and the flavor is tasty.

Calabaza—A small handful of the seeds, either toasted or raw, eaten on an empty stomach along with a few leaves of *yerba buena*, is believed to expel parasites.

Chaparro amargoso is not always easy to find, but it has a reputation for really wiping out amebic dysentery and giardiasis, eliminating both the adult and formative parasites as well as alleviating the unpleasant symptoms. It should be taken as a cold infusion, made by soaking bits of the clean, dried stems in water, or as a tincture, made by soaking the wood bits in cane alcohol. The herbalist Michael Moore makes a very strong case for it in his book *Medicinal Plants of the Desert and Canyon West*. Moore recommends taking twenty-five to fifty drops of the tincture several times a day. He also suggests using the herb as a preventative measure and even adds half a dropperful of the tincture to dubious drinking water when traveling.

Cuasia chips are used to treat amebic dysentery and roundworms. Make a cold infusion by soaking a teaspoonful of the chips in a cup of water for twelve hours before straining. The recommended dosage is three or four cups a day. To expel pinworms, the same infusion is administered as an enema.

Epazote is the classic cure for roundworms and hookworms. These are some of the many home recipes for the remedy: Add one stem and two or three small roots to a liter of water. Boil until the liquid is reduced by half, strain, and drink in place of water throughout the day until the worms are expelled. Make a tea by simmering *epazote* leaves with Mexican chocolate, sugar, and water. Make an infusion with a spoonful of *epazote* leaves mixed with a few leaves of *orégano, tomillo,* and *yerba buena.* Drink three cups a day on an empty stomach.

A laxative, such as a spoonful castor oil, or a tea made with *cáscara sagrada,* is usually recommended after three or four consecutive days of the *epazote* treatment.

Estafiate tea, made by infusing the fresh leaves, sometimes combined with a little *epazote,* is often used to expel roundworms and pinworms. It has a reputation for effectiveness, but it also has a nasty flavor and must be used consistently every day for a couple of weeks.

Granada is another classic cure for intestinal tapeworms. One version of the remedy calls for soaking one part of the root bark in ten parts of water overnight, then boiling the mixture until the liquid is reduced by two-thirds before straining and drinking. First thing in the morning, on an empty stomach, three half-cup doses of the tea are taken at half-hour intervals. This treatment is repeated for three days. On the third day, after drinking the tea, a good dose of castor oil is taken. The tea can cause nausea and vomiting, especially on the first day of treatment.

Jalapa has been used as a purgative since the days of the Aztec empire. Add no more than half a teaspoonful of fresh or dried powdered root to a glass of water. (Larger doses can cause nausea.) Take on an empty stomach.

Papaya is used to treat intestinal parasites in both children and adults. One remedy calls for drinking a tea of the leaves on an empty stomach several times a day for three days, while also eating the fruit. Another remedy calls for eating the poached seeds along with a little of the sap collected from incisions in the unripe fruit.

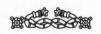

Other infusions sometimes used to treat parasites:

> The papery skin that envelops the pit of an avocado, along with a little
> of the peel from the fruit
> Peach leaves, especially for roundworms and hookworms
> Lemon leaves and seeds
> Horehound leaves and flowers
> Mexican oregano leaves and flowers

HERBS FOR THE URINARY TRACT, KIDNEY, AND LIVER

WATER RETENTION AND URINARY TRACT DISORDERS

aceitilla (burr marigold)
barba de maíz (corn silk)
cola de caballo (horsetail)
colita de rata (flat-top buckwheat)
diente de león (dandelion)
enebro (juniper)
gobernadora (creosote)
linaza (flax)
malva (mallow)
nopal (prickly pear cactus)
perejil (curly parsley)
pingüica (uva ursi)

Herbs with Diuretic Properties

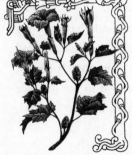

Some herbs are effective diuretics. They can be wonderful for the bloating of PMS and are used to treat the ailment that Mexican Americans call *mal de orín*, which refers to painful, burning urination often a symptom of "honeymoon cystitis." If you suspect that you have a urinary infection though, it's a good idea to see a doctor.

Aceitilla is a traditional remedy for urinary tract infections and inflammations or for clearing cloudy urine. Combine the herb with equal parts of *barba de maíz* and *manzanilla*. Boil two big spoonfuls of the mixture in a quart of water for ten to fifteen minutes. Allow to stand overnight. Strain and drink by the glassful three or four times a day. Continue this treatment for a few days after the symptoms are relieved.

Barba de maíz makes a remedy for cystitis, water retention, and even geriatric incontinence. It's considered to have both anti-inflammatory and diuretic properties. Pour half a liter of boiling water over two rounded teaspoons of the corn silk. Drink three times a day as needed.

Cola de caballo is widely used for its effectiveness as a diuretic. Many health food stores sell it packaged in tea bags. It's also often used in combination with other diuretic herbs like *pingüica*. A very effective diuretic tea can be made combining equal parts of *cola de caballo, diente de león, perejil,* and *malva*. The *malva* is soothing to the urinary tract, and the other herbs have diuretic action. Pour a cup of boiling water over a rounded teaspoonful of the herb mixture. Steep for ten minutes before straining.

Diente de león and *pingüica* combined make an excellent diuretic tea. The dandelion replaces some of the potassium lost by the diuretic action and has anti-inflammatory properties. The *pingüica* has diuretic, astringent, and antimicrobial properties. Mix equal parts of the herbs and steep a spoonful in a cup of boiling water for ten or fifteen minutes before straining.

Enebro is considered to have both diuretic and antiseptic properties. A simple infusion of dried leaves and berries is used to treat inflammations of the urinary tract.

Gobernadora is considered an effective diuretic. It has antimicrobial properties and may work to help decongest the urinary tract. An infusion of the leaves is cooled to room temperature and taken throughout the day in place of water.

Nopal—The juice of the paddles is an effective diuretic and has soothing properties. To make *nopal* juice, peel one of the paddles, chop it coarsely, and whir it in the blender until liquefied. The juice can be kept in the refrigerator and used as needed for about a week. *Nopal* paddles are sold in the produce section of many supermarkets. Canned *nopal* is also available in some markets, but it may be less potent than the fresh paddles.

For men with prostate problems, Socorro Vázquez recommends an infusion made with equal parts of *cola de caballo* stems, silky hairs of *barba de maíz*, and *retama* leaves. She instructs her clients to put the infusion in a large jar and drink it like water.

Herbs Used in Treating Urinary Tract Inflammations Because of Their Emollient Properties

Colita de rata—An infusion of the flowers.

Linaza—A big spoonful of the seeds boiled in a liter of water until the liquid is reduced by half. The tea is strained and drunk in place of water throughout the day. A little lemon may be added.

Malva—A heaping spoonful of the leaves steeped in a cup of boiling water can be taken as needed to relieve burning urination.

KIDNEY PROBLEMS

abedul (white birch)
barba de maíz (corn silk)
cola de caballo (horsetail)
copalchí (copalchí)
damiana (damiana)
inmortal (milkweed)
ortiga (stinging nettle)
palo azul (kidneywood)
pingüica (uva ursi)
popotillo (Mormon tea)
ruda (rue)
tejocote (Mexican hawthorn)
yerba del golpe (evening primrose)
yerba del sapo (button snakeroot)

In traditional Mexican and Mexican-American medicine, kidney problems are often treated by flushing the kidney with infusions of diuretic herbs.

Diuretic Remedies

Barba de maíz works as a diuretic and is soothing. One remedy calls for a small handful of corn silk along with a heaping tablespoon each of alfalfa leaves and barley grains simmered in about a quart of water. The recommended dosage is three or four glasses a day of the cooled liquid.

Cola de caballo is considered highly effective in treating kidney problems. In addition to its usefulness as a diuretic, it may also help dissolve kidney stones. It has a high silicone content and may be irritating if taken for more than a day or two. It's a good idea to mix two parts of *cola de caballo* stems with one part of a soothing herb like *malva* or *yerba mansa* leaves.

Copalchí is a bitter herb, so *piloncillo*, brown sugar, or honey is added to cut the taste. An infusion is made with a rounded spoonful of the bark in half a cup of water and taken three or four times a day.

Inmortal in the form of infusion made with a teaspoonful of powdered root in a glass of cool water is taken first thing in the morning on an empty stomach.

Ortiga is thought to have diuretic and astringent properties. An infusion made with one or two teaspoons of the herb in a cup of boiling water can be taken up to three times a day.

Palo azul is considered to have diuretic, anti-inflammatory, and disinfectant properties. A big pinch of wood chips is added to a quart of water. The mixture is simmered, covered, for fifteen minutes, then strained and allowed to cool to room temperature. The resulting liquid is taken in place of water throughout the day.

Pingüica is a good diuretic and is thought to "clear" the kidneys. An infusion is made with a rounded spoonful of the leaves and berries steeped in a cup of boiling water. Three cups of the tea are taken throughout the day.

Popotillo has diuretic and astringent properties. An infusion made with a spoonful of the leaves steeped in a cup of boiling water is taken three or four times a day.

Tejocote's roots are considered the most potent part, but the leaves and bark can also be used. A simmered tea made with the chopped roots or an infusion of the leaves, using two teaspoons to a half cup of boiling water, is taken three times a day—first thing in the morning and between meals.

Yerba del sapo can be taken as an infusion—a handful of herbs in a quart of water. One small glassful on an empty stomach first thing in the morning is the recommended dose.

Soothing and Antispasmodic Remedies

Abedul is taken to soothe an inflamed kidney and to prevent kidney stones from forming. An infusion is made with equal parts of the crushed bark and young leaves or the leaves alone, using one part of the plant to ten parts of boiling water.

Damiana is considered a gentle but effective diuretic and a soothing tea for kidney or bladder inflammation. An infusion of the leaves is taken first thing in the morning and as many as three more times during the day.

Yerba del golpe is considered to have anti-inflammatory and antispasmodic properties. An infusion is made with the leaves and flowers.

Fidela Gutiérrez uses pineapple juice to cleanse the kidneys, and watercress in a salad to cleanse the liver. She recommends an infusion of *ruda* for both kidney pain and high blood pressure.

ADULT-ONSET DIABETES

matarique (Indian plantain)
nopal (prickly pear cactus)
prodigiosa (bricklebush)
salvia real (butterfly bush)
tronadora (trumpet bush)

Adult-onset diabetes, also known as Type II or non-insulin-dependent diabetes, is the third biggest health problem globally, right behind cancer and heart disease. It particularly plagues Mexicans and Mexican Americans due to a combination of genetic predilection to the disease and a starch-heavy diet. Researchers have been surprised to discover that indigenous healers in Mexico today prescribe many remedies for Type II diabetes. In addition to the herbs listed here, a particular species of *cola de caballo* (*Equisetum myriochaetum*) has recently been studied by scientists Adololfo Andrade and Helmut Wiedenfeld. Working with a native healer in the state of Oaxaca, they discovered that the herb had active hypoglycemic properties. Further research now taking place in Germany may result in a commercially available herbal product in the near future. Diabetes is a life-threatening condition and requires medical attention. *If you are taking any of these herbs, it is imperative that you tell your doctor.*

Matarique is considered an effective remedy for the early stages of adult-onset diabetes, particularly in cases where the diabetic is overweight. A recommended remedy is a cold infusion made with a level teaspoonful of the ground root soaked overnight in three-quarters of a cup of water. It is taken first thing each morning on an empty stomach for four or five days. The treatment is suspended for a few days, then repeated.

Nopal juice exuded from the paddles is also used to treat diabetes. A piece of peeled paddle is liquefied in the blender. The resulting slush is added to water along with any sugar-free flavoring that might make it more palatable. This drink should be made fresh and taken daily.

Prodigiosa is widely used as a remedy for the symptoms of adult-onset diabetes. An infusion of the leaves and flowers taken in the morning and another cup in the evening is considered useful in lowering blood sugar.

Salvia real doesn't help the body manage its blood sugar level, but a tea made by simmering the root is used to treat the frequent urination often associated with insulin-resistant diabetes. In his book *Plantas Curatives de Mexico*, Dr. Luis G. Cabrera also recommends making a tincture by covering the powdered leaves with cane alcohol and steeping for forty-eight hours before straining. The dosage is about a teaspoonful taken with water three times a day.

Tronadora is used by many Mexican Americans to treat symptoms of diabetes and has been shown to have hypoglycemic activity. A suggested formula is three or four dried leaves infused in a cup of boiling water. Doses of half a cup are taken up to three times a day.

BILIS

ajenjo (wormwood)

albahaca (basil)

alcanfor (camphor tree)

epazote del zorillo (wormseed)

estafiate (mugwort)

fresno (evergreen ash)

guayaba (guava)

hinojo (fennel)

manzanilla (German chamomile)

marrubio (white horehound)

nopal (prickly pear cactus)

orégano (Mexican oregano)

prodigiosa (bricklebush)

romero (rosemary)

simonillo (horseweed)

verbena (vervain)

yerba buena (spearmint)

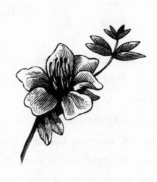

Bilis is an infirmity specific to Mexican and Mexican-American culture. It is caused by an attack of *coraje*, of rage, which is so powerful it affects the body. Literally translated, *bilis* is simply the Spanish word for bile. When we say someone is bilious, we mean that he is ill-tempered, but what we are literally saying is that he is filled with bile.

Both the disease *bilis* and the English word "bilious" are rooted in humoral theory. According to the tenets of ancient Greek medicine, yellow bile was one of the four humors, along with blood, phlegm, and black bile. Health could be maintained only so long as these four humors were in balance. This theory continued to be held through the Middle Ages and was brought to the New World by the Spanish friars. The disease *bilis* is a holdover of humoral theory, an excess of yellow bile triggered by an emotional upset.

Bilis is also rooted in Aztec religious-medical theory which held that the liver was one of the three centers of energy. Human passions were centered in the liver, which would swell with an excess of rage.

The symptoms of the disease begin to show up in the days following an angry outburst. They can include intestinal inflammation, gas, constipation, a bad taste in the mouth, a coated tongue, a yellowish tone to the complexion or to the whites of the eyes, vomiting, nervousness, and sleeplessness.

The treatment is designed to get rid of the excess bile. This frequently involves the use of a laxative, such as *cáscara sagrada*, a massage of the abdomen, and herbal poultices. Sometimes fasting is recommended or the avoidance of certain foods. Frequently, a period of rest is advised.

If the symptoms of *bilis* persist, they may actually point to gall bladder disease and should be treated by a doctor.

These are just a few of the many herbal remedies for *bilis:*

A sprig of fresh **estafiate** is chewed to remedy the stomach disorders associated with *bilis*.

An interesting remedy calls for a tea made with a bit of **nopal** root, plus some leaves of **albahaca, tomato, estafiate, yerba buena,** and **orégano**. The combined herbs are simmered in water for ten minutes, then strained. One cup a day is taken on an empty stomach for nine consecutive days.

Hinoja is used in many remedies for *bilis*. One recipe calls for an infusion combining a spoonful of *hinojo* leaves and flowers with a **guayaba** leaf and pinch of **marrubio** leaves, all steeped in a cupful of water. Another combines the *hinojo* with a **fresno** leaf, yet another with a pinch of **romero** leaves.

An infusion of **prodigiosa** leaves, flavored with ground cinnamon and salt, is taken to help the body expel excess bile. This is also considered a good preventative tea against the formation of gallstones or the onset of a gall bladder attack.

Other herbs used to make infusions for *bilis* are **epazote de zorillo** leaves, **ajenjo** leaves, and **simonillo** leaves and flowers.

The Oaxacan *curandera* Hermilia Diego Gonzales recommends a treatment for *bilis* that begins with massaging the stomach from the center down. The massage is followed with doses of the juice of fresh **verbena** leaves or an infusion of the dried leaves. She uses the same treatment to calm an overactive or "hot" liver.

HERBS FOR THE RESPIRATORY TRACT, FEVER, FLU, AND SORE THROAT

ASTHMA

amapola (field poppy)
estafiate (mugwort)
florifundio (angel's trumpet)
jojoba (jojoba)

Traditionally, asthma is often treated by smoking a dried leaf from one or another of the herbs, either rolled up in a cigarette or stuffed into a pipe.

Estafiate is one of the most popular herbs smoked for asthma, but it may be more beneficial to inhale the fumes in a steam. The leaves are boiled in water on the stove, and a tent is made by placing a towel over the pot. Some people add a few eucalyptus leaves or a spoonful of VapoRub. The *estafiate* is believed to be antispasmodic and to help break up chest congestion.

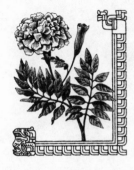

Florifundio is also smoked to calm the spasms of asthma, or the leaves can simply be burned in an ashtray and the fumes inhaled.

Asthma is also treated with these herbs:

Amapola is considered to have sedative properties and may help calm asthmatic spasms. A rounded spoonful of the petals is steeped in a cup of boiling water for fifteen minutes. One to three cups a day is taken as needed.

Jojoba has emollient properties which may be soothing to inflamed bronchial tubes. A rounded spoonful of the leaves is steeped in a cup of boiling water for fifteen minutes. Three cups a day are taken.

(Also see the remedies for bronchial congestion, pages 255–58.)

BRONCHIAL CONGESTION, CHEST COLDS, AND COUGH

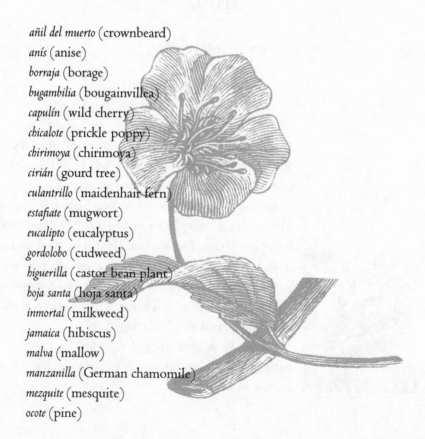

añil del muerto (crownbeard)
anís (anise)
borraja (borage)
bugambilia (bougainvillea)
capulín (wild cherry)
chicalote (prickle poppy)
chirimoya (chirimoya)
cirián (gourd tree)
culantrillo (maidenhair fern)
estafiate (mugwort)
eucalipto (eucalyptus)
gordolobo (cudweed)
higuerilla (castor bean plant)
hoja santa (hoja santa)
inmortal (milkweed)
jamaica (hibiscus)
malva (mallow)
manzanilla (German chamomile)
mezquite (mesquite)
ocote (pine)

orozús (licorice)

pingüica (uva ursi)

pirú (pepper tree)

poleo de monte (poleo de monte)

salvia real (butterfly bush)

saúco (elder flowers)

tamarindo (tamarind)

tejocote (Mexican hawthorn)

tomillo (garden thyme)

trébol morado (red clover)

tusilago (western coltsfoot)

yerba del buey (gum weed)

yerba mansa (swamp root)

Soothing and Expectorant Remedies

Gordolobo is the herb of choice for all sorts of chest ailments. Considered an effective expectorant and emollient, it is used to break up congestion and soothe irritated bronchial tubes. The herb can be taken by itself as a hot tea, but there are many interesting recipes for *gordolobo* tea made with a combination of herbs:

Mix two parts of *gordolobo* flowers with one part each of **bugambilia** blossoms, **eucalipto** leaves, and **tejocote** leaves. Boil a handful of the combined herbs in a quart of water and simmer for a few minutes before straining. Add a little lemon and honey to taste. Sip the tea throughout the day. All four herbs are considered expectorants and are traditionally used to treat coughs. The cooked fruit of *tejocote* is also eaten to help alleviate a cough.

Another recipe made in the same way calls for two parts of *gordolobo* with one part each of **bugambilia, manzanilla,** and **jamaica** blossoms, one part of **tomillo** leaves, and just a sprinkle of ground cinnamon. The *manzanilla* and *tomillo* have antispasmodic properties to help calm the cough.

Yet another remedy calls for two parts of *gordolobo* flowers with one part each of **chirimoya** bark and **añil del muerto** leaves. The *chirimoya* may have antiseptic qualities, and the *añil del muerto* is considered an anti-inflammatory.

Gordolobo and *bugambilia* blossoms can also be mixed with the juice of **tamarindo** fruit, flavored with cinnamon, and sweetened with honey.

Estafiate sometimes helps coughing children. They are given a rag to suck on, filled with fresh *estafiate* leaves mashed in water. It may help them stop coughing, but nobody likes the taste.

Ocote is recommended by Dr. Luis Cabrera in his book *Plantas Curativas de Mexico.* He prescribes six drops of pine resin on a sugar cube to eliminate bronchial catarrh, reduce inflammation, and destroy the microbes that cause infection. The resin can be added to a pot of boiling water and the steam inhaled to loosen phlegm. A simple tea of clean pine needles has a similar effect. Pine needle oil has been shown to be an effective expectorant.

Dr. Cabrera also suggests a tea made by combining the leaves of *eucalipto* and *borraja* with a bit of *pingüica* leaves or berries to help eliminate phlegm.

Other Herbal Expectorants

Anís, in an infusion made with a few lightly crushed seeds, is sipped to alleviate lung congestion and fever. A little *anís* can also be added to any of the other teas recommended for respiratory ailments.

Capulín bark makes a good expectorant and may also have antispasmodic properties to help calm a cough. The remedy calls for a teaspoon or two of clean ground bark steeped in a cup of boiling water. Some people add a few *bugambilia* petals.

Cirián is used for chronic cough, bronchitis, and asthma. A syrup is made by boiling down the pith of the fruit with sugar, straining, and taking as needed by the spoonful.

Culantrillo is made into an expectorant cough syrup by simmering a handful of the leaves in half a liter of water, straining it, and then returning it to the heat. Honey or brown sugar is added, and the mixture is stirred constantly, to get the desired consistency. An infusion, using one rounded spoonful of herb for half a cup of water, is also recommended for chest colds.

Hoja santa is used as an expectorant. Several cups of an infusion of the leaves can be sipped throughout the day.

Inmortal is considered an effective expectorant. Half a spoonful of the powdered root is added to a glass of cool water and taken first thing in the morning. The Aztecs used this herb as a purgative, so you don't want to overdo it. Larger doses can cause nausea and vomiting.

Pirú is used as an expectorant and may also have soothing emollient properties. A weak infusion is made by steeping half a spoonful of the leaves in a cup of boiling water.

Trébol morado is used to loosen phlegm and calm coughing spasms. An infusion of the flowers flavored with lemon and honey is sipped—up to three cups a day.

Yerba del buey is used as an expectorant and antispasmodic. A tea is made by simmering the leaves and flowers. This is a bitter herb that needs to be sweetened with honey.

Soothing Teas

Chicalote is used as a sedative and antispasmodic. An infusion of the leaves, sipped at bedtime, is recommended for a cough that keeps you up all night.

Malva leaves make a soothing tea, emollient for the mucous membranes. The herbs can also be added to an expectorant tea such as *gordolobo*.

Mezquite tea is sipped for irritated bronchial tubes or gargled for a sore throat. A weak infusion is made of the leaves, twigs, or bark and steeped only briefly.

Salvia real is used to diminish the secretion of mucus. The leaves are simmered in water, strained, and flavored with honey and lemon to taste.

Tusilago tea is used as an antispasmodic and sedative for cough sufferers. A mild infusion made from the dried leaves is sweetened with honey.

Yerba mansa tea is soothing for a cough. An infusion can be made from the ground roots and then flavored with honey and lemon. It can also be combined with *gordolobo*, along with a little *orozús*, to make a soothing and expectorant infusion.

Liniments and Poultices for Chest Congestion

Higuerilla leaves are warmed and placed on the chest and the back. Along with this treatment, a tea is made by simmering a bit of *ocote* bark, two *eucalipto* leaves, and three *bugambilia* flowers in two cups of water. One cup is taken in the morning and another at night. This remedy is also used for fever.

Poleo de monte is covered with alcohol in a jar. The jar is sealed with a tight lid and kept in a dark place for a few days. The resulting liniment is rubbed on the chest for congestion. A tea made from the leaves and sweetened with sugar or honey can also be sipped for a cough.

(Please see directions for making liniments and poultices on pages 224 and 226.)

HEAD COLD AND STUFFY NOSE

eucalipto (eucalyptus)
inmortal (milkweed)
limón (lemon tree)
linaza (flax)
marrubio (white horehound)
orégano (Mexican oregano)
pericón (Mexican marigold)
yerba del pasmo (desert broom)

Head congestion and stuffy nose are sometimes treated by sniffing a pow-dered dry herb or drinking an infusion:

Inmortal—Sniff the powdered root.

Limón juice is diluted in a little salted water and sniffed.

Marrubio is sniffed to break up mucus and soothe inflamed membranes. A rounded spoonful of the leaves is simmered for ten minutes in half a cup of water and allowed to cool before straining. The same tea can be sipped hot.

Yerba del pasmo in an infusion made with the leaves is sniffed for stuffy nose and hay fever. The infusion is also sipped for headaches associated with sinus congestion.

Teas sipped for head colds:

Eucalipto should be sipped lukewarm. About two tablespoons of leaves are simmered for ten or fifteen minutes in a quart of water and then strained.

Linaza can be sipped throughout the day for cold symptoms. To prepare it, add one tablespoon of seeds to a liter of water, bring to a boil, and simmer until the liquid is reduced by half.

Orégano, in an infusion of the leaves or ground roots, can be sipped throughout the day. For chest colds and cough, the steam from the same tea can be inhaled.

Pericón, in an infusion made with a small handful of leaves simmered in a quart of water and strained, can be sipped throughout the day.

COLDS WITH FEVER AND FLU

borraja (borage)
canela (cinnamon)
cenizo (purple sage)
copal (elephant tree)
eucalipto (eucalyptus)
gordolobo (cudweed)
manzanilla (German chamomile)
orégano (Mexican oregano)
oshá (Porter's lovage)
saúco (elder flower)
tila (linden)
verbena (vervaine)
yerba buena (spearmint)
yerba de la víbora (snakeweed)
yerba del indio (Indian root)

Most of us have childhood memories of days when we stayed home from school, all stuffed up and feverish. Our mothers wrapped us in blankets and fed us hot tea until we "sweated it out." Many generations of Mexican-American mothers have used the following herbs to brew fever-breaking teas. They can be mixed with *yerba buena* or sprinkled with cinnamon to add flavor and sweetened with brown sugar, honey, or the Mexican dark sugar cones called *piloncillo.*

Borraja is considered soothing to the mucous membranes and is used popularly to treat fever. One recipe calls for *borraja* leaves combined with equal parts of *gordolobo* flowers and *eucalipto* leaves, both expectorants, and *saúco* flowers, which is used to induce perspiration and to soothe mucous membranes.

Another tasty recipe uses equal parts of *gordolobo* flowers and *borraja* leaves, spiked with a sprinkle of cinnamon and a squeeze of lemon.

Cenizo tea is a popular cold remedy in the southwestern United States. The leaves have mildly sedative properties and induce perspiration, which helps lower fever.

Copal is used to lower fever. It's considered an effective expectorant, and it may have properties that help boost the immune system. One recommended remedy is a handful of the leaves simmered in a quart of water. The resulting liquid is strained and taken throughout the day.

Manzanilla tea has anti-inflammatory and sedative properties and soothes mucous membranes.

Orégano helps with the aches and pains of fever and flu. A simmered tea of the leaves and stems is taken first thing in the morning and again during the day as needed.

Oshá acts as an expectorant, loosening phlegm. It's an effective anti-inflammatory and an immune system booster, and is suspected of having antiviral properties. It also induces perspiration, helping to lower fever. The remedy calls for a tea made by simmering the ground root. Half a cup is taken three or four times a day.

Saúco flowers are considered effective in reducing inflammation and lowering fevers by inducing perspiration. Two teaspoons of dried or fresh flowers, sometimes blended with mint or other herbs, is steeped in a cup of boiling water. In Morelos the remedy is prepared by simmering the flowers in milk.

Tila tea made from the flowers is delicious and mildly sedative. It is said to induce perspiration if the infusion is brewed strong, using two or three spoonfuls per cup. A leaf each of *borraja* and *eucalipto* is added to the *tila* if there is bronchial congestion.

Verbena leaf is considered especially useful at the beginning of a bad cold or flu. The infusion induces perspiration to lower fever, helps settle the stomach, and is mildly sedative.

Yerba buena is the ultimate comfort tea, perfect for colds and flu. It induces perspiration, loosens phlegm, and soothes the stomach.

Yerba del indio appears to be an effective remedy for early stages of the flu. The finely chopped roots are simmered to make a fairly weak tea, taken every three hours.

Yerba de la víbora is used to treat a feverish cold. Bonnie Ochoa recommends adding a little whiskey or brandy to the infusion.

Also see remedies for fever, pages 261–63, and bronchial congestion, pages 255–58.

FEVER

álamo (cottonwood)

altamisa mexicana (feverfew)

azafrán (safflower)

chamiso (four-wing saltbrush)

espinosilla (hummingbird flower)

estafiate (mugwort)

fresno (evergreen ash)

incienso (brittle bush)

malva (mallow)

pericón (Mexican marigold)

plumajillo (yarrow)

poleo chino (pennyroyal)

quina roja (Peruvian bark)

rosa de castilla (French rose, red rose)

saúco (elder flower)

sáuz (white willow)

yerba de la víbora (snakeweed)

Many of these herbs have properties that effectively lower body temperature by inducing perspiration. The teas are often flavored with *piloncillo*, honey, or sugar to taste and perhaps a bit of lemon rind. Ginger or cinnamon can be added for flavor and is useful for inducing perspiration.

Altamisa mexicana is known to have anti-inflammatory properties. An infusion of the leaves and flowers has been traditionally used to treat fever, as its English name, feverfew, suggests.

Children with fever are often given an infusion made with the leaves and flowers of *malva,* an exceptionally nontoxic and mild herb.

Rosa de castilla is mildly astringent and anti-inflammatory. An infusion is made with the petals.

Yerba de la Víbora has a long history as a fever remedy, and it is also considered beneficial for a stomachache or cold. An infusion of the leaves is brewed with honey and lemon.

Other herbs used to brew fever-reducing teas:

Álamo—An infusion of the fresh or dried leaves.

Azafrán—An infusion of the flower petals.

Chamiso—An infusion of the fresh leaves.

Espinosilla—A handful of the herb simmered in a liter of water, strained and flavored with lemon.

Estafiate—An infusion of the fresh leaves.

Fresno—An infusion of the dried leaves.

Incienso—A tea made by simmering the leaves and stems.

Pericón—A tea made by simmering the stems, leaves, and flowers.

Plumajillo—An infusion of the flowers combined with an equal part of *manzanilla*.

Poleo chino—A tea made by simmering the leaves and stems.

Quina roja—A tea made by simmering the bark.

Saúco—An infusion of the flowers.

Sáuz—An infusion of the bark contains acetylsalicylic acid, which is the ingredient in aspirin.

Also see the remedies for colds with fever and flu, pages 259–60.

A classic Mexican-American remedy for fever is to slather tomatoes on the soles of the feet. Ofelia Esparza told me this story: "I remember when I was about four years old, I had a high fever. My mother cooked up some tomatoes. Then she tore an old sheet into strips, filled a strip with the tomatoes, and wrapped them around my feet like plasters. She tied my feet up tight with lots of rags, and I wasn't allowed to move from the bed. In the morning when she took off the plasters, the tomatoes were all dried up and cooked to a crisp, and my fever was gone."

Concha Talavera recommended another classic remedy: *papas en vinagre.* Potato slices sprinkled with vinegar are placed on the temples to cure fever and headache. These remedies may be survivals of the ancient European theories of humoral medicine, which were brought to Mexico by the Spanish friars. According to humoral theory, foods and herbs were classified as either hot or cold. Tomatoes, potatoes, and vinegar would be considered cold, and would therefore draw out the heat of a fever.

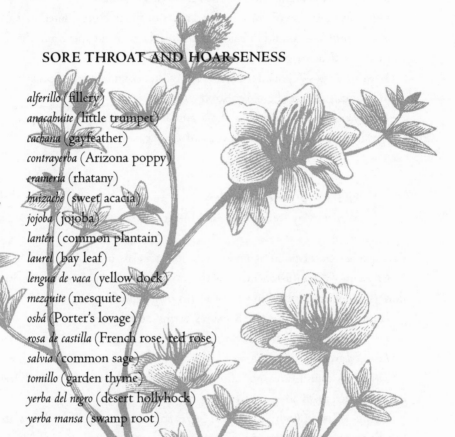

SORE THROAT AND HOARSENESS

alferillo (fillery)
anacahuite (little trumpet)
cachana (gayfeather)
contrayerba (Arizona poppy)
crameria (rhatany)
huizache (sweet acacia)
jojoba (jojoba)
lantén (common plantain)
laurel (bay leaf)
lengua de vaca (yellow dock)
mezquite (mesquite)
oshá (Porter's lovage)
rosa de castilla (French rose, red rose)
salvia (common sage)
tomillo (garden thyme)
yerba del negro (desert hollyhock)
yerba mansa (swamp root)

These herbs can be made into herbal gargles, which are simply cool teas. Some of these herbs have a bitter flavor and can be sweetened with honey. Adding a squeeze of lemon helps eliminate excess phlegm.

Anti-inflammatory Gargles that Soothe the Mucous Membranes

Alferillo—A tea is made by simmering the leaves, flowers, and stems.
   Anachuite—A tea is made by simmering bits of clean wood.
   Cachana—A tea made by simmering the roots and flowers.

Caléndula—An infusion of the petals.

Jojoba—An infusion made with a few leaves.

Lantén—A strong tea made by simmering the leaves.

Malva—An infusion of the leaves.

Mezquite—A weak infusion of the leaves, twigs, or bark.

Oshá—An infusion of the powdered roots or the tincture diluted in water.

Rosa de castilla—A mild infusion of the petals. Some people claim that red roses are particularly good for this purpose.

Yerba del negro—A boiled tea of the leaves, stems, and flowers. Sprigs of the fresh herb can also be chewed to soothe the throat.

Yerba mansa—An infusion of the ground roots or leaves, or a teaspoon of the ground root soaked in half a glass of cool water.

Herbs with Astringent Properties and Which May Reduce Excess Phlegm

Contrayerba—A teaspoon of powdered root in a glass of cool water.

Crameria—An infusion made with two heaping teaspoons of the dried flowers and stems steeped in three-fourths of a cup of boiling water.

Huizache—An infusion of the leaves, stems, and flowers.

Laurel—A tea made by simmering the leaves.

Lengua de vaca—An infusion of the leaves.

Salvia—A rounded teaspoonful of dried leaves or two spoonfuls of fresh leaves steeped in a half cup of boiling water.

Tomillo—Two spoonfuls of dried leaves steeped in a cup of boiling water. *Tomillo* has antiseptic properties.

HERBS FOR THE EARS AND EYES

EARACHE

albahaca (basil)
ruda (rue)

The traditional treatment for earache involves soaking a cotton ball in warm vegetable oil infused with the herb and placing it in the ear. The herbs most commonly used for this purpose are **ruda** and **albahaca** (rue and basil).

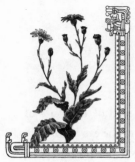

For "stuffed" ears an old treatment is to make a funnel from paper, put the narrow end just inside the ear, and light the wide end, creating suction. This is followed with an application of the herbal oil-soaked cotton ball. Hollow wax candles can also be used for this purpose. The practice of ear "candling" to clean out the ears has recently become popular among some practitioners of alternative medicine, and ear candles can now be found in some health food stores.

SORE, IRRITATED EYES

caléndula (English marigold)
chía (sage)
contrayerba (Arizona poppy)
lantén (common plantain)
manzanilla (German chamomile)
mezquite (mesquite)
rosa de castilla (rose petals)

These herbs make soothing compresses for irritated eyes. Cotton balls soaked in the cool infusion are placed over closed eyelids.

The eyes can also be gently washed with cotton balls soaked in the cool liquid. When making herbal infusions for eyewashes, add a little salt to the water before boiling. Fresh infusions should be made daily and kept refrigerated.

Caléndula—An infusion of the blossoms.

Contrayerba—A teaspoonful of the powdered root dissolved in a glass of cool water.

Lantén—The leaves added to rose water, brought to a boil, and allowed to cool.

Manzanilla—An infusion of the blossoms.

Mezquite can be used to make a soothing eyewash. In parts of northern Mexico and the southwestern United States, the gum of the mesquite bush is added to distilled water in a jar, which is then sealed and shaken. The mixture is allowed to macerate until the gum dissolves. An infusion of mesquite leaves is also used as an eyewash.

Rosa de castilla—A mild infusion of the petals.

To remedy sticky eyes caused by irritation, a tiny black seed of a species of sage called *chía (Salvia hispanica)*, sold in *botánicas,* is placed in the eye before going to bed. It reputedly absorbs excess mucus while you sleep, although placing anything in the eye can be irritating.

HERBS FOR THE MOUTH, TEETH, AND GUMS

alacrán (plumbago)
cardo santo (Mexican thistle)
clavo (clove)
florifundio (angel's trumpet)
orégano (Mexican oregano)
yerba del indio (Indian root)

TOOTHACHE

Despite the advent of modern dentistry, these remedies have endured in rural areas where dentists are hard to find. They won't fix a decayed tooth, but they can help you through a painful night or weekend.

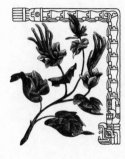

Alacrán—A few drops of juice from the mashed leaves is collected on a piece of cotton and placed where it hurts. *This herb should be used cautiously because it can be toxic if ingested.*

Cardo santo tea is made by simmering a little of the root in water and straining. Swish the liquid in the mouth, holding it over the painful area for a few minutes. The herb is considered to have both anti-inflammatory and astringent properties.

Clavo seems to "stun" the tooth, acting as a counter-irritant. A cotton ball is moistened with a drop of clove oil (available in health food stores) and placed on the problem tooth for temporary relief.

Florifundio is used for emergency relief of a toothache. A petal is placed directly over the problem area. Ground petals mixed with lard or oil can be used in the same way. The flower is a topical analgesic. *Be very careful with this plant because it can be toxic if ingested.*

Orégano is an ancient toothache remedy. Oregano oil, which is available in some health food stores, is used in the same way as *clavo*, clove oil.

Yerba del indio tea is made by simmering the grated root. It is also used in a compress placed over the painful tooth. The root itself is sometimes heated and placed directly on the tooth.

Fidela Gutiérrez recommends peeling the stem of a *cempasúchil* flower and using it as a poultice on an aching tooth.

GUM INFLAMMATION

cañaigre (red dock)
cilantro (coriander)
contrayerba (Arizona poppy)
copal (elephant tree)
crameria (rhatany)
encino (oak)
granada (pomegranate)
huizache (sweet acacia)
incienso (brittle bush)
lengua de vaca (yellow dock)
linaza (flax)
nopal (prickly pear cactus)

pirú (pepper tree)

rosa de castilla (French rose, red rose)

salvia (common sage)

sangre de drago (limberbush)

siempreviva (stonecrop)

yerba mansa (swamp root)

These mouthwashes are simply teas—used warm, not hot—swished over the gums and held in the mouth for a few minutes before spitting out.

Mouthwashes Made with Simmered Teas

Cañaigre's dry tubers make an astringent mouthwash.

Cilantro leaves make a soothing mouthwash.

Encino tea, made strong with the fresh or dry bark, is an astringent mouthwash. Some people add a little rosemary.

Granada peel is used to make an astringent mouthwash for sore gums.

Lengua de vaca leaves make a soothing mouthwash. The roots are also chewed to strengthen the teeth.

Linaza seeds make a soothing mouthwash.

Mouthwashes Made with Steeped Teas

Huizache—The leaves, flowers, and stems make a wash that is particularly soothing to the mucous membranes, and has astringent properties as well. The dried herb can also be applied directly to the sore spot.

Incienso—An infusion of the leaves is used as a mouthwash. Some people use the gummy resin of the bush directly on the sore spot, as an antiseptic, and analgesic.

Rosa de castilla—Rose petal tea is used as a soothing and lightly astringent wash.

Yerba mansa—An infusion of the leaves makes a soothing wash for inflamed gums and mouth sores. The crushed root can also be placed directly on the sore spot as a poultice.

Mouthwash Made with a Cold Infusion

Contrayerba is considered an effective antiseptic mouthwash. A teaspoon of powdered root is added to a cup of cool water.

Herbs Applied Directly to the Gums
or Chewed to Strengthen the Teeth

Crameria root is chewed or the powdered root is applied to the gums. The herb has astringent properties.

Copal's astringent resin is applied directly to painful gums.

Nopal—Small pieces of peeled paddle are placed directly on inflamed gums.

Pirú berries are eaten or applied topically for mouth ulcers or sore gums. They have emollient properties.

Salvia leaves are rubbed on sore gums for their astringent qualities. Sage tea is also used as a mouthwash, and the dry leaves are used as a tooth powder.

Sangre de drago sap is rubbed directly on the gums or chewed. A tea made by simmering either a bit of the sap or a few leaves can also be used as a wash to treat inflammations. It is held in the mouth and swirled around the sore spot for a minute or two before spitting out.

Siempreviva's succulent leaves, which have anti-inflammatory properties, are chewed to alleviate gum problems.

CANKER SORES AND COLD SORES

achiote (annatto)
añil del muerto (crownbeard)
caléndula (English marigold)
granada (pomegranate)
lantén (common plantain)
malva (mallow)
nopal (cactus)
rosa de castilla (French rose, red rose)

The herbs listed below, used as poultices or ointments, or applied directly to the skin, have astringent properties to help dry up the blister or soothing properties to help reduce the inflammation.

Ointments

Achiote, añil del muerto, caléndula, and *malva,* used singly or in combination, make a soothing ointment for cold sores. *(Please see directions for making salves and ointments, page 223.)*

Herbs Applied Directly to the Sore

Nopal paddles, parboiled and skinned, can be applied directly to the sore to bring down irritation and inflammation. *Nopal* is available in the produce department of many markets.

Granada—A little piece of pomegranate peel placed on the sore may help dry it up.

Rosa de castilla has a mildly astringent quality. Some people simply place a fresh rose petal over the sore spot or sprinkle on dried powdered rose petals.

Teas Used to Make a Soothing Compress

Achiote—A handful of leaves are simmered for ten minutes in a liter of water, strained, and allowed to cool.

Lantén—A half cup of leaves are simmered in two cups of water.

Malva—A round teaspoonful of leaves are steeped in a cup of water.

HERBS FOR ACHES AND PAINS

HEADACHES

acacia (gum arabic)
aguacate (avocado)
azahares (orange blossom)
barbasco (Texas croton)
boldo (bold)
florifundio (angel's trumpet)
fresno (evergreen ash)
geranio (geranium)
lantén (common plantain)
lengua de vaca (yellow dock)
malva (mallow)
passiflora (passion flower)
ruda (rue)
tila (linden)

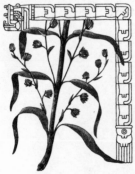

In traditional medicine, headaches are often treated topically with cool compresses or poultices placed on the forehead or with liniments that are massaged into the temples.

Compresses and Poultices

Boldo leaves are used in an infusion. A cloth is soaked in the warm tea, then wrung out and bound to the head.

Fresh *florifundio* leaves are dampened, then applied directly to the forehead.

Fresh *fresno* leaves are mixed with wine and applied directly to the forehead.

Geranio leaves are mashed with vinegar and salt, and applied directly to the forehead.

Fresh *lantén* leaves are mashed, salted, and bound to the head.

Fresh *lengua de vaca* leaves are mashed, salted, and bound to the head with a cloth.

Fresh *malva* leaves are mashed, mixed with salt and vinegar, then bound to the head in a poultice.

Liniments

Acacia flowers, used fresh or dry, are mixed with cold cream.

Fresh *aguacate* leaves are steeped in alcohol for at least one day.

Barbasco leaves, fresh or dried, are soaked in alcohol, vinegar, or wine, then used as a rub.

Ruda has antispasmodic properties, which could be especially helpful for headaches brought on by tension. Its leaves and stems are steeped in alcohol. The crushed leaves are also sometimes rubbed directly on the forehead. It is thought that *ruda* "lets the air out" of the head.

Calming Teas for Headaches

Azahares, passiflora, and *tila* are used for headaches brought on by stress. An infusion of any of these herbs, singly or in combination, will have a lightly sedative effect.

Socorro Vázquez gave me a classic recipe for chronic headaches: hot chocolate laced with an infusion of *ruda* (rue). Sufferers are advised to drink one cup every evening for fifteen days, then one cup every morning for fifteen days more. Señora Vázquez believes that headaches are caused by a chill, by *mal aire*, bad air. "You have to cover your head at night," she warns. It may be possible to trace this fear of the cold evening air, which is very common among Mexicans and Mexican Americans, to the notion—shared by the Aztecs, Tarahumaras, Maya, Zapotecs and Otomies—that invisible dangers float in the night breezes. In Nahuatl it was called *ehecatl cocoliztle*, ill winds. According to Aztec beliefs, these diseases were perpetrated by the invisible messengers of the water god Tláloc who came from the cold mountains. So Señora Vázquez tells her patients to keep warm. She is particularly careful to protect the head, which the Aztecs and other Mesoamerican people believed was the center of the essential warmth of life, the spirit called *tonalli*.

MIGRAINES

altamisa (feverfew)
barba de chivo (clematis)
chicalote (prickle poppy)
yerba buena (spearmint)

In 1985 the City of London Migraine Clinic published the results of a study which showed that regularly drinking *altamisa* tea reduced the frequency of severe migraine headaches. These results were further substantiated by a study conducted in 1988 at the University of Nottingham in England.

Altamisa tea, made by infusing a few sprigs of the herb in a cup of boiling water, is also a traditional Mexican-American remedy for headache. This herb tastes lousy, so it's often added to hot chocolate, along with a little *ruda*.

Barba de chivo has a big reputation as a headache remedy, but *it can be toxic if used in excess.* The recommended treatment is an infusion made with a rounded teaspoonful of the dried leaves and flowers steeped in a cup of boiling water for twenty to thirty minutes and sipped only by the spoonful.

Chicalote tea, made with a spoonful of *chicalote* leaves steeped in a cup of boiling water, may bring some relief. The plant has lightly sedative and anti-spasmodic properties.

The essential oils in *yerba buena* contain cooling menthol. A sprig of the fresh herb or a scant spoonful of dried leaves is combined with a few leaves of *romero* and steeped in a cupful of boiling water.

Ofelia Esparza told me that her mother used to cure migraine headaches with a tea she made from sprigs of *romero* and a little *yerba buena.* In addition to the tea, her mother crushed a little *ruda* and rubbed it on her forehead, so she inhaled the aroma.

ARTHRITIS AND RHEUMATISM

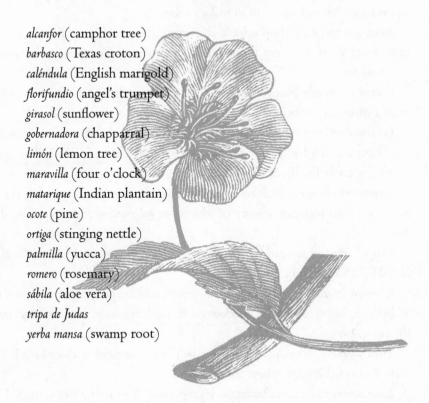

alcanfor (camphor tree)
barbasco (Texas croton)
caléndula (English marigold)
florifundio (angel's trumpet)
girasol (sunflower)
gobernadora (chapparral)
limón (lemon tree)
maravilla (four o'clock)
matarique (Indian plantain)
ocote (pine)
ortiga (stinging nettle)
palmilla (yucca)
romero (rosemary)
sábila (aloe vera)
tripa de Judas
yerba mansa (swamp root)

Liniment Remedies

Florifundio makes perhaps the most acclaimed liniment for all sorts of sore or swollen joints and muscles. The flowers, leaves, and stems (sometimes along with an equal amount of fresh marijuana plant) are infused in rubbing alcohol. The herb contains analgesic properties.

Socorro Vázquez gave me this liniment recipe: "*Florifundio*, a little bit of *marijuana,* a stem of *ruda, romero,* and *alcanfor.* These five herbs are used in equal parts. Put them in the cane alcohol from Mexico, because the one they sell here is wood alcohol and is bad. You leave the herbs in until you see that the alcohol turns *el colorcito tiernito,* a delicate pale color. Then you rub it on, and it's incredible. It's *buenisimo,* really good."

Other Liniments

Maravilla roots are macerated in alcohol for a few days or dried and ground to a powder and mixed with lard to make a salve.

Matarique roots are chopped and then steeped in alcohol for three days to make an analgesic liniment for arthritis, rheumatism, neuralgia, and swollen sore muscles.

Girasol stems and leaves are steeped in alcohol for three days and then used as an anti-inflammatory rub.

Gobernadora leaves are steeped in alcohol for a few days to make an analgesic liniment. A salve can also be made by frying the leaves in olive oil or lard over a low flame for about four hours. Cool and strain.

Trementina de ocote, pine resin, is dried and ground to a powder, then combined with an equal amount of *alcanfor* or *gobernadora* and steeped in alcohol.

Ortiga leaves are steeped for two days to make a liniment rubbed on the affected joints at bedtime.

A *romero* branch is steeped in alcohol, or a few drops of rosemary oil are added to rubbing alcohol. A rubdown with this tincture is used to stimulate the circulation.

Tripa de Judas stems are steeped for two hours in alcohol to make a liniment that is believed to relieve inflammation.

Yerba mansa has anti-inflammatory properties. A soothing rub is made by steeping the ground roots in alcohol for a few days.

Herbs Used to Make Salves or Ointments

Caléndula petals or leaves are simmered in olive oil, or the powdered dried leaves are mixed with petroleum jelly or cold cream. The herb has soothing properties.

Barbasco leaves are mixed with Vaseline or cold cream to make an analgesic ointment.

Limón makes a refreshing liniment. Two parts of lemon juice are mixed with one part almond oil and one part rubbing alcohol.

Alcanfor sap is steeped in alcohol or simmered in oil or lard and rubbed on the affected parts.

Herbs Taken Internally to Relieve the Discomfort of Swollen Joints

Palmilla tea is made by simmering the chopped peeled roots. It is used to reduce inflammation, but *it should be taken cautiously because the plant can also have a laxative effect.* Take up to three cups a day.

Sábila gel taken internally first thing in the morning is believed to relieve pain in the joints. A little of the fresh aloe vera gel is added to a glass of orange juice or diluted with a little lemon juice.

Yerba mansa tea is made from the ground roots or leaves, or both. It may help reduce the pain of swollen joints by eliminating excess uric acid, especially when combined with one of the diuretic herbs such as *cola de caballo* or *pingüica.*

SCIATICA AND BACKACHE

florifundio (angel's trumpet)
ruda (rue)
siempreviva (stonecrop)

Florifundio leaves and flowers make an effective topical analgesic. They can be brewed and added to the bathwater for a soothing soak or steeped in alcohol to be used as a liniment.

Ruda makes a liniment for alleviating muscle spasms. Bruised leaves are rubbed directly onto the sore areas or steeped in alcohol.

Siempreviva leaves are warmed and then mashed to make a poultice that may help soothe inflamed muscles.

SORE MUSCLES

aguacate (avocado)
anís (anise)
árnica mexicana (camphor weed)
boldo (bold)
caléndula (English marigold)
chirimoya (custard apple)
estafiate (mugwort)
piru (pepper tree)
uña del gato (cat claw)

Liniments

The following herbs, steeped in alcohol for two or three days, make soothing liniments:

Anís—A handful of the lightly toasted seeds. Used for sore chest or shoulder muscles.

Arnica mexicana—A handful of the leaves and a cinnamon stick.

Aquacate—A handful of the leaves.

Boldo—A handful of the leaves. Used for strained muscles, rheumatic joints, and throbbing temples

Caléndula—A handful of the flowers.

Poultices and Compresses

Chirimoya—An infusion of the leaves is applied in a warm compress to strained shoulder muscles.

Estafiate—A warm infusion of the leaves is used as an analgesic and anti-inflammatory compress for sore muscles.

Pirú leaves are ground and mixed with warm cooking oil or lard to make a poultice for backache.

Uña del gato pods are ground and made into a paste with warm water. It is plastered onto inflamed muscles. A cloth or plastic is wrapped over the area to keep it warm.

(Also see arthritis remedies on pages 276–77.)

BRUISES

aguacate (avocado)
cancerina (Mexican heather)
higuerilla (castor bean plant)
orégano (Mexican oregano)
saúco (elder flower)
sueldo (common comfrey)
yerba del golpe (evening primrose)

SOOTHING COMPRESSES

Aguacate liniment, which is used as an astringent, is made by placing a handful of avocado leaves in a jar and covering with rubbing alcohol. The jar is sealed and the mixture is allowed to steep in a cool dark place for twenty-four hours.

Cancerina is traditionally used to treat all sorts of inflammations. A compress is made with an infusion of the leaves.

Orégano—An infusion of the leaves is used to make a compress for soreness when there is also swelling.

Soothing Poultices

Wet *higuerilla* leaves are mashed and applied directly to the sore spot to reduce inflammation.

Saúco reduces inflammation. The mashed wet leaves are placed directly on the bruise or an ointment is made by warming the leaves in petroleum jelly and straining.

Sueldo is used to speed healing. A poultice is made with an infusion of *sueldo* leaves.

Yerba del golpe is regarded as an anti-inflammatory and antispasmodic. The mashed wet leaves are used to make a poultice or the flowers are simmered in water to make a soothing wash.

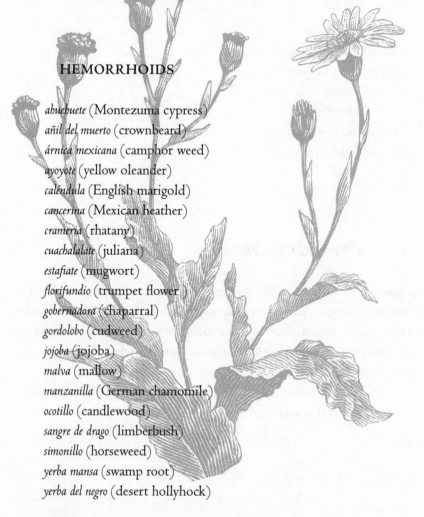

HEMORRHOIDS

ahuehuete (Montezuma cypress)
añil del muerto (crownbeard)
árnica mexicana (camphor weed)
ayoyote (yellow oleander)
caléndula (English marigold)
cancerina (Mexican heather)
crameria (rhatany)
cuachalalate (juliana)
estafiate (mugwort)
florifundio (trumpet flower)
gobernadora (chaparral)
gordolobo (cudweed)
jojoba (jojoba)
malva (mallow)
manzanilla (German chamomile)
ocotillo (candlewood)
sangre de drago (limberbush)
simonillo (horseweed)
yerba mansa (swamp root)
yerba del negro (desert hollyhock)

Topical Treatments

Ahuehuete tea, made by simmering the twigs and needles, is used to bathe hemorrhoids or make a compress. The tree contains properties that may act as a vasoconstrictor to shrink the swollen veins.

Ayoyote seeds are mashed and mixed with lard, oil, or petroleum jelly to make an analgesic ointment that is a very popular treatment for hemorrhoids.

Caléndula makes a soothing salve. Simmer the flowers in olive oil.

Gordolobo salve is made by mixing the flowers with warm butter, lard, or oil.

Jojoba is used to soothe the membranes. Commercially prepared jojoba oil is applied, or an infusion of the leaves is used as either a compress or a wash.

Simonillo was used by the ancient Aztecs to treat hemorrhoids. A strong infusion of the leaves and stems can be used to make a compress. If you can find some of the fresh plant, the mashed leaves can also be used as a poultice.

VapoRub is mixed with various herbs to make a salve. The powdered dry leaves and flowers of *añil del muerto* are added to the ointment to help soothe inflammation. and the fresh or dried leaves of *florifundio* add analgesic properties. Fresh damp *florifundio* leaves can also be applied as a poultice.

Sitz Baths and Soaks

Any of these herbs, used singly or in combination, can be added to a sitz bath for a soothing soak. Use about a half cup of the dried herb in a liter of boiling water. Add the liquid to the bath.

Añil del muerto—An infusion of the leaves and flowers is soothing.

Arnica—An infusion of the leaves is soothing.

Cancerina—An infusion of the leaves and flowers is soothing and astringent.

Cuachalalate—A tea made by simmering the bark has astringent properties.

Florifundio—An infusion of the leaves and flowers makes an analgesic bath.

Gobernadora—An infusion of the leaves is lightly analgesic.

Malva—An infusion of the leaves is soothing.

Sangre de drago—A decoction made by simmering the chopped roots and twigs is considered to have anti-inflammatory and astringent properties.

Soothing Washes

The following herbs are used to make a soothing wash. Infusions used externally are generally brewed stronger than teas. A half liter of boiling water is poured over four well-rounded teaspoons of herb and the mixture is allowed to steep for at least fifteen minutes.

Crameria—The ground root.

Estafiate—The leaves and stems.

Malva—Two round teaspoons of the dried leaves steeped in half a liter of boiling water. This infusion is used both as a wash and an enema.

Manzanilla—The flowers.

Yerba mansa—An infusion of the ground roots or leaves makes a soothing wash. The herb can also be simmered in olive oil and applied as a warm poultice.

Yerba del negro—A strong tea made by simmering the fresh or dried leaves is soothing and emollient. The herb can also be fried in butter, lard, or vegetable shortening to make a suppository.

Teas Taken Internally

Ocotillo root or boiled bark is taken internally to reduce varicose veins and is effective in certain cases of hemorrhoids, which are, after all, just varicose veins in a particularly unfortunate location.

A friend in Zihuatenejo, Guerrero, gave me this remedy for hemorrhoids, which she insists is remarkably effective: Heat a clean, smooth, flat stone in the sun, cover it with VapoRub, and place it where the sun never shines. Reheat the stone and reapply as needed.

SORE, SWOLLEN, OR TIRED FEET

abrojo (puncture vine)
golondrina (spurge)
guayaba (guava)
lantén (common plantain)
yerba mansa (swamp root)

Soothing Foot Baths

Add about half a cup of any of these herbs to a liter of water: chopped roots of *abrojo;* leaves and chopped twigs of *golondrina;* leaves and chopped bark or roots of *guayaba;* leaves and stems of *yerba mansa.* Bring to a boil, cover tightly, and simmer for ten or fifteen minutes. Allow the liquid to cool before straining. Pour the tea into a bucket or pan, add more hot water, and soak your tootsies.

Poultice

Mashed fresh *lantén* leaves are applied directly to sore feet to reduce inflammation.

CHILBLAINS

alhucema (lavender)
eucalipto (eucalyptus)
marrubio (white horehound)
romero (rosemary)
ruda (rue)

These remedies were surely intended for a hardworking *ranchero* or *vaquero* riding the wintry plains, but they might work just as well for a guy out shoveling the snow off his driveway.

For a warming bath, simmer a handful each of *eucalipto, marrubio, alhucema, romero,* and *ruda* leaves in three liters of water. Strain and add to the bathwater.

A handful of *marrubio* leaves and stems simmered in half a liter of water can be added to a bucket or pan to make a soothing soak for frozen feet.

A traditional home remedy for chilblains is to simply apply hot roasted onions to the skin.

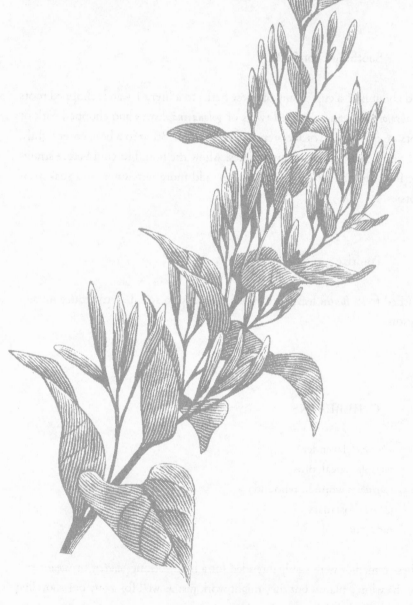

HERBS FOR THE SKIN

Sores, wounds, and other skin problems are treated in a variety of ways:

by applying an herbal salve or ointment

by applying an herbal poultice

by applying an herbal compress

by washing the area with a cool herbal tea

by cleaning the area and then sprinkling a powdered dried herb over it

SKIN IRRITATIONS AND RASHES

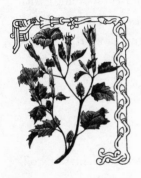

acacia (gum arabic)

aceitilla (burr marigold)

achiote (annatto)

aguacate (avocado)

álamo (cottonwood)

alferillo (fillery)

árnica mexicana (camphor weed)

barba de chivo (clematis)

caléndula (English marigold)

cancerina (Mexican heather)

gobernadora (chaparral)

huizache (sweet acacia)

lengua de vaca (yellow dock)

mimbre (desert willow)

papaya (Mexican papaya)

sábila (aloe vera)

saúco (elder flower)

sueldo (common comfrey)

tabachín (Mexican bird of paradise)

yerba buena (spearmint)

yerba mansa (swamp root)

yerba mora (black nightshade)

Most of these herbs have been used for generations simply because they have anti-inflammatory or astringent properties, so they're soothing to the skin. **Yerba mora, tabachín, mimbre,** and *saúco* have antifungal properties, and **gobernadora** and **árnica mexicana** have antimicrobial properties, which could explain their long history of use for certain rashes. Use as needed.

Powders

Apply these powdered dry herbs to areas that have been cleaned with mild soap and water and allowed to air dry: *acacia* leaves (soothing); **alferillo** leaves (soothing); *cancerina* leaves and flowers (soothing and astringent); *huizache* leaves (soothing and astringent); *lengua de vaca* root or leaves (soothing); **mimbre** leaves and stems (antifungal and antiseptic). Leaves can be crumbled by hand. Roots can be powdered with a cheese grater or given a whirl in a coffee grinder.

Washes

Infusions can be brewed double strength for topical use. A half liter of boiling water is poured over four well-rounded teaspoons of herb and the mixture is allowed to steep for at least fifteen minutes. A clean, soft cloth or cotton ball is dipped in the cooled infusion and sponged over the affected area.

Aceitilla—An infusion of the leaves is soothing and astringent.

Achiote makes a soothing wash. Put a handful of leaves into a clear glass jar, cover with water, and allow to sit in the sun all day before straining.

Alferillo—An infusion of the leaves, stems, and flowers is soothing.

Arnica mexicana—An infusion of the leaves and flowers is soothing, antiseptic, and antimicrobial.

Lengua de vaca—A soothing tea is made by simmering the chopped roots.

Saúco—An infusion of the leaves is soothing and antifungal.

Tabachín —An antifungal wash is made by steeping the leaves or flowers in boiling water or by simmering the roots.

Yerba buena—An infusion of the leaves is lightly antiseptic and analgesic.

Yerba mansa—An infusion of the leaves or powdered roots is soothing.

Yerba mora—An infusion of the leaves is soothing and antifungal.

Poultices

These herbs are applied directly to the skin as poultices to reduce inflammation: the mashed fresh leaves of *álamo;* the pulpy gel from the inside of a freshly slit leaf of *sábila;* the mashed pulp of the ripe fruit of *aguacate;* the mashed pulp of the ripe *papaya* fruit or the fruit juice.

Ointments

These herbs can be made into ointments using the methods on page 223:

caléndula—The petals have soothing properties.

gobernadora—The leaves have analgesic and antimicrobial properties.

huizache—The leaves and petals have soothing and astringent properties.

sueldo—The leaves have soothing properties.

WOUNDS AND ABRASIONS, CUTS AND SCRATCHES

caléndula (English marigold)
cancerina (Mexican heather)
cempasúchil (Aztec marigold)
colita de rata (flat-top buckwheat)
encino (oak)
gobernadora (chaparral)
golondrina (spurge)
guayaba (guava)
huizache (sweet acacia)
lantén (common plantain)
limón (lemon tree)
matarique (Indian plantain)
mezquite (mesquite)
mimbre (desert willow)
oshá (Porter's lovage)
plumajillo (yarrow)
sábila (aloe vera)
sueldo (common comfrey)
yerba mansa (swamp root)
yerba mora (black nightshade)
yerba del pollo (Mexican dayflower)

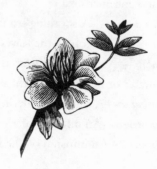

These remedies have been used for generations in rural areas, where to the knowledgeable eye the terrain provides a living first aid kit. They can be especially useful to campers, hikers, and outbackers.

Powders

The affected area should be thoroughly cleaned and allowed to air dry before any herbal preparation is applied.

Golondrina is soothing and lightly antiseptic. The powdered dried leaves are dusted onto wounds, or a wash is made by infusing the leaves.

Huizache's powdered dried leaves and flowers are astringent and soothing.
Mimbre's powdered dried leaves or twigs are antifungal and antiseptic.

Plumajillo's powdered dried leaves are anti-inflammatory, antiseptic, and astringent.

Yerba mansa's powdered dried roots are soothing.

Compresses and Poultices

(Please see directions for making compresses and poultices on pages 225–26.)

Caléndula or *cempasúchil*—A compress made with an infusion of the flowers is soothing to fresh wounds and mildly antiseptic.

Limón is astringent, antiseptic, and will help stop bleeding. It will also sting like crazy. The cut side of half a lemon is placed on the affected area.

Matarique is lightly antiseptic and analgesic. Mashed fresh leaves are applied directly to the wound.

Plumajillo's flower heads or fresh leaves are mashed and pressed against a wound to stop bleeding. An infusion of the leaves is used later as a compress to speed healing.

Sábila—The cut side of a freshly sliced aloe vera leaf is soothing, promotes healing, and is mildly antibacterial.

Sueldo, in the form of a poultice of mashed fresh leaves or a compress made from an infusion of the leaves, is used to speed healing.

Yerba mansa leaves are dampened and applied as a poultice to reduce inflammation and promote healing.

Yerba mora leaves are mashed and applied as a soothing poultice.

Yerba del pollo leaves contain properties that effectively stop bleeding. They are mashed and placed directly on the wound.

Washes

These herbal infusions are used to clean sores and skin irritations. They should be prepared double strength, using about two spoonfuls for each cup of boiling water and applied cool or tepid, not hot.

Barba de chivo's dried leaves are used to make a wash for skin irritations and scratches.

Cancerina leaves, stems, and flowers are soothing and astringent.

Colita de rata is simmered to make a soothing and lightly antiseptic wash. All parts of the plant can be used.

Encino tea, made by simmering bits of the bark and twigs, is astringent.

Gobernadora leaves are used as an antiseptic wash for scratches and abrasions.

Guayaba bark is simmered to make a wash. Guava was used in an ancient Aztec remedy for scabies and sores.

Lantén leaves are used as a soothing wash. A poultice of the fresh leaves can also be used to close clean wounds.

Mezquite leaves or finely chopped bark or twigs are astringent, antiseptic, and soothing.

Oshá root is ground, and steeped in alcohol, or brewed as a tea, and used as an antiseptic, antiviral, and anti-inflammatory wash.

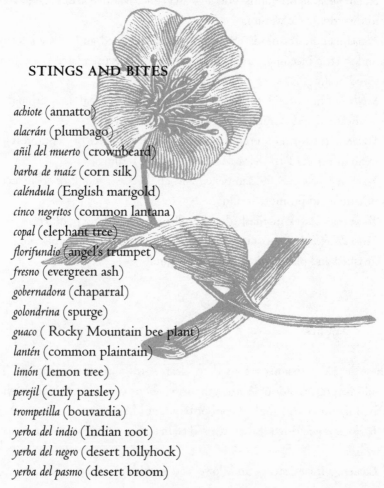

STINGS AND BITES

achiote (annatto)
alacrán (plumbago)
añil del muerto (crownbeard)
barba de maíz (corn silk)
caléndula (English marigold)
cinco negritos (common lantana)
copal (elephant tree)
florifundio (angel's trumpet)
fresno (evergreen ash)
gobernadora (chaparral)
golondrina (spurge)
guaco (Rocky Mountain bee plant)
lantén (common plaintain)
limón (lemon tree)
perejil (curly parsley)
trompetilla (bouvardia)
yerba del indio (Indian root)
yerba del negro (desert hollyhock)
yerba del pasmo (desert broom)

Soothing Washes

Añil del muerto tea is made by simmering the leaves and flowers. This wash is soothing.

Barba de maíz—An infusion of corn silk is used to bring down inflammation.

Golondrina tea is made by simmering a big handful of leaves in a liter of water. It makes a soothing, lightly antiseptic wash. This herb is used to treat all sorts of insect bites, snakebites, and scorpion stings. The mashed leaves can also be applied directly to the bite.

Trompetilla tea is made by simmering a handful of the stems and leaves in water to cover. It is used to wash snakebites and insect stings.

Yerba del pasmo leaves and stems are made into an infusion used as a topical astringent.

Ointments

Achiote—A pinch of the powdered leaves mixed with olive oil is soothing and astringent.

Alacrán leaves are infused with olive oil and applied to the bite. The plant is considered to have astringent and antiseptic properties. (*Please see directions for making infused oils on page 222.*) The mashed leaves can also be applied directly to the skin. The plant is used to treat scorpion stings.

Caléndula flowers are used to make an ointment, or fresh petals can be rubbed over the bitten spot. (*Please see directions for making salves and ointments on page 223.*)

Gobernadora salve is made by simmering the leaves in lard or oil. It is used for insect bites, ringworm, and skin sores.

Poultices

Cinco negritos's fresh leaves are crushed and applied to insect bites and snakebites.

Copal resin is rubbed directly on scorpion stings and spider bites.

Florifundio's crushed leaves are applied as a topical analgesic.

Fresno's fresh leaves are crushed and applied to spider bites.

Guaco's fresh leaves are crushed or powdered and applied to insect bites and skin irritations.

Lantén's fresh leaves are crushed and applied to insect bites and snakebites.

Limón—The cut side of half a lemon applied to bee stings acts as an astringent.

Perejil's fresh leaves are applied to help take the sting out of insect bites.

Yerba del indio is considered an especially effective poultice for snakebites and scorpion stings. The crushed plants are dampened with a bit of warm water. In addition to the poultice, a hot infusion made with one leaf of the herb in a cup of hot water is taken at three-hour intervals.

Yerba del negro is made into a poultice by mixing the leaves with warm water. It is considered soothing and emollient. The dried leaves can also be powdered and sprinkled over the affected area.

Growing up on a ranch, Concha Talavera used heated *golondrina* leaves on insect bites. Spider webs served as bandages for cuts and scratches.

BOILS AND ABSCESSES

> *florifundio* (trumpet flower)
> *higuerilla* (castor bean plant)
> *linaza* (flax)
> *malva* (mallow)
> *nopal* (prickly pear cactus)

Florifundio's damp leaves or ground seeds are applied as a poultice over a boil to draw out the pus and to numb the pain.

Higuerilla—Mashed damp leaves make a soothing and emollient poultice.

Linaza seeds are ground to a coarse powder and mixed with a little cornmeal and hot water to make a paste. Sometimes a little *malva,* which is soothing, is also added. The hot mixture is spread on a clean rag and covered with another rag. This plaster is applied to the boil and changed for a new one as soon as it has cooled. Flaxseed plasters are used to bring a boil or abscess to a "head," drawing the pus to the surface of the skin.

Nopal's freshly peeled paddles are placed directly on the boil or abscess to draw out the infection.

BURNS

achiote (annatto)
caléndula (English marigold)
lantén (common plaintain)
linaza (flax)
nopal (prickly pear cactus)
sábila (aloe vera)
sueldo (common comfrey)

Ointments

Achiote, caléndula, and *sueldo* all have anti-inflammatory properties. They can be simmered in petroleum jelly or olive oil to make a soothing ointment, using the directions on page 223.

Linaza oil, mixed with a little lime water, has long been used to treat burns, particularly those caused by acid.

Washes

Lantén tea is made by simmering the leaves in water. It is used as a soothing wash.

Poultices

Sábila's fresh leaves are split and applied, cut side down, directly on the burn. The plant has properties that speed healing, and the juice is an emollient that helps to keep the burned skin from drying out.

Nopal paddles work in much the same way as aloe vera to reduce swelling and to soothe and soften the skin. Apply a peeled slice, cut side down, over the burn and wrap the whole thing with gauze for a few hours.

SUNBURN

chicalote (prickle poppy)
papaya (Mexican papaya)
sábila (aloe vera)
sueldo (common comfrey)

Chicalote seeds are crushed and mixed with olive oil or petroleum jelly to make a soothing analgesic ointment.

Papaya juice is applied directly to the irritated area to reduce inflammation.

Sábila gel is a well-known soothing agent and has been shown to encourage healing.

Sueldo, simmered in petroleum jelly or olive oil, is thought to speed healing. *(Please see the directions for making herbal salves and ointments on page 223.)*

HERBS TO SOOTHE THE SPIRIT

NERVOUSNESS AND INSOMNIA

amapola (field poppy)
azahares (orange blossom)
cedrón (lemon-scented verbena)
cilantro (coriander)
damiana (damiana)
eneldo (dill)
flor de manita (handflower tree)
jazmín (Mexican mock orange)
manzanilla (German chamomile)
passiflora (passion flower)
poleo (brook mint)
salvia (common sage)
tila (linden)
toronjil (giant hyssop)
tumba vaqueros (morning glory)
valeriana (garden heliotrope)
yerba buena (spearmint)
zapote blanco (white sapote)

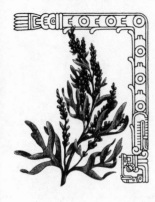

Many kitchen cabinets contain a box or tin of *siete azahares,* seven-blossom tea. A mix of dried flowers, the tea is a time-honored remedy for ruffled nerves and sleeplessness. There is no single recipe for *siete azahares,* and every recipe doesn't necessarily include seven different blossoms. One commercially packaged brand lists six ingredients: *tila, azahares de naranjo, passiflora, toronjil, zapote blanco,* and *flor de manita.* Another lists only five, two of which are plucked from the same tree and three of them are not blossoms at all: *tila, tila estrella* (linden flowers), *passiflora, valeriana,* and *yerba buena.*

You can invent your own calming tea by combining any of the herbs listed above. The majority of the mixture should be herbs with sedative properties, but you can experiment with the proportions, adding a little bit of a stomach-settling herb, or throwing in a little something just for flavor. Some examples follow.

Sleepy Tea Formula #1

Flor de manita with *azahares de naranjo, toronjil, hinojo,* and *yerba buena.* The *flor de manita* and *azahares de naranjo* are lightly sedative. The *toronjil* has sedative and antispasmodic properties, and the *hinojo* and *yerba buena* add an interesting flavor and are soothing to the digestive system.

Sleepy Tea Formula #2

Tila with *valeriana, azahares de naranjo,* and *damiana.* This tea should really put you to sleep. These herbs all have sedative properties. Damiana is calming to the nervous system and is considered an antidepressant.

More Good Choices for Sleepy Tea Formulas

Azahares de naranjo makes a fragrant, calming tea. A sprinkle of cinnamon can be added for additional flavor.

Cedrón, a lovely lemon-scented herb, calms the digestion and helps induce sleep.

Cilantro leaves are used to make a soothing and sedative tea.

Eneldo is lightly sedative and works to calm a gassy stomach.

Jazmín tea is used to treat insomnia combined with nervous indigestion. One recipe for the infusion calls for ten or fifteen blossoms steeped in half a liter of boiling water.

Manzanilla, the ultimate comfort tea, is mildly sedative and settles the stomach.

Passiflora on its own is the sedative of choice for many people. Concha Talavera told me that when her husband died she was unable to sleep and tried everything until a *botánica* owner recommended *passiflora* tea.

Poleo tea is calming and soothes the digestion. It is often given to restless children.

Salvia, in combination with other herbs or on its own, flavored with lemon and honey, is used in cases of insomnia accompanied by indigestion.

Tumba vaqueros is considered an effective long-lasting sedative and is used to treat hysteria as well as insomnia. One formula calls for simmering chopped *tumba vaqueros* roots combined with a few orange leaves or *tila* leaves.

Valeriana is a world-famous sedative and is often used in combination with other sedative herbs such as *tila* and *passiflora.*

Zapote blanco was called "sleep fruit" by the Aztecs who used it as a sedative. Today an infusion of the leaves is used to remedy insomnia, especially if the sleeplessness is associated with pain.

DEPRESSION

Damiana tea is used to lift the spirits. An infusion is made by steeping a rounded spoonful of the dried herb in a cup of boiling water. This tea is taken on an empty stomach first thing in the morning. The effects are supposedly noticeable only after the tea has been used daily for two or three weeks.

HERBS FOR WOMEN

PREMENSTRUAL SYNDROME

barba de maíz (corn silk)
cola de caballo (horsetail)
diente de león (dandelion)
ortiga (stinging nettle)
perejil (curly parsley)
pingüica (uva ursi)

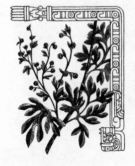

PMS is a modern woman's dilemma. It is unlikely that Aztec ladies noticed that their *huipiles* grew a little snug at a certain time of the month, and the rural Mexican woman struggling with her daily chores hardly has the luxury of worrying about PMS. If she is particularly irritable one day, she has plenty of things to blame it on. These remedies are contemporary adaptations of the old herbal knowledge, aimed primarily at combating water retention and bloating. The herbal diuretics are mild and can be very effective.

Any of the diuretic herbs listed on page 245 can

be useful for PMS. One good choice is a tea made with *diente de león* leaves combined with *pingüica, barba de maíz* or *cola de caballo.*

Marrubio in a mild tea made with the fresh leaves and flowers, taken two days before the expected onset of menstruation, is considered helpful. The recommended dose is half a spoonful of the herb steeped in half a cup of boiling water.

Ortiga is considered useful for relief of premenstrual bloating. Pour a cup of boiling water over one or two teaspoons of dried herb and steep for ten minutes. Take up to three cups a day.

Perejil tea, made by boiling the grated roots of curly parsley, is thought to be an effective remedy for the bloating of PMS. The recommended dosage is one cup a day, three to five days before menstruation is expected to start. Parsley oil capsules, sold in health food stores, have a similar effect.

When her daughters complain of PMS, Fidela Gutiérrez gives them a thick shake she makes in the blender with chopped pineapple, apple, carrot, and parsley.

DELAYED MENSTRUATION AND CRAMPS

aguacate (avocado)
albahaca (common basil)
anís (anise)
árnica mexicana (camphor weed)
canela (cinnamon)
cedrón (lemon-scented verbena)
cilantro (coriander)
culantrillo (maidenhair fern)
epazote (American wormseed)
estafiate (mugwort)
hinojo (fennel)
inmortal (milkweed)

manzanilla (German chamomile)

nochebuena (poinsettia)

nogal (walnut shells)

orégano (Mexican oregano)

poleo chino (pennyroyal)

romero (rosemary)

rosa de castilla (French rose, red rose)

ruda (rue)

sábila (aloe vera)

salvia (common sage)

tila (linden)

toronjil (giant hyssop)

tumba vaqueros (morning glory)

yerba buena (spearmint)

Most of these herbs are thought to ease menstrual discomfort by promoting the flow. Some of them have antispasmodic properties which may help to relieve cramps. The infusions are usually sipped three or four times a day for two or three days.

These teas are prepared as infusions. Use about a spoonful of the dried herb in a teacup or a couple of sprigs of the fresh herb. Fill the cup with boiling water and steep for ten or fifteen minutes before straining.

Anís's bruised seeds, in an infusion flavored with cinnamon and nutmeg, are used as an antispasmodic.

Arnica mexicana leaves in a mild infusion are used to soothe menstrual cramps.

Cedrón leaves in an infusion are used to soothe menstrual cramps.

Culantrillo leaves in an infusion are used to stimulate the menstrual flow.

Estafiate, in an infusion of three or four fresh leaves with a little cinnamon and honey to mask the nasty taste, is used to stimulate menstrual flow.

Hinojo and *sábila* are combined. Bruised *hinojo* seeds are infused in boiling water, and then a little *sábila* juice and some cinnamon are added to the cup. *Hinojo* has antispasmodic properties to calm cramps, and the *sábila* is soothing.

Manzanilla tea works to calm cramps.

Orégano leaves in an infusion are used to bring on delayed menstruation.

Poleo chino leaves, stems, and flowers in an infusion are used to bring on delayed menstruation.

Romero leaves in a strong infusion are used to bring on delayed menstruation and ease cramps.

Ruda, albahaca, epazote, and *yerba buena* are sometimes combined. Rue is an antispasmodic and is often used to bring on delayed menstruation. It has been used to induce abortion and *can be dangerous if taken in large doses.* The infusion is made by combining half a spoonful each of dried *ruda, yerba buena,* and either *albahaca* or *epazote,* and steeping the mixture in a cup of boiling water.

Salvia has no known properties that might promote menstruation, but it is often used for that purpose. The tea is flavored with honey and lemon.

Tila and *toronjil* are considered antispasmodic and mildly sedative. They are used separately or in combination to make a soothing tea for menstrual cramps.

Fidela Gutiérrez recommends an infusion of *nochebuena* to regulate menstruation. "Use just the flowers, not the leaves," she cautions. *Parts of the plant are toxic.*

To bring on delayed menstruation, Fidela makes a tea by boiling walnut shells, *nogales.* She says that drinking a cup every night will bring on a period within three or four days.

These teas are prepared by simmering the herbs in a covered pot for ten or fifteen minutes:

Aguacate is used to promote menstrual flow. A handful of the leaves is simmered in half a liter of water. The recommended dosage is three cups a day, taken lukewarm, not hot.

Tumba vaqueros is considered antispasmodic and mildly sedative. A teaspoonful of the chopped roots is simmered in a cup of water. *This herb loses its potency when heated, so it should be prepared as a cold infusion.*

Inmortal is used to promote menstrual flow. A teaspoonful of powdered root is added to a glass of cool water and taken in the morning. Stronger doses are used for labor pains and to induce abortion.

A soothing sitz bath for menstrual cramps:

Altamisa mexicana is brewed double strength—about half a cup of dried herb steeped in a liter of boiling water. Most of it is added to the bathwater, but a little is saved so it can be sipped while soaking in the tub. The tea is diluted with more hot water and flavored with lemon, honey, or cinnamon.

EXCESSIVE MENSTRUAL BLEEDING

escoba de la víbora (snake broom)
plumajillo (yarrow)
poleo (brook mint)
salvia (common sage)

In his Aztec Herbal of 1552, Martín de la Cruz describes this elaborate recipe to stanch menstrual blood: A poultice is made with salt, ashes of a deer and a frog, egg white, rabbit hair, oak acorns, papyrus burned with deer's horn, pure gold, iron scrapings, the roots of willow, and an unidentified herb called *ahuiyacxihuitl,* which means "agreeable plant." The mixture was to be strained with river water and the liquid used to make a poultice placed where the blood flowed. Then a lizard was captured; its head was amputated and the viscera extracted and allowed to dry out in a cold place. When the viscera had dried, it was burned, and the woman was anointed with the ashes that were mixed with pulque liquor and white honey.

Nowadays, nobody wants to go to that much trouble. The remedies below rely on hot teas and compresses.

Escoba de la víbora—An infusion of the flowering tops and stems is sipped as a simple tea. A cloth soaked in the hot tea can also be applied directly to the abdomen as a compress.

Plumajillo—Yarrow is used to stop excessive bleeding externally, and an infusion of the herb is sometimes taken internally for heavy menstrual periods.

Poleo, salvia—Equal parts of the leaves of the two herbs are combined to make a soothing tea for heavy menstruation.

MENOPAUSE

muicle (Mexican honeysuckle)
passiflora (passion flower)

Muicle is considered particularly helpful for the irregular menstrual cycles of perimenopause. In his book *Plantas Curativas de México*, Dr. Luis Cabrera recommends a tea made with a rounded teaspoonful of the leaves and flowers boiled in three-fourths of a cup of water, taken three times a day between meals for menstrual cramping as well as symptoms such as hot flashes and headaches.

Passiflora, taken in an infusion of the flowers, is recommended for the sleeplessness and restlessness associated with menopause.

VAGINAL INFLAMMATIONS

escoba de la víbora (snake broom)
hoja santa (hoja santa)
huizache (sweet acacia)
lantén (common plaintain)
malva (mallow)
mimbre (desert willow)
sangre de drago (limberbush)
yerba mansa (swamp root)
yerba del indio (Indian root)
yerba mora (black nightshade)

Teas used for douches can be brewed a bit on the strong side. They should always be used warm, not hot. These herbs can also be used in a sitz bath for external inflammations.

Escoba de la víbora—A simple infusion, made by steeping the flowering branches in boiling water and allowing to cool to a comfortably warm temperature, is used as a soothing douche or sitz bath.

Hoja santa—An infusion of the leaves is used to make a soothing douche.

Huizache—The leaves and flowers or the chopped roots are simmered to make a soothing douche or sitz bath. The dried, powdered herb can also be dusted over the affected parts if the problem is external.

Lantén—A strong tea made by simmering the leaves is used as a soothing douche.

Malva—An infusion made with a big spoonful of leaves for each cup of boiling water is used as a soothing douche or sitz bath. The herb is considered to be especially beneficial to inflamed mucous membranes.

Mimbre—A strong infusion of the leaves and twigs is used as a douche for yeast infections.

Sangre de drago—A tea made by simmering the chopped roots or twigs is used as a wash or douche to calm inflamed mucous membranes.

Yerba del indio—This herb may be hard to find, but it's considered to be an especially effective douche for vaginal infections. It has antiseptic and antibiotic properties, and may also help reduce inflammations. An infusion is made using one or two leaves for each half cup of water.

Yerba mansa—An infusion of the leaves can be used either as a wash or a douche. The herb is soothing to inflamed mucous membranes and has antimicrobial properties.

Yerba mora—A douche made with an infusion of the leaves may be useful in relieving yeast infections. The plant has anti-inflammatory and antifungal properties.

INFERTILITY

Damiana is believed to enhance fertility in both men and women. The infusion is used as both a tea and a douche to remedy *frío de matriz*, or cold in the womb, which is traditionally thought to be a leading cause of female infertility. The *damiana* tea supposedly "warms" the womb, restoring it to the proper state for impregnation.

According to traditional beliefs, failure to conceive may also be caused by *caída de matriz*, a womb that has fallen or is twisted, perhaps as a result of having been chilled after childbirth. A practiced *curandera* will attempt to correct this condition by massaging the lower abdomen to manipulate the womb into the correct position.

CHILDBIRTH

The Aztec midwife first visited her client two months before the baby was expected. Together they crawled into the *temezcal*, the steam bath, where the midwife examined the pregnant woman's belly, palpating it to determine the position of the fetus. If necessary, the midwife massaged the woman's belly to turn the baby around. They still say that a good *partera*, midwife, can see inside a pregnant woman's belly with her hands as though she were looking through a clear glass bottle.

During labor the Aztec midwife administered a tea to hasten the birth; it was made with *tihuapatli (zoapatle)*, woman's medicine. In the sixteenth century, Fray Bernardino de Sahagún reported that the tea was taken when the first "blood comes, which shows that the baby is about to follow." The Aztec midwives believed that a good labor is quick, with strong contractions. The medicines lessened the woman's suffering by speeding things up, not by numbing the pain. If delivery did not quickly ensue, a second dose of the tea was administered, and if the woman still had not given birth, she was given a drink made with a bit of ground possum's tail. If the labor was long and the woman was very tired, she might be given a noxious drink, or a feather or some other object might be inserted into her throat to provoke vomiting.

In rural Mexico today, much of this tradition has continued, although many women give birth without even the help of a *partera*, relying only on the expertise of a female relative or friend. In many places the *temezcal* is still a part of life. To speed the contractions, the woman still sips hot chocolate laced with *zoapatle*, or a good strong infusion of rue. Other herbs are used in teas during labor: *manzanilla, cardo santo, estafiate, epazote, cempasúchil, pericón, guaco, albahaca, yerba del sapo*, or *yerba buena* laced with cinnamon. Herbs are sometimes burned or boiled, and the woman is helped to squat over the fire or the pot so that the vapors reach her cervix and help to speed dilation.

The woman's belly may also be washed with a warm infusion of herbs. Combinations of *pericón, zapote blanco*, and *higueroa* may be used, or onions fried in lard with *manzanilla*. As delivery approaches, ground *inmortal* root soaked in water may be rubbed on the abdomen to ease labor pains.

Above all, it is considered essential that the woman stay warm, both during the birth process and in the following days while she is recuperating. A fire is often kept burning in the room where the birth takes place. The Aztecs kept a fire burning for four days after the birth. They believed that the newborn baby needed the heat to strengthen its vital spirit, its *tonalli*.

This notion of a need for warmth is still very widespread and persistent. Socorro Vázquez told me that she thinks it's very dangerous for women to give birth in the air-conditioned rooms of modern hospitals. "All that cold goes inside you, and before you know it, this hurts, that hurts." A chill can cause *fría de matriz*, a cold womb, or *caída de matriz*, a fallen womb, which will make it difficult for the woman to become pregnant again.

Traditionally, women give birth kneeling, with their knees spread apart. The father, a friend, or a family member takes the part of the *tenedor*, the holder, supporting the woman from behind and holding her under her arms. The *partera*, the midwife, positions herself to pull the baby out, and she might assist the woman by pressing down on her belly with each contraction.

After the birth, a tea made with *epazote* or a little ground *inmortal* root dissolved in a glass of water might be administered to help expel the afterbirth.

POSTPARTUM DISCOMFORT

> *canela* (cinnamon)
> *escoba de la víbora* (snake broom)
> *hinojo* (fennel)
> *manzanilla* (German chamomile)
> *rosa de castilla* (French rose, red rose)
> *yerba del pollo* (Mexican dayflower)

Following childbirth, a woman will traditionally rest and be kept warm. Three or four days after the birth, she will begin a series of visits to the *temezcal*, taking ritual healing baths with her midwife who may massage her or flay her with branches of medicinal plants to stimulate her circulation. Healing teas and compresses are used to reduce swelling and discomfort.

Boldo—Fidela Gutiérrez recommends *boldo* tea for postpartum bleeding.

Canela, rosa de castilla, manzanilla—An infusion made with equal parts of the three herbs is soothing.

Escoba de la víbora—An infusion of the stems and flowers is sipped and also used as a compress that is applied to the lower abdomen.

Hinojo—An infusion of the leaves is used to soothe the stomach.

Yerba del pollo—The Aztecs applied the leaves of this plant as a poultice to stop the bleeding of battle wounds. In some places it is still used as a tea to stop internal bleeding, particularly after childbirth.

NURSING

Not Enough Milk

angélica (angelica)
epazote (American wormseed)
hinojo (fennel)

Mexicans and Mexican Americans use a number of herbs to increase lactation, although there have been no scientific studies to prove that they work or to explain why they might.

Angelica—In Morelos, midwives prescribe a tea made by simmering chopped angelica root.

Epazote—An infusion of the leaves, sweetened with sugar.

Hinojo—An infusion of the leaves or crushed seeds, alone or in combination with other herbs, is used to promote lactation, and a compress made with the same infusion is applied to swollen breasts.

Too Much Milk

Nursing mothers drink three cups of *salvia* (sage) tea a day to help dry up their milk supply while they are weaning. A little of the tea is also applied to the nipples. Sage has astringent properties, and some studies have shown that the herb may be slightly estrogenic.

Sore Nipples

árnica (Mexican arnica)
caléndula (English marigold)
crameria (rhatany)

sábila (aloe vera)

yerba mansa (swamp root)

Arnica, caléndula, and **yerba mansa,** used singly or in combination, can be made into a soothing infusion.

Crameria, which has astringent properties, is a traditional remedy for sore nipples. The nipples are washed with a cool tea made by pouring half a liter of boiling water over two heaping teaspoons of the crushed bark. The infusion is allowed to steep for ten or fifteen minutes before straining.

Sábila—Some Mexican women dab a little *sábila* juice on their nipples when they are weaning their babies. It has a bitter taste that the babies find quite nasty; at the same time, its emollient and healing properties are nice for the mother.

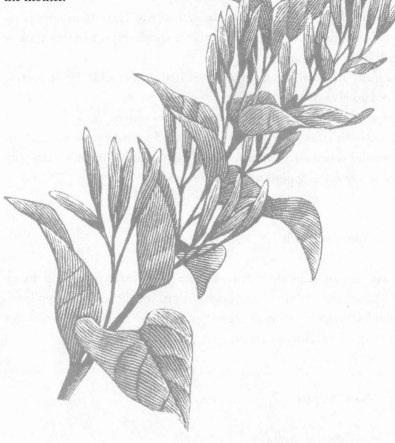

HERBS FOR BABIES

CAÍDA DE MOLLERA
(FALLEN FONTANELLE)

estafiate (mugwort)
albahaca (common basil)
manzanilla (German chamomile)

Caída de mollera, which means "fallen fontanelle," is an old folk illness, but people still talk about it. When the fontanelle, the soft spot on a baby's head, forms a depression, the baby is believed to be suffering from this condition. The cause can be a fall or pulling the nipple out of the baby's mouth too abruptly while it is still sucking. Newborn babies are not supposed to be held upright for fear that this will cause the soft spot to fall. A baby with *caída de mollera* will also have diarrhea and may be vomiting. A lump or knob may develop on the baby's hard palate, and the baby might not be able to nurse properly.

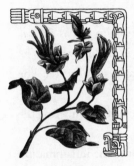

The traditional remedies for this condition are mechanical. A *curandera* may wet the baby's head and then attempt to suck the soft spot back up with her mouth. She may put her fingers into the baby's mouth and push up on the palate while pulling on the baby's hair over the soft spot. Sometimes egg white is plastered over the spot or the baby is held upside down by the feet in the hope that the soft spot will fall back into place. If the baby is able to suckle, it is fed plenty of liquids in the form of weak infusions of *estafiate, albahaca,* or *manzanilla*—herbs that soothe the digestive system.

The modern explanation for this condition is dehydration caused by diarrhea, which results in the depression of the fontanelle.

DIAPER RASH

malva (mallow)
rosa de castilla (French rose, red rose)
yerba del índio (Indian root)
yerba mora (black nightshade)

Many Mexican Americans refer to a rash they call *"chincual,"* which afflicts newborns and nursing infants. The word comes from the Nahuatl *tzin,* meaning buttocks, and *cualli,* meaning hot. It is essentially the same thing as diaper rash, but according to traditional beliefs the problem stems not only from the irritation of wet diapers, but also from "hot" foods in the mother's diet. Pregnant and nursing mothers are instructed to avoid chiles as well as hot coffee, peanuts, and pumpkin seeds.

Washes

Malva and **rosa de castilla**—For diaper rash, or the condition known as *chincual,* a soothing herbal wash is made by infusing *malva* leaves in boiling water. The remedy calls for a heaping teaspoonful of the herb for each cup of water. The resulting liquid is used at room temperature.

Yerba del indio—An infusion of the flowers or a tea made by simmering the roots is used as a soothing and antiseptic wash.

Yerba mora—An infusion of the leaves is used to soothe the inflammation of diaper rash. The plant also has antifungal properties.

COLIC AND DIARRHEA

albucema (lavender)

eneldo (dill)

hinojo (fennel)

poleo (brook mint)

rosa de castilla (French rose, red rose)

saúco (elder flower)

tila (linden)

Herbal teas for babies should be very weak. Use only a scant quarter teaspoonful of the herb for each cup of water.

Albucema—A tea of dry lavender leaves, sweetened with a little *piloncillo* or sugar is fed to newborns who are thought to be suffering from colic caused by drinking the mother's first milk. The infusion is also used in bottles or sprinkled on the nipples of the breasts when the mother's milk is delayed.

Eneldo, hinojo—Colicky babies are sometimes given bottles of *"gripe* water," a mild tea made with crushed dill or fennel seeds that helps dispel stomach gas.

Poleo, saúco, yerba buena—A diluted infusion of *poleo* or *yerba buena* leaves, sometimes mixed with *saúco* flowers, is used to relieve the pain of colic.

Rosa de castilla—Because rose petals have no toxic properties and are mildly astringent, a weak rose tea is used to treat infantile diarrhea, although the rose hips or petals in stronger doses actually have a slight laxative effect.

Tila—A mild infusion of the flowers is used to treat colic caused by teething. It's also considered mild enough to be used as a sedative tea when the baby is restless and can't seem to fall asleep.

For babies, Ofelia Esparza advises making an infusion of **poleo** that can be kept in a jar to be diluted as needed. She uses no more than two ounces of the infusion in a bottle, and the rest is warm water. If the poleo doesn't work, she recommends adding a little infusion of **cedrón**. *"Cedrón* was a lifesaver with my kids," she told me. "I have a little *cedrón* bush in the yard. It's also very soothing and pleasant if you can't sleep."

STICKY EYES

As the tear ducts and sinuses develop, babies can have sticky eyes. A cool *manzanilla* (German chamomile) tea is used to gently wash away the goo.

TEETHING

Teething babies are given the stem and leaves of an onion plant to chew. It is believed that chewing the plant alleviates the pain and swelling of the baby's gums.

BATHING

Aztec babies were bathed in water scented with *pericón* (Mexican tarragon) leaves soon after they were born.

Fidela Gutiérrez recommends bathing cranky babies in an infusion of romaine lettuce leaves.

HERBAL TONICS

alegría (amaranth)
boldo (bold)
copal (elephant tree)
cuasia (quassia)
damiana (damiana)
diente de león (dandelion)
lengua de vaca (yellow dock)

Tonic herbs are often very bitter and can be flavored with cinnamon, brown sugar, *piloncillo*, or honey.

Alegría tea, made by simmering amaranth flowers, is used as a heart tonic particularly favored by older people in the Southwest. One cup of the tea is taken each morning.

Boldo leaves, in a simple infusion, are used to rebuild strength after a long illness.

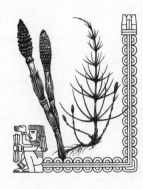

Copal tea, made by simmering the leaves and bark, is used to give a tonic boost to the immune system.

Damiana, the "love tea," is nature's Viagra. It is popularly believed to enhance the male sex drive and combat impotency. It is used as a general tonic for weakness in the rest of the body as well. The remedy calls for an infusion of the leaves and stems to be taken each morning.

Cuasia is used to make a tonic tea. Clean wood chips are soaked in cold water rather than brewed. One level teaspoon of the chips is used for each cup of cold water. The mixture is allowed to steep for twelve hours, then strained. One cup of the liquid is taken first thing in the morning on an empty stomach, and a second cup in the evening. This dose is repeated for several days to fortify the body after an illness.

Diente de león is a time-honored tonic, taken in the spring to revitalize the body after the long hard winter. Two teaspoons of the leaves or dried root, or a combination of the two, are infused in a cup of boiling water and drunk twice a day for several weeks. If you have a juicer and access to clean, non-pesticide-ridden leaves, you can also drink freshly squeezed dandelion juice. Look for very young leaves on plants that have not yet begun to show buds. Wash the leaves well and soak overnight before juicing.

Lengua de vaca tea, made by simmering the chopped root, is used as a tonic to "strengthen the blood" after an illness.

In Ofelia Esparza's family, *maguey* sap was taken as a tonic. She remembers this story: "Oh, *maguey*! I call it the tree of life. A man used to come and cut the top off our *maguey* tree and then scrape it and cover it, and he'd get the *agua miel* of the *maguey*, a saplike honey. Eventually, of course, that gets fermented to make the *pulque* liquor. He'd give us half a gallon of it. Mother kept it in the refrigerator, and we'd drink it in the morning as a tonic. They called it *agua miel* (honey water), but it wasn't sweet; it was sour. We didn't like it!

HERBS FOR DETOXIFYING

alcachofa (artichoke)
alfalfa (alfalfa)
berro (watercress)
boldo (bold)

diente de león (dandelion)

lengua de vaca (yellow dock)

pingüica (uva ursi)

Traditional Mexican and Mexican-American medical beliefs hold that cleansing the body is the road to good health. Kidney and liver ailments are often thought to be the result of some blockage that needs to be washed out. There are many popular recipes for teas used to decongest the organs, and the list of general purgatives is a long one. (*Also see remedies for constipation, page 234.*)

Alcachofa leaves make a diuretic drink used to decongest the liver. They lose potency when heated, so the remedy should be prepared as a cold infusion, not a tea. The leaves are covered with cold water and allowed to steep for at least twelve hours. The strained liquid is taken in place of water throughout the day.

Alfalfa is a mild diuretic used to cleanse the kidneys and colon. The plant loses its potency when dried, so it is always used freshly picked. Three teaspoons of lightly mashed leaves are steeped in a cup of boiling water.

Berro is a natural diuretic used to stimulate the liver and lymph glands. It loses potency when heated, so it's eaten raw in salads or taken as a juice or a cold infusion.

Boldo is considered a good kidney cleanser, among its many other uses. An infusion is made with the dried leaves.

Diente de león is regarded as an excellent liver decongestant and general tonic. A simple infusion can be made with the dry leaves, but a tea made by simmering the chopped roots is considered more potent. The tea is taken first thing in the morning on an empty stomach for several days.

Lengua de vaca tea is made by simmering the chopped root. It is considered a particularly effective kidney cleanser as well as a tonic. The tea is also taken three or four times a day to clear the complexion.

Pingüica, an effective diuretic, is used to cleanse the bladder and kidneys. One remedy calls for a cold infusion made according to these directions: Soak a big handful of the berries in water to cover for an hour or until they get soft and mushy. Remove them from the water and mash them in a bowl to extract the juice. Strain the liquid. A half cup is taken in the morning, and another at night.

HERBS FOR HANGOVERS

The Aztecs brewed potent *pulque* liquor from the *maguey* cactus, but they had very strict rules about who was allowed to drink it and when. *Pulque* was given to members of the nobility, the ill, and to captives who were soon to be sacrificed. The general citizenry was permitted to drink *pulque* only for special celebrations and religious rituals. Since drunkenness interfered with a citizen's duty to contribute to society, it was a crime. Nobles and priests, who had the heaviest obligation to serve the community, were executed if they were found inappropriately imbibing even once. Commoners were given a second chance, but habitual drunkenness was a capital offense for everyone. Only the elderly, who had reached an age when they were relieved of their worldly duties, were permitted to drink *pulque* to their heart's content

After the conquest, when the structure of Aztec society was destroyed, indigenous Mexicans drank *pulque* much more freely, perhaps to escape from the misery of the often harsh treatment they received by exploitative Spanish masters. Drunkenness became a widespread problem, attacked by the Church and the government without success. *Maguey*, previously not much of a crop, began to be grown on a large scale by *pulque*-producing *haciendas*.

The following remedies, of a more recent vintage, are used to treat the aftereffects of overindulgence in beer or tequila more often than *pulque*.

> *canela* (cinnamon)
> *clavo* (clove)
> *damiana* (damiana)
> *guayaba* (guava)
> *nuez moscada* (nutmeg)
> *té de monte* (savory)
> *tronadora* (trumpet bush)
> *yerba buena* (spearmint)

Damiana—The traditional cure for the awful headache that comes with a hangover is *damiana* tea, three cups on an empty stomach or between meals, taken throughout the "day after." In his book *Plantas Curativas de México,* Dr. Luis G. Cabrera speculates that the infusion may stimulate cerebral circulation.

Guayaba—Fidela Gutiérrez told me that a tea made with *guayaba* leaves helps a hangover.

Té de monte—An infusion of *té de monte,* which is also known as *té de borracho,* drunk's tea, is used to treat an alcohol-abused digestive system.

Tronadora—An infusion of the flowers and leaves is a traditional hangover remedy.

Yerba buena—For the queasy stomach associated with a hangover, the traditional remedy is a spoonful of *yerba buena* leaves steeped in a cup of boiling water, topped with a spicy sprinkle of cinnamon, nutmeg, and cloves.

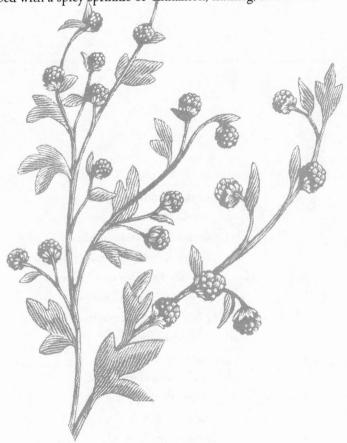

HERBS FOR BATHS AND SOAKS

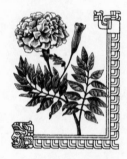

albahaca (common basil)
alferillo (fillery)
cancerina (Mexican heather)
chamiso hediondo (basin sagebrush)
cinco negritos (common lantana)
florifundio (angel's trumpet)
gobernadora (chaparral)
golondrina (spurge)
hoja santa (hoja santa)
jarilla (willow groundsel)
linaza (flax)
malva (mallow)
ocotillo (candlewood)
ruda (rue)
saúco (elder flower)
tila (linden)
verbena (vervain)
yerba del indio (Indian root)
yerba del negro (desert hollyhock)
yerba mansa (swamp root)

Aztec homes were built with an adjacent steam bath, called a *temezcal*, a dome-shaped adobe hut heated by a wood-burning fireplace and entered by crawling through a low tunnel-like entrance. Water sprayed on the hot walls and floor of the bath produced steam. Healers treated the ill and the infirm inside the *temezcal*, using massage or smacking the patient with branches to stimulate the circulation.

The word *temezcal* comes from the name of the Aztec god Temazaltoci, who learned the art of bathing from the water goddess Ayauh. Images of Temazaltoci adorned the walls of ancient Aztec bathhouses.

The tradition of the *temezcal* has survived in rural Mexico and is currently being revived by Mexicans and Mexican Americans who are becoming increasingly interested in exploring their heritage. The many therapeutic herbal baths prescribed by some of the most modern urban *curanderas* are survivors of the ancient *temezcal*. Many of the infusions added to bathwater have anti-inflammatory or emollient properties. Others may be soothing because of their aroma. A number of remedies specify that a little of an infusion should be sipped and the rest added to the bathwater.

TO PREPARE AN HERBAL BATH

Brew the tea at double the strength you would use if you were going to drink it. Use about half a cup of dried herb in a liter of water.

Infusions are prepared by pouring the boiling water over the tea in a pan, covering, and steeping for fifteen or twenty minutes before straining and adding to the bathwater.

Simmered teas are made by adding half a cup of dried herb to a liter of water in a pot, bringing the mixture to a boil, covering tightly, and simmering over low heat for fifteen minutes. The mixture should be allowed to cool slightly before straining and adding to the bathwater.

SOOTHING SOAKS FOR ARTHRITIS, RHEUMATISM, ACHES, AND PAINS

Alferillo—An infusion of *alferillo* for the discomfort of rheumatism.

Cancerina—An infusion of the leaves, stems, and flowers for muscle pains and arthritis. Some people add a few *malva* leaves.

Cinco negritos—An infusion of the leaves, stems, and flowers for muscle pain and arthritis.

Chamiso hediondo—An infusion of the leaves for rheumatism.

Florifundio—An infusion of the flowers, or the flowers and leaves, for arthritis, strained muscles, aches, and pains. To make an infusion with fresh leaves or flowers, add a big handful to a liter of water and steep. *This herb should not be taken internally.*

Gobernadora—An infusion of the leaves for rheumatism, sore muscles, saddle sores, and bruises. Some people add a few *florifundio* or *árnica* leaves.

Hoja santa—An infusion of the leaves for aches and pains.

Jarilla—An infusion of the leaves for arthritis and rheumatism.

Ocotillo—The chopped root of this plant is boiled in water for thirty minutes before cooling and straining to make a soak for soreness, bruises, and general fatigue.

Tila—An infusion of the leaves for cramped muscles. Some of the tea, diluted with an equal part of boiling water, can be sipped while soaking.

Verbena—An infusion of the leaves for nervousness or rheumatism.

Yerba del indio—An infusion of the flowers and stems or a simmered tea made with the roots for arthritis or rheumatism.

Yerba mansa—A strong infusion of the ground roots or the leaves for arthritis, swollen feet, and sore muscles.

SOOTHING BATHS FOR IRRITATED SKIN

Linaza, the source of linseed oil, makes a soothing anti-inflammatory bath. Three teaspoons of seeds are used for each half cup of water. The mixture of seeds and water is brought to a boil and then simmered over low heat, covered, for ten or fifteen minutes. The pan is removed from the heat, and the mixture is allowed to infuse for ten minutes more before it is strained and added to the bathwater.

Malva leaves or the leaves and flowers are used in an infusion for inflammations. Some people add a little *romero* to the *malva* before infusing. It will give the bath a nice aroma and has slightly astringent properties.

Saúco flowers add a lovely fragrance to bathwater and have soothing emollient properties. Traditionally, the herb is used to make a soak for children with measles, but it can also be used for any sort of skin irritation and to ease sore muscles. Make an infusion using four teaspoons of fresh or two teaspoons of dried blossoms for each cup of boiling water. Pour the water over the flowers and allow them to infuse for ten minutes before straining.

Yerba del negro has emollient and soothing properties. An infusion of the leaves, stems, and flowers is added to the bath water to treat skin irritations.

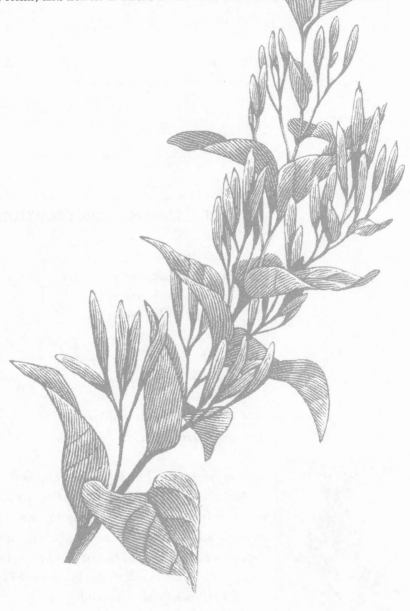

HERBS FOR BEAUTY AND HAIR

PIMPLES AND SKIN ERUPTIONS

árnica (árnica)
bugambilia (bougainvillea)
cáscara sagrada (bearberry)
diente de león (dandelion)
jarilla (willow groundsel)
mastuerzo (garden nasturtium)
plumajillo (yarrow)
sábila (aloe vera)
salvia real (butterfly bush)
saúco (elder flower)

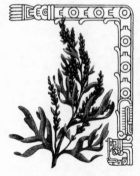

Infusions should be made fresh daily and kept refrigerated.

Arnica is used to make a lotion for drying up pimples. It is brought to a boil in water to cover. The resulting liquid is allowed to cool before straining and then blended with an equal part of rubbing alcohol. Because of the alcohol content, this lotion can be kept in a cool dark place for several months.

Cáscara sagrada is used to make a cleansing wash. Add

a rounded spoonful of the crushed bark to a cup of water. Bring the mixture to a boil, lower the heat, and simmer for ten or fifteen minutes. Cool and strain. The resulting liquid can be dabbed over the area with a cotton ball.

Diente de león juice from freshly squeezed leaves is applied to skin eruptions.

Jarilla leaves are mashed and applied directly to the area to reduce redness.

Mastuerzo, which has astringent properties, is mixed with a little *sábila* juice and applied to the face before going to bed. In the morning, the face is washed with a mild soap.

Plumajillo is considered both astringent and anti-inflammatory, and may be useful in treating breakouts. Three or four leaves are steeped for ten or fifteen minutes in a cup of boiling water. The cooled, strained liquid is dabbed on the skin several times a day and allowed to air dry.

Salvia real leaves are used as a poultice to dry up pimples.

Saúco flowers are used to make an infusion that is dabbed on clean skin to reduce the redness and inflammation. A spoonful of dried flowers is steeped in a cup of boiling water for twenty minutes, strained, and then allowed to cool before using.

Fidela Gutiérrez uses a cool infusion of *bugambilia* blossoms as a topical treatment for acne.

SKIN CREAMS AND FRESHENERS

caléndula (English marigold)
papaya (Mexican papaya)
sábila (aloe vera)
sueldo (common comfrey)

Caléndula oil is soothing to the skin and makes a good hair conditioner, It will keep for at least a year if it is kept in a sealed jar in a cool dark closet. Place dry flower heads in a jar and cover with a good, cold-pressed vegetable oil; sesame oil is especially light and odorless. Close the jar tightly and leave it in a dark closet for four to six weeks, shaking the jar once a day, then strain it into a clean dark glass bottle or jar. Cool *caléndula* tea can also be used as a soothing skin freshener.

Papaya sap, which is collected from making incisions in the skin of an unripe fruit, is applied to warts and freckles. The mashed ripe fruit can be used as a facial mask to soften the skin.

Sábila—Fresh aloe vera juice is applied directly to the skin. It is an effective moisturizer. The cut side of the leaves can also be applied directly to the face as a moisturizing mask.

Sueldo leaves, in a cool infusion, make a soothing and astringent skin freshener. The tea can be kept in the refrigerator for a couple of days and used as needed.

HAIR CARE

> *caléndula* (English marigold)
> *cola de caballo* (horsetail)
> *encino* (oak)
> *espinosilla* (hummingbird flower)
> *guayaba* (guava)
> *higuerilla* (castor bean plant)
> *jojoba* (jojoba)
> *manzanilla* (German chamomile)
> *palmilla* (yucca)
> *plumajillo* (yarrow)
> *romero* (rosemary)
> *salvia* (common sage)
> *yerba del negro* (desert hollyhock)

Caléndula, manzanilla, romero, and *salvia* are used to make a rinse for body and shine. The four herbs are combined and steeped in boiling water for twenty minutes before straining. Use about three rounded teaspoons of the herb mixture in a pint of water.

Cola de caballo has a high silicone content, so drinking an infusion of the herb is believed to promote healthy hair and nails.

Encino and *romero* are combined to make a rinse for dandruff. Add three rounded teaspoons of the herb mixture to a pint of water and bring to a boil. Lower the heat and simmer for ten or fifteen minutes before cooling and straining.

Jojoba oil is used as a treatment for dandruff. A tea made by simmering the leaves can also be used as a hair rinse. Follow the instructions for *encino* and *romero* above.

Plumajillo tea is used as an astringent rinse for oily hair and dandruff. Steep a rounded spoonful of the leaves and flowers in a cup of boiling water for ten or fifteen minutes. Strain and allow to cool before using.

Yerba del negro is used to make a rinse that adds body to the hair. Bring three rounded teaspoons of the herb to a boil in a pint of water. Lower the heat until the liquid barely simmers. Cover tightly and continue simmering for about an hour. Remove from the heat and let the mixture cool until it is just tepid, then strain.

Yucca roots are used to make a shampoo. Cover chopped roots with water and bring to a boil. Stir over heat until the water looks foamy. Cool and strain. The plant adds shine and body to the hair.

Ofelia Esparza told me: "Mother's *guayaba* tree is still growing here outside by the front door. The fruit is big and white inside. In Mexico they made an infusion from the leaves of the *guayaba* tree to rinse the hair. Women from the neighborhood used to come over to collect leaves from my mother's tree. They said it made their hair thicker and darker. Well, it makes sense, because when those leaves fall, they stain the sidewalk."

HAIR LOSS

encino (oak, leaves)
espinosilla (hummingbird flower)

nogal (walnut tree)
orégano (Mexican oregano)
romero (rosemary)
salvia (common sage)

Encino, espinosilla, nogal, orégano, and *romero* are combined in equal parts to make an infusion used as a rinse to combat hair loss. Some people also wash the scalp with a shampoo made by boiling mashed *espinosilla* leaves.

Salvia has astringent qualities that may be good for the scalp. A strong *salvia* tea is used as an after-shampoo rinse to darken the hair.

DEODORANT

Gobernadora, which doesn't smell so good itself, is nevertheless one of nature's deodorants. Raunchy rustlers on the range dust the powdered, dried leaves on smelly feet and armpits.

WEIGHT LOSS AIDS

cáscara sagrada (bearberry)
barba de maíz (corn silk)
cocolmeca (greenbrier)
cola de caballo (horsetail)
hinojo (fennel)
hojasen (senna)
palo azul (kidneywood)
pingüica (uva ursi)

Most of the "diet" teas sold in *botánicas* are just a combination of herbs with astringent and diuretic properties. *Pingüica, cola de caballo, palo azul,* and *barba de maíz* are among the herbs often included in these teas. Some diet tea formulas also include an herbal laxative such as *hojasen* or *cáscara sagrada.*

In southern New Mexico, Bonnie Ochoa told me that she recommends *co-colmeca* for weight loss. "It makes you give off a lot of water," she said.

On the other hand, *hinojo* may actually have some value as an appetite suppressant. In the Middle Ages, fennel seeds were chewed by those too poor to buy food in the belief that their hunger would be relieved. Some modern-day dieters chew the seeds for the same reason.

HERBS FOR
INSECTICIDES

alhucema (lavender)
barbasco (Texas croton)
cola de caballo (horsetail)
pericón (Mexican tarrigon)
poleo chino (pennyroyal)
ruda (rue)
tanceto (tansy)

Barbasco is dried and thrown on hot coals in a closed room to fumigate for bedbugs. It is also sometimes placed under the mattress or hung from the rafters for the same purpose.

Cola de caballo, in a cooled infusion, is sprayed on roses to kill leaf fungus.

Alhucema sprigs are placed among the clothes in closets and drawers to keep moths away.

Pericón is dried, then burned outdoors to ward off flies and mosquitoes.

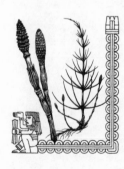

Poleo chino is hung in the house in bunches to discourage flies and other flying intruders.

Ruda plants are placed on windowsills to keep bugs out of the kitchen. Sprigs of *ruda* are placed under bed pillows as a fumigant.

Tanceto, tied in bunches, is hung from windows to repel ants and flies.

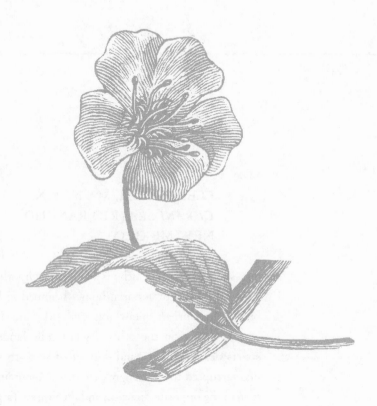

PROFILE:
A MODERN CURANDERA

ELENA AVILA, M.S.N., R.N.,
***CURANDERA* (RIO RANCHO,**
NEW MEXICO)

The suburb of Rio Rancho is a family neighborhood, a peaceful enclave of modern homes hemmed in by Albuquerque's urban sprawl on one side and by the Sonora desert on the other. Its tastefully landscaped streets dead-end into sand dunes that seem to stretch uninterrupted to the Sangre de Cristo Mountains. But turn in the opposite direction and the nearest Target superstore is only half a mile away.

There is nothing unusual about Elena Avila's house. She is simply the *curandera* next door. But her personal style is a blazing expression of her inner culture clash: feathers woven into her long loose hair, an embroidered Mexican *huipil* and skirt worn over a stretch lace body suit.

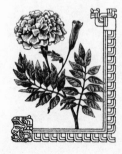

In the comfortable den where she meets clients, the late afternoon sun is reaching across the room to meet the dim glow of the votive candles on the altar. The residual aroma of smoldering rosemary and sage persists in the air. Elena invites me to make myself comfortable on the couch, offers me a cool glass of *yerba buena* tea. Looking up from my notebook, I lock into her black eyes. She sits opposite me in an armchair, leaning forward, her expression open, expectant, like a shrink with a new patient.

Vibrant, darkly beautiful at fifty-three, she is the poster girl for modern *curanderismo*. While many *curanderas* practice their art discreetly, even surreptitiously, she actively promotes her work, her heritage, herself. She has published collections of her poetry, written a book about her life as a *curandera* (*Woman Who Glows in the Dark*), and she makes frequent appearances on the conference circuit. Her presentations—part lecture, part performance art— are heavily dosed with ritual. She is in demand not only because she puts on a good show but because people are intrigued by a woman with a master's degree in psychiatric nursing, trained to use the resources of modern science, who prefers to practice an ancient folk medicine.

"The nursing degree really helps," she admits. "Not that many people are interested in just talking to a *señora* about her knowledge, which is a shame. But health professionals are very interested in what my day-to-day practice is. I talk about the folk diseases. I treat a lot of *susto, envidia, bilis.* I do a lot of *pláticas*, soul retrievals. There were some good things I learned in nursing school, and some things I've had to unlearn. I still keep up my nursing license. I don't know why, but I do."

The transition from nursing to *curanderismo* was slow and painful. It was as though she had managed to truly assimilate, to finally achieve the American dream after years of struggle, only to discover that she couldn't bear it and had to fight her way back to her Mexican roots. "I was born and raised in El Paso, first generation Chicana. My first language was Spanish. Even when I was a child, I was a little healer, taking care of the kids in the neighborhood." She was a high school dropout, married at sixteen, and a mother at seventeen. For a long time she put all thoughts of healing aside. Then her marriage ended. A single mother with no education and four children to raise, one of them mentally disabled, she had to fight hard. She finished her high school diploma, put herself through nursing school, then graduate school. She was the first person in her family to graduate from college.

"In nursing school I was asked to get up and talk about *curanderismo*, and it really made me very angry that they would want me to do that. I was feeling that push to assimilate. I just wanted to be like everybody else. But I thank them for that now because it woke me up to my culture. I started going across the border to Juarez, to the *indio* market, talking to the señoras in the stalls selling the *yerbas.* They would give me *limpias* and treat me for *susto.*

"So my *desarrollo*, my training, in *curanderismo* was going in one direction, and my *desarrollo* in nursing was going in another. I was always studying and practicing *curanderismo*, but on the side." Gradually she began to try to introduce elements of traditional healing into her professional life. She wanted to use all her skills, including the traditional rituals she was sure would work.

She spent a year at the UCLA Neuropathic Institute, where her patients were emotionally disturbed children. Many of them had been sexually abused. To Elena they were suffering from *susto*, a Mexican folk disease that is the physical and emotional reaction to a traumatic experience. "I would ask, 'Can we incorporate the concept of *susto* in our therapy, in our teamwork? Can I do some ceremony to help the child?'" But she was always emphatically refused.

"Finally, it became clear to me that I had to drop the structure of institutions and practice *curanderismo* full time. I had to ask myself if I was willing to let go of everything I'd accomplished, all those hard years of being poor while I worked on my degrees." She quit her job and bought the house in Rio Rancho. It takes courage to live by the motto she likes to repeat: "We go into the unknown for unknown reasons." She was afraid that she'd lose it all, end up a homeless bag lady, but she took the plunge.

Twelve years later she has a full schedule of clients, lectures, and personal appearances, and a devoted flock of apprentice *curanderas*. For the past two years she has been training nineteen women, not all of them Mexican American but most of them health care professionals who, like Elena, have become frustrated by the limitations of the modern medical system. They have traveled together to Mexico to meet with native healers, lived in the field, learned how to participate in the Aztec rituals, and been given Nahuatl names. This *desarollo* is serious work. Not one of the apprentices is ready to call herself a *curandera*.

Elena Avila hasn't really changed careers but merely switched one set of tools for another, still using the same talents that enabled her to become an effective psychiatric nurse. She feels she can be more effective working as a *curandera*. "It's wonderful to be able to help people in a way that's not so fragmented," she explains.

"I guess if you had to categorize me, I'm a spiritual healer. When people come to me, I see the whole picture. I don't go too much by Western standards of diagnosis, which can be very structured and, I believe, very rigid. Instead, I listen to their stories, to what they think is making them sick. I can sense their energy fields. And pretty soon what is going on with the person manifests itself. The person may be talking about physical problems, but the root of it could be spiritual. I might suggest an herb, we might do a couple of *limpias*, and then I might send them to a doctor for some other aspect of the problem. I don't put myself in a place where I say that I can take care of everything.

"*Curanderismo* starts with heart and intuition. I always tell people that they themselves are medicine. I help them activate their own healing potential. Healing begins with an acceptance of what is."

WHEN THE REMEDY IS A *LIMPIA*

Because Elena Avila is a spiritual healer, one of her primary remedies is the *limpia*, an ancient ritual still practiced throughout Mexico and in Mexican-American communities. The name comes from the Spanish word *limpiar*, to clean. The *curandera* cleanses the patient's spirit, removing the source of suffering.

Folk diseases such as *susto*, which is caused by fright or trauma; *envidia*, which is caused by jealousy; *desasombra*, a more serious form of *susto*; and, most serious of all, *espanto*, the loss of the spirit, are treated with *limpias*. A *limpia* can remedy an infirmity caused by evil-doing, such as *mal puesto*, or *mal de ojo*, a curse or a spell inflicted by another person or by a *bruja*, a witch. Although the sources of these illnesses may be purely emotional or even magical, they can all manifest real physical symptoms such as exhaustion, weight loss, diarrhea and nervousness that do not respond to medical treatment.

It may be possible to trace the origins of the *limpia* to the Aztec belief in *tonalli*. *Tonalli* is the spirit, the source of strength. It defines a person's destiny. The *tonalli* resides in the head. In pre-Hispanic drawings, the Aztecs are shown dragging captives away by their hair, to illustrate that they had captured the *tonalli* of these prisoners. Hair protects the *tonalli*. An Aztec punishment for drunkenness was a shaved head. The *limpia* is a ceremony in which the spirit, the *tonalli*, is cleansed and strengthened.

There are as many variations of the *limpia* ritual as there are *curanderos*. Each region, each pueblo has its own traditions. But *limpias* always include the use of some element that attracts whatever is polluting the spirit and draws it out. The most commonly used tools for this are an egg and branches of aromatic herbs.

Elena Avila always begins with a *plática*, a heart-to-heart talk, during which the nature of the patient's problem is revealed. This can be accomplished in one session, or a whole series of *pláticas* may be required. Once a date for the *limpia* has been decided on, she instructs her clients to prepare by taking a bath scented with chamomile, rosemary, and rose petals. For three days before the *limpia* they are restricted to a vegetarian diet, taking "only foods from the earth and no drugs except important prescriptions such as blood pressure medications." Both Elena and her client dress in white. They begin in her garden where the client is asked to choose the branches of herbs that will be used during the ritual. "I have them say a prayer," she explains. "I want them to thank the plant, to connect with it."

These aromatic herbs are passed over the patient's body in a ritual sweeping, the *barranda*. The Aztecs believed that pleasant aromas attracted *tonalli* and repelled negative underworld spirits. Fragrant oils may also be rubbed on the patient's forehead and temples. Sometimes a cross is drawn with the oil on each of the patient's major joints: the neck, knees, elbows. At the conclusion of the ritual, the patient may be fumigated with incense and given an herbal tea to drink.

The Aztec patron of cleansing ceremonies was Tlazoltécotl, the goddess of filth, immoral behavior, and carnal love, who was depicted holding handfuls of herbs similar to those used today. The goddess was attracted to pollutants, and if properly invoked, she would devour the contaminating source of the patient's problem. After the conquest, Tlazoltécotl was replaced by the Virgin Mary and the Catholic saints, and to some extent the ritual Aztec herbs such as *cempasúchil, pericón*, and *estafiate* were replaced by those more acceptable to the Spanish friars, such as rosemary and sage.

Usually an egg is rubbed over the patient's body, starting with the head. Then the *curandera* breaks the egg in a glass of water and examines it for evidence of the patient's problem. The egg is both a diagnostic tool and a remedy, pulling the pollutant out of the patient. In some rituals the broken egg is placed under the bed overnight, positioned directly beneath the patient's head, under the *tonalli*.

Elena Avila trained seriously in the art of the *limpia*. Her mentor is an Aztec healer in Mexico City. "I've passed *romero, ruda,* and an egg over a person's body thousands of times. I have some sort of knowledge of that. It comes from experience. I pick up some things about the energy. I can drop the egg in water and I can look at it, and there are things that I know. So if somebody wants a *limpia*, they'll be sent to Elena."

WHERE TO FIND MEXICAN-AMERICAN HERBS

Because I live in southern California, I can grow most of the herbs at home, using very little garden space. I grow them in four big shallow pots on a shelf in my backyard, drying some of each herb and rotating the crops. I keep *yerba buena* in its own pot because it tends to take over. Other pots contain some combination of rue, chamomile, feverfew, sage, *estafiate, epazote,* and basil. Once a year I plant borage and chamomile, and dry them for future use. All these plants can also be grown indoors on a sunny windowsill.

Bigger plants such as *florifundio (Datura), cancerina (Cuphea), tabachín (Caesalpinia), espinosilla (Loeselia), muicle (Justicia), romero (Rosmarinus), alhucema (Lavendula), cenizo (Leucophyllum),* and the various bush sages are sold as ornamental plants in southwestern nurseries. If your local nursery doesn't carry these plants, they may be willing to order them for you.

Many of the herbs on our list are not carried by the average health food store. If you live in the southwestern United States or near an area with a substantial Mexican-American population, you can easily find a *botánica* or market that sells these remedies by looking in the yellow pages under "herbs" or "*botanica.*"

Once you've found a resource for the herbs, how do you know what you're getting? Because there can be many names for each herb, and in some cases many herbs for each name, unless you can find an herb resource that will verify the botanical name, you can't be sure exactly which plant you're buying.

Even if you know what an herb looks like, it can be difficult to identify those dried bits in the cellophane packet.

And there's something else to consider: Many of these herbs are collected in the wild, not grown. That means you're trusting a mysterious chain of collectors, distributors, and importers. There's no guarantee that the plant is reasonably fresh or that it was plucked from a pristine forest nurtured by clean breezes—and not from the side of a highway polluted by exhaust fumes. Sometimes you may not even be getting the right plant.

So it's important to find a reliable, knowledgeable resource. Look for packaged herbs that have retained their color and shape. Make sure that what's in the package corresponds to the correct plant part. If you're buying chamomile, expect to find flowers in the package. *Cáscara sagrada* should be bits of clean bark. *Yerba de la víbora* should be small green leaves. Look for established labels. I feel comfortable buying herbs from some of the better known Mexican herb companies. Tadin and Therbal are two reputable labels carried by shops in the United States.

A safe and easy solution is to order the plants by mail from a knowledgeable supplier. The following directory includes just a few of the many responsible herbalists:

Carol Mason
Wise Woman Herbals
161 Bridge Street
Las Vegas, New Mexico 87701
800-994-1664

A student of author and herbalist Rosemary Gladstar, Carol Mason has also gotten to know the indigenous medicines used by her Native American and Mexican-American neighbors. She personally wildcrafts or grows most of the herbs she sells through her mail order catalog.

Deborah Brandt, R.N.
From the Ground Up
2137 N. Main Street
Las Cruces, New Mexico 88001
505-523-7510

Deborah Brandt studied with Michael Moore, who literally wrote the book on southwestern medicinal herbs. She sells more than one hundred species of herbs, which she wildcrafts in New Mexico or imports from reliable sources, including most of the Mexican-American favorites such as *yerba mansa, oshá, gobernadora, epazote, florifundio, damiana,* and *pingüica.* Phone orders are accepted. No minimum purchase required

Daniel Gagnon
Herbs Etc.
1340 Rufina Circle
Sante Fe, New Mexico 87501
800-634-3727
505-471-6488

Formerly owned by the herbalist Michael Moore, this store carries a wide selection of reliably crafted southwestern herbs. Mail order catalog available.

Dorothy Marietta
The Natural Life Center
305 Mistletoe Avenue
Bosque Farms, New Mexico 87068
505-869-3285

Dorothy Marietta has studied with local *curanderas,* Native Americans, and herbalists. She wildcrafts, grows her own, and trades with other herb growers around the country. She carries a good selection of Mexican-American herbs that are available by phone order.

Alven and Robert Cervilla
Yerbas de México
3903 Whittier Boulevard
Los Angeles, California 90023
323-261-2521

These suppliers carry the largest selection of Mexican and Mexican-American herbs we've found. Their catalog lists the herbs by their many common Spanish and English names. They claim to use organically grown herbs whenever possible. Twenty-five-dollar minimum purchase.

Herb Products Company
11012 Magnolia Boulevard
North Hollywood, California 91601
818-761-0351
Fax: 818-508-6567
888-339-HERB (credit card orders only)
www.herbproducts.com

This catalog of nearly three hundred herbs includes many Mexican-American favorites such as *boldo, gobernadora, chía* seed, *barba de maíz, damiana, jamaica, malva, hojasen, passiflora, tila, yerba mansa,* and *zapote blanco.* Minimum order four ounces.

Mountain Rose Herbs
20818 High Street
North San Juan, California 95960
800-879-3337
Fax: 530-292-9138

These suppliers work with wildcrafters and organic farmers. Their catalog of products includes several of the Mexican-American herbs, including *damiana, saúco, linaza, cola de caballo, tila, oshá, passiflora, poleo, lantén, ortiga,* and *inmortal.* Other herbs can be special-ordered but require a one-pound minimum.

Star West Botanicals
11253 Trade Center Drive
Rancho Cordova, California 95742
800-800-HERB
Fax: 916-853-9673

This glossy catalog lists all kinds of herb products including several of the Mexican-American standards: *estafiate, yerba santa, plumajillo, capulín, sáuz, pengüica, berro, encino, cola de caballo, hojasen, cuasia, azafrán, fitolaca, lantén, passiflora, orégano, tila, damiana, barba de maíz, saúco, gobernadora,* and powdered aloe, *papaya,* and artichoke leaf. The herbs are listed by common name. The company guarantees the purity of its products through laboratory testing. Minimum purchase is $50.

The following *bótanica* owners were among those consulted for this book. Visit them when you are in the area.

TEXAS

John Cazares
La Botánica Green & White
1201 E. Seventh Street
Austin, Texas 78702-3222
512-472-0675

Lee and Mary Lou Cantu
Cantu's Mexican Imports
1500 South First Street
Austin, Texas 78704-3043
512-448-2677
Fax: 512-448-3432

Evelia and Sabas Guajardo
Casa Guajardo
5223 South Flores
San Antonio, Texas 78214
210-922-8949

Papa Jim
5630 South Flores
San Antonio, Texas 78214
210-922-6665

NEW MEXICO

Bonnie Ochoa
El Viajio Herb Shop
4885 S. Highway 28
Las Cruces, New Mexico 88005
505-526-8946
Or visit her at the Las Cruces Downtown mall on Wednesdays and
Saturdays from 9 A.M. to 12 noon

CALIFORNIA

Victoria Vazquez
Botánica Vazquez
4518¾ S. Rosemead Boulevard
Pico Rivera, California 90660
562-692-9509

Aguilar, Contreras, Alfaro Martínez, and Miguel Angel. "Los Herbarios Medicinales de México." In *La Investigación Científica de la Herbolaria Medicinal Mexicana.* Mexico City: Secretaría de Salud, 1993.

Anonymous. *A Medieval Herbal.* San Francisco: Chronicle Books, 1994.

Antol, Marie Nadine. *Healing Teas: How to Prepare and Use Teas to Maximize Your Health.* Garden City Park, NY: Avery Publishing Group, 1996.

Argueta, Arturo, and Leticia Cano. "El Atlas de las Plantas de la Medicina Tradicional Mexicana." In *La Investigación Científica de la Herbolaria Medicinal Mexicana.* Mexico City: Secretaría de Salud, 1993.

Arvigo, Rosita, and Michael Balick. *Rainforest Remedies, One Hundred Healing Herbs of Belize.* Twin Lakes, WI: Lotus Press, 1993.

Ascencio, Domingo. *Tés Curativos Mexicanos.* Mexico City: Selector, S.A. de C.V., 1994.

Aviles, Margarita, and Guillermo Suárez. *Catálogo de Plantas Medicinales Jardín Etnobotánico.* Morelos: Centro Instituto Nacional de Antropología e Historia, Proyecto Etnobotánico, 1994.

Baytleman, Bernardo. *Acerca de Plantas y de Curanderos.* Mexico City: Instituto Nacional de Antropología e Historia, 1993.

Blumenthal, Mark, et al., eds. *The Complete German Commission E Monographs; Therapeutic Guide to Herbal Medicines.* Austin, TX: American Botanical Council, 1998.

Cabrera, Dr. Luis G. *Plantas Curativas de México.* Mexico City: Ediciones Ciceron, 1943.

Campos-Navarro, Roberto. *Nosotros los Curanderos.* Mexico City: Editorial Patria, 1977.

Carvajal, P. A. *Plantas que Curan, Plantas que Matan.* Mexico City: Editorial Pax México, 1988.

Chiej, Roberto. *Guia de Plantas Medicinales.* Barcelona: Grijalbo Mondadori, 1983.

Clark, Margaret. *Health in the Mexican-American Culture.* Berkeley: University of California Press, 1959.

Cline, S. L. "Revisionist Conquest History: Sahagún's Revised Book II." In J. Jorge Kor de Alva et al., eds., *The Work of Bernardino de Sahagún,* Albany: Institute for Mesoamerican Studies, University of Albany, State University of New York, 1988.

Crosswhite, Frank S. and Carol D. "Spanish-Named Medicinal Plants Used in Arizona." Boyce Thompson Arboretum, Superior, Arizona, 1997.

Curtin, L. S. M. *Healing Herbs of the Upper Rio Grande,* revised and edited by Michael Moore. Sante Fe, NM: Western Edge Press, 1997.

Davies, Nigel. *The Aztecs.* Norman: University of Oklahoma Press, 1973.

De la Peña Páez, Ignacio. "El Estudio Formal de la Herbolaria Mexicana y la Creación del Instituto Médico Nacional: 1888–1915." In *La Investigación Científica de la Herbolaria Medicinal Mexicana.* Mexico City: Secretaría de Salud, 1993.

Díaz del Castillo, Bernal. *Historia Verdadera de la Conquista de la Nueva España.* Mexico City: Editorial Porrúa, 1968 (orig. 1568).

Dodson, Ruth. *The Faith Healer of Los Olmos: A Biography of Don Pedrito Jaramillo.* Falfurrias, TX: Brooks County Historical Survey Committee 1972.

Duke, James A., Ph.D. *CRC Handbook of Medicinal Herbs.* Boca Raton, FL: CRC Press, 1985.

Emmart, Emily Wolcott. *The Badianus Manuscript.* Baltimore: Johns Hopkins University Press, 1940 (orig. 1552).

Engstrand, Iris H. W. *Spanish Scientists in the New World.* Seattle: University of Washington Press, 1981.

Espinosa, Lydia Veronica. *Pregnancy and Childbirth in Chicano Culture: Changing Customs and Beliefs.* N.p.: 1976.

Esteyneffer, Juan de. *Florilegio Medicinal de Todas las Enfermedades,* ed. by Carmen Anzures y Bolaños. Mexico City: Academia Nacional de Medicina, 1978 (orig. 1719).

Estudillo, Rigoberto López, and Alicia Hinojosa García. *Catálogo de Plantas Medicinales Sonorenses.* Hermosilla, Mexico: Universidad de Sonora, 1988.

Ford, Karen Cowan. *Las Yerbas de la Gente: A Study of Hispano-American Medicinal Plants.* Ann Arbor: University of Michigan Press, 1975.

Foster, George M. *Hippocrates' Latin American Legacy.* Amsterdam, Holland: Gordon and Breach Science Publishers, 1994.

Gali, Dr. Hero. *Las Hierbas del Indio.* Mexico City: Impresora Lorenzana, 1996.

Gardner, Dore, and Kay F. Turner. *Niño Fidencio, a Heart Thrown Open.* Albuquerque: Museum of New Mexico Press, 1992.

Gates, William. *The De la Cruz Badiano: Aztec Herbal of 1552.* Baltimore: Maya Society, 1939 (orig. 1552).

Grieve, M. *A Modern Herbal,* 2 vols. New York: Dover Publications, 1971 (orig. 1931).

Gryj, Arturo Warren, et al. *Flora Medicinal Indígena de México.* Mexico City: Instituto Nacional Indigenista, 1994.

Health Services and Mental Health Administration, Community Health Service, U.S. Department of Health, Education and Welfare. "Handbook for Public Health Nurses Working with Spanish-Americans." Sante Fe, NM: 1964, 1970.

Hernández, Francisco. *Historia de las Plantas de Nueva España.* Mexico City: Universidad Nacional Autónoma de México, 1959 (orig. 1577).

Holden, William Curry. *Teresita.* Owings Mills, MD: Stemmer House, 1978.

Kay, Margarita Artschwager. *Healing with Plants in the American and Mexican West.* Tucson: University of Arizona Press, 1996.

———. "Health and Illness in a Mexican Barrio." In E. H. Spicer, ed., *Ethnic Medicine in the Southwest.* Tucson: University of Arizona Press, 1977.

Las Casas, Fr. Bartolomé de. *Los Indios de México y Nueva España.* Mexico City: Editorial Porrúa, S.A., 1987 (orig. 1564).

LaTorre, Dolores L. *Cooking and Curing with Mexican Herbs.* Austin, TX: Encino Press, 1977.

Legorreta, Xavier Lozoya. *Plantas, Medicina y Poder: Breve Historia de la Herbolaria Mexicana.* Mexico City: Procuraduría Federal del Consumidor, Editorial Pax México, 1994.

———. *Los Señores de las Plantas.* Mexico City: Consejo Nacional para la Cultura y las Artes, Panagea Editores, 1990.

Léon-Portilla, Miguel. *Aztec Thought and Culture.* Jack Emory Davis, trans. Norman: University of Oklahoma Press, 1963.

Linares, Edelmira. *Selección de Plantas Medicinales de México.* Mexico City: Editorial Limusa, 1988.

López-Austin, Alfredo. *Tamoanchan y Tlalocan.* Mexico City: Fondo de Cultura Económico, 1994.

————. *Textos de Medicina Náhuatl.* Mexico City: Universidad Autónoma de México, 1975.

López Piñero, José M., et al. *Medicinas, Drogas y Alimentos Vegetales del Nuevo Mundo.* Mexico City: Ministerio de Sanidad y Consumo, 1992.

Lust, John. *The Herb Book.* New York: Bantam, 1974.

Madson, William. *Mexican-Americans of South Texas.* New York: Holt, Rinehart and Winston, 1964.

————. *The Virgin's Children.* Austin: University of Texas Press, 1960.

Martínez, Jose. *Yerbario Medicinal Mexicano.* Mexico City: Editores Mexicanos Unidas, S.A., 1986, 1994

Martínez, Maximino. *Catálogo de Nombres Vulgares y Científicos de Plantas Mexicanas.* Mexico City: Fondo de Cultura Económica, 1979.

————. *Plantas Utiles de México.* Mexico City: Ediciones Botas, 1936.

Martínez, Ricardo Arguijo. *Hispanic Culture and Health Care.* St. Louis, MO: C. V. Mosby Company, 1978.

Mason, Charles T., and Patricia B. *A Handbook of Mexican Roadside Flora.* Tucson: The University of Arizona Press, 1987.

McGuffin, Michael, et al., eds. *American Herbal Products Association's Botanical Safety Handbook.* Boca Raton: CRC Press, 1997.

Mendieta, Fray Gerónimo de. *Historia Eclesiástica Indiana.* Mexico City: Cien de México, Dirección General de Publicaciones, Consejo Nacional para la Cultura y las Artes, 1997.

Monardes, Nicolás. *Joyfull Newes Out of the Newe Founde Worlde, Englished by John Frampton.* New York: Alfred A. Knopf, 1925 (orig. 1596).

Moore, Michael. *Medicinal Plants of the Pacific West.* Sante Fe, NM: Red Crane Books, 1993.

————. *Los Remedios, Traditional Herbal Remedies of the Southwest.* Sante Fe, NM: Red Crane Books, 1990.

————. *Medicinal Plants of the Desert and Canyon West.* Sante Fe: Museum of New Mexico Press, 1989.

————. *Medicinal Plants of the Mountain West.* Sante Fe: Museum of New Mexico Press, 1979.

Nuttall, Zelia. "The Gardens of Ancient Mexico." In *Annual Report of the Smithsonian Institution,* 1923.

Ortiz de Montellano, Bernard R. *Aztec Medicine, Health, and Nutrition.* New Brunswick, NJ: Rutgers University Press, 1990.

Pesman, M. Walter. *Meet Flora Mexicana.* Flagstaff, AZ: Northland Press, 1962.

Prescott, William Hickling. *A History of the Conquest of Mexico.* New York: Heritage Press, 1949 (orig. 1843).

Rätch, Dr. Christian. *The Dictionary of Sacred and Magical Plants.* London: Prism Press, 1992.

Rivas, Heriberto García. *Plantas Curativas Mexicanas.* Mexico City: Panorama Editorial, 1991.

Rodríguez, Richard, and Gloria Rodríguez. "Teresa Urrea: Her Life as It Affected the Mexican–U.S. Frontier." *El grito del sol,* no. 4 (1972).

Roeder, Beatrice A. *Chicano Folk Medicine from Los Angeles, California.* Los Angeles: University of California Publications, Folklore and Mythology Studies, 1989.

Roman, Octavo. "Don Perditio Jaramillo: The Emergence of a Mexican-American Folk-Saint." Ph.D. dissertation, University of California at Berkeley. Ann Arbor, MI: University Microfilms, 1964.

Ruiz de Alarcón, Hernando. *Treatise on the Heathen Superstitions That Today Live Among the Indians Native to This New Spain 1629.* Trans. and ed. by J. Richard Andrews and Ross Hassig. Norman: University of Oklahoma Press, 1984 (orig. 1629).

Sahagún, Fray Bernardino de. *Florentine Codex: General History of the Things of New Spain, Book II—Earthly Things.* Trans. from the Aztec into English by Charles E. Dribble and Arthur J. O. Anderson. Sante Fe, NM: The School of American Research and the Museum of New Mexico, 1963 (orig. 1793).

Sanfilippo B., José. "La Aculturación de las Plantas Medicinales Mexicanas a la Medicina Europea." In *La Investigación Científica de la Herbolaria Medicinal Mexicana.* Mexico City: Secretaría de Salud, 1993.

Schendel, Gordon. *Medicine in Mexico from Aztec Herbs to Betatrons.* Austin: University of Texas Press, 1968.

Siméon, Rémi. *Diccionario de la Lengua Náhuatl o Mexicana.* Trans. from French into Spanish by Josefina Oliva de Coll. Mexico City: Siglo Veintuno Editores, 1977 (orig. 1885).

Soustelle, Jacques. *Daily Life of the Aztecs on the Eve of the Spanish Conquest.* Trans. by Patrick O'Brien. Stanford, CA: Stanford University Press, 1961.

Standley, Paul C. *Trees and Shrubs of Mexico.* Washington, D.C.: Smithsonian Press, 1920–1926.

Steck, Francis Borgia, O.F.M., Ph.d., trans. *Motolinia's History of the Indians of New Spain.* Washington, D.C.: Academy of American Franciscan History, 1951.

Tenney, Louise. *Cáscara Sagrada.* Pleasant Grove, UT: Woodland Publishing, 1996.

Toor, Frances. *A Treasury of Mexican Folkways.* New York: Bonanza Books, 1985 (1947).

Torres, Eliseo. *The Folk Healer: The Mexican-American Tradition of Curanderismo.* Kingsville, TX: Nieves Press, 1984.

Trotter, Robert T. II, and Juan Antonio Chavira. *Curanderismo: Mexican-American Folk Healing.* Atlanta: University of Georgia Press, 1981, 1997.

Turner, R. J., and Ernie Wasson. *Botanica.* Milsons Point: Random House Australia, 1997.

Velasco, Guillermo Espinosa, et al. *Flora Medicinal Indígena de México II.* Mexico City: Instituto Nacional Indigenista, 1994.

Viesca Treviño, Carlos. "La Herbolaria Medicinal en México Prehispanico." In *La Investigación Científica de la Herbolaria Medicinal Mexicana.* Mexico City: Secretaría de Salud, 1993.

Villacis, Dr. Luis R. *Plantas Medicinales de México.* Mexico City: Editorial Epoca, S.A., 1978.

West, Tommy. "The Power of Don Pedrito." *San Antonio Express-News Magazine,* September 26, 1993.

Zoller, Carlos, et al. *Diccionario Enciclopédico de la Medicina Traditional Mexicana.* Mexico City: Instituto Nacional Indigenista, 1995.

In addition, the following Web sites are among those consulted:

Agricultural Research Service
Dr. Duke's Phytochemical and Ethnobotanical Databases:
http://www.ars-grin.gov/duke/

The American Botanical Council:
http://www.herbalgram.org

The Autonomous University of Nayarit:
http://www.uan.mx

CLNet Library, Latino Research Collections:
http://clnet.ucr.edu/library/rescoll.html

The Ethnobotany Café on the Web:
http://countrylife.net/ethnobotany

The Herb Research Foundation:
http://www.herbs.org

The Mexican Biodiversity Commission:
http://www.conabio.gob.mx

Mexico Desconocido Virtual:
http://www.mexicodesconocido.com.mx/hierbas

The National Library of Medicine, Medline via Paperchase:
http://www.paperchase.com

The Southwest School of Herbal Medicine:
http://www.chili.rt66.com/hrbmoore

The University of Guadalajara:
http://www.udg.mx:81

The University of Michoacán Museum of Natural History:
http://www.ccu.umich/museo/hist-natural

Please visit our Web site:

www.infusionsofhealing.com

English Name	Spanish Name	Botanical Name	Other Names
Alfalfa	Alfalfa	Medicago sativa	Purple Medic, Lucerne
Aloe Vera	Sábila	Aloe barbadensis, Aloe vulgaris, Aloe mexicana	Zábila
Amaranth	Alegría	Amaranthus spp.	Chile Puerco, Pig Weed, Cockscomb, Chichilquiltic
American Wormseed	Epazote	Chenopodium ambrosioides syn. Teloxys ambrosioides	Epasote, Ipazote, Pazote, Quinoa, Mexican Tea, Goosefoot
Angelica	Angélica	Angelica archangelica, Angelica atropurpurea	Raíz de Angélica
Angel's Trumpet	Florifundio	Datura stramonium, Datura arborea, Dantura spp.	Floripondio, Toloache, Trombita, Estramonio, Campana, Campanilla, Jimson Weed, Thorn Apple
Anise	Anís	Pimpinella anisum	
Annatto	Achiote	Bixa orellana	Lipstick Tree
Apple Mint	Mastranso	Menta rotundifolia	
Arizona Poppy	Contrayerba	Kallstroemia californica, Kallstroemia grandiflora; also Dorstena contrayerva	Varbulilla, Caltrop, California Poppy, Summer Poppy
Arnica	Arnica	Arnica montana	
Artichoke	Alcachofa	Cynara scolymus	
Avocado	Aguacate	Persea americana, Persea gratissima	Ahuacate
Aztec Marigold	Cempasúchil	Tagetes erecta	Flor de Muerto, African Marigold, American Marigold
Basin Sagebrush	Chamiso Hediondo	Artemisia tridentata	Chamizo, Big Sagebrush
Bay Leaf	Laurel	Laurus nobilis, Litsea glauscens	
Bearberry	Cáscara Sagrada	Rhammus purshiana, Rhammus californica	Buckthorn
Birch	Abedul	Betula alba, Alnus acuminata, Betula pubescens	Alamo Blanco, White Birch
Black Nightshade	Yerba Mora	Solamum nigrescens, Solamum nigrum	Malabar, Solano Negro, Buena Mujer, Mariola, Chichiquelite, Garden Nightshade, Pretty Morel

English Name	Spanish Name	Botanical Name	Other Names
Bold	Boldo	Peumus boldus	
Borage	Borraja	Borago officinalis	
Bougainvillea	Bugambilia	Bougainvillea glabra, Bougainvillea spectabilis	Camelina
Bouvardia	Trompetilla	Bouvardia ternifolia syn. Bouvardia triphylla	Cantaris, Cerillito, Contrayerba, Yerba del Indio, Yerba del Pasmo, Mirto
Brazilwood	Brasil	Haematoxylum brasiletum	Logwood, Palo de Brasil, Palo Rojo, Palo de Tinto, Brasilillo, Marismeño
Bricklebrush	Prodigiosa	Brickellia cavanillesii, Brickellia grandiflora, Brickellia californica	Rodigiosa, Hamula, Amula, Mala Mujer, Atanasia
Brittle Bush	Incienso	Encelia farinosa	Rama Blanca, Verba del Vaso, Palo Blanco
Brook Mint	Poleo	Mentha arvensis, Mentha pulegium	Poleo Casero
Buffalo Gourd	Calabacita	Cucurbita foetidissima	Calabazilla Loco, Calabacilla Armarga, Chilicoyote
Burr Marigold	Aceitilla	Bidens pilosa, Bidens spp.	Té de Coral, Té de Milpa, Beggar's Ticks, Tickseed, Spanish Needles
Burrobush	Yerba del Burro	Hymenoclea sp.; also Spigelia longiflora	Romerillo, Sangre de Toro
Butterfly Bush	Salvia Real	Buddleia americana, Buddleia wrightii, Buddleia cordata, Buddleia perfoliata, Buddleia spp.	Salverial, Cantue, Cantuesa, Lengua de Buey, Salvia de Bolita, Tepozan
Button Snakeroot	Yerba del Sapo	Eryrrgium sp.	Sea Holly
Camphor Tree	Alcanfor	Cinnamomum camphora	
Camphor Weed	Arnica mexicana	Heterotheca inuloides, Heterotheca spp.	Falsa árnica, Arnica del país, Telegraph Weed
Candlewood	Ocotillo	Fouquieria splendens	Mariola
Canyon Ragweed	Chícura	Ambrosia ambrosioides syn. Franseria ambrosioides	Yerba del sapo
Castor Bean Plant	Higuerilla	Ricimus communis	Ricino
Cat Claw	Uña del Gato	Acacia gregii	Catclaw, Acacia
Celery	Apio	Apium graveolens var. dulce	
Century Plant	Maguey	Agave salmiana, Agave americana, Agave lechuguilla, Agave spp.	Lechuguilla, Mescál
Chaparral	Gobernadora	Larrea tridentata	Hediondilla, Goma de Sonora, Creosote Bush

English Name	Spanish Name	Botanical Name	Other Names
Chaste Tree	Aceitunillo	Vitex mollis, Vitex agnus-castus	Uvalama, Ahuilote
Cinnamon	Canela	Cinnamomum zeylanicum	
Clematis	Barba de Chivo	Clematis virginiana, Clematis lasiantha, Clematis spp.	Virgin's Bower, Old Man's Beard
Clove	Clavo	Syzgium aromatic syn. Eugenia aromatica	
Cockspur	Espino Blanco	Acacia cornigera	Cornezuelo, Carnizuelo, Velo de Novia, Velo de Viuda
Common Basil	Albahaca	Ocimum basilicum, Ocium spp.	Albahacar, Albácar
Common Comfrey	Sueldo	Symphytum officinale	Consueldo, Knitbone
Common Fig	Higueroa	Ficus carica	Amate
Common Juniper	Enebro	Juniperus communis, Juniperus spp.	Bellota de Sabina, Sabino, Guata, Drooping Juniper, Mexican Juniper
Common Lantana	Cinco Negritos	Lantana camara	Siete Negritos, Yerba de Cristo, Confiturilla, Alfombrilla, Shrub Verbena
Common Plantain	Lantén	Plantago major	Llantén, Planten, Pastorcito, Broad-leafed Plantain
Common Sage	Salvia	Salvia offinalis, Salvia lavanduloides	Alhucema de la Costa, Té de Mar, Yerba de Santa María
Copalchí	Copalchí	Coutarea latiflora; also Croton niveus, Croton tiglium, Croton reflexifolius	Colapchín, Quina Blanca, Falsa Quina, Garañona
Coriander	Cilantro	Coriandrum sativum	
Corn silk	Barba de Maíz	Zea mays	Barba de Elote, Cabelo de Elote, Estilos de Maíz
Cottonwood	Alamo	Populus angustifolia, Populus alba, Populus wislizeni, Populus spp.	Poplar
Crownbeard	Añil del Muerto	Verbesina enelioides, Verbesina crocata	Capitaneia, Goldweed
Crucifixion Thorn	Chaparro Amargoso	Castela emoryi, Castela texana, Holocantha emoryi	Chaparro Amargo, Corona de Cristo
Cudweed	Gordolobo	Gnaphalium spp.	Manzanilla del Rio, Everlasting
Curly Parsley	Perejil	Petroselinum crispum syn. Carum petroselinum	
Custard Apple	Chirimoya	Annona cherimola	Chirimolla, Cheremoya
Damiana	Damiana	Turnera diffusa var. aphrodisiaca, Turnera ulmifolia	Mexican Damiana, Agüita de Damiana, Yerba del Pastor, Pastorcita

English Name	Spanish Name	Botanical Name	Other Names
Dandelion	Diente de León	Taraxacum officinale	Chicória, Chinita, Wild Endive
Deerweed	Yerba del Venado	Porophyllum spp.	Odora, Maravilla
Desert Broom	Yerba del Pasmo	Baccharis multiflora, Baccharis spp.; also Haplopappus sonorensis	Escoba Ancha, Romerillo, Yerba del Carbonero, Escobilla, Tepopote, Raíz del Indio
Desert Hollyhock	Yerba del Negro	Sphaeralcea angustifolia, Sphaeralcea spp.	Yerba de la Negrita, Mal de Ojo, Negrito, Plantas Muy Malas, Globemallow
Desert Willow	Mimbre	Chilopsis linearis	Jano, Flor de Mimbres
Dill	Eneldo	Anethum graveolens	
Drake's Foot	Contrayerba Blanco	Psoralea pentaphylla, Psoralea glandulosa, Psoralea tenufolia	Prairie Potato
Elder Flower	Saúco	Sambucus mexicana, Sambucus nigra, Sambucus racemosa	Flor Sáuco, Azumiate, Guarico, Nigrito, Tápiro
Elephant Tree	Copal	Bursera jorullensis, Bursera microphyllia, Bursera spp.	Palo Mulato, Torote, Cuajiote
English Marigold	Caléndula	Calendula officinalis	Mercadela, Coronilla, Virreyna, Caléndula, Pot Marigold
Eucalyptus	Eucalipto	Eucalyptus globulus	Dolár, Gum Tree
Evening Primrose	Yerba del Golpe	Oenothera kunthiana, Oenothera pallida, Oenothera rosea	Flor de San Juan, Rose of Mexico
Evergreen Ash	Fresno	Fraxinus udhei, Fraxinus cuspidata, Fraxinus berlandieriana	
Fennel	Hinojo	Foeniculum vulgare, Foeniculum officinale	Hinojo de Castillo, Cilantrillo
Feverfew	Altamisa mexicana	Tanacetum parthenium syn. Chrysanthemum parthenium	Santa Maria, Yerba de Santa María, Featherfoil
Field Poppy	Amapola	Papaver rhoeas	Adormideros, Corn Poppy, Flanders Poppy
Fillery	Alferillo	Erodium cicutarium	Alfilaria, Storksbill, Heronsbill
Flat-top Buckwheat	Colita de Rata	Eriogonum fasciculatum	
Flax	Linaza	Limum usitatissimum	Linasa, Lino, Linseed
Four-O'Clock	Maravilla	Mirabilis multiflora, Mirabilis jalapa, Mirabilis longiflora	Amarilla, Chuyem
Four-Wing Saltbrush	Chamiso	Atriplex canescens	Chamizo, Costilla de Vaca, Cenizo
French Rose, Red Rose, etc.	Rosa de Castilla	Rosa gallica, Rosa chinensis, Rosa spp.	
Garden Heliotrope	Valeriana	Valeriana ceratophylla, Valeriana officinalis, Valeriana mexicana	Yerba del Gato
Garden Nasturtium	Mastuerzo	Tropaeolum majus	Indian Cress, Mexixi
Garden thyme	Tomillo	Thymus vulgaris	

English Name	Spanish Name	Botanical Name	Other Names
Garlic	Ajo	Allium sativum	
Gayfeather	Cachana	Liatris punctata	Blazing Star
Geranium	Geranio	Pelargonium spp.	
German Chamomile	Manzanilla	Matricaria chamomila syn. Matricaria recutita; also Anthemis nobilis	Camamilla, Roman Chamomile
Giant Hyssop	Toronjil	Agastache mexicamum syn. Cedronella mexicana; also Melissa spp.	Toronjil Morado, Toronjil Rojo, Toronjil Blanco, Té de Menta
Ginger	Jengibre	Zingiber officinale	Ajenjibre, Jenjibre
Gourd Tree	Cirián	Crescentia alata	Cuatecomate, Tecomate, Aval, Calabash
Green Gentian	Cebadilla	Swertia radiata	Indiana Caustic Barley, Deer's Horn
Greenbrier root	Cocolmeca	Phaseolus spp.	Gotoko, Cocolmecate, Kidney Bean Vine
Guava	Guayaba	Psidium spp.	Guayabilla
Gum Arabic	Acacia	Acacia senegal	
Gum Weed	Yerba del Buey	Grindelia phanactis	Pegapega, Tripa de Judas
Handflower Tree	Flor de Manita	Chiranthodendron pentadactylon	Arbol de las Manitas, Mano de Dragón
Hibiscus	Jamaica	Hibiscus sabdariffa	Flor de Jamaica, Tulipán
Hoja Santa	Hoja Santa	Piper auritum, Piper sanctum	Acoyo, Momo, Cordoncillo, Yerba Santa
Hop Tree	Cola de Zorrillo	Ptelea trifollata	Swamp Dogwood, Wafer Ash
Horsetail	Cola de Caballo	Equisetum arvense, Equisetum hyemale, Equisetum spp.	Cañutillo del Llano, Carricillo, Shave Grass, Scouring Rush
Horseweed	Simonillo	Conyza confussa, Conyza filaginoides, Conyza canadensis	Pazotillo, Texiote Canadian, Fleabane
Hummingbird Flower	Espinosilla	Loeselia mexicana	Chuparrosa, Huachichilel, Huizache
Indian Paintbrush	Santa Rita	Castilleja arvensis, Castilleja spp.	Flor de Santa Rita, Garañona, Enchiladas, Yerba del Cancér, Cola de Borrego
Indian Plantain	Matarique	Psacalium decompositum, Cacalia decomposita, Odontotrichum decompositum	Buffalo Root
Indian Root	Yerba del Indio	Aristolochia mexicana, Aristolochia watsonii, Aristolochia wrightii	Raíz del India, Inmortal, Comino, Guaco, Yerba del Pasmo, Birthroot, Snakeroot, Dutchman's Pipe
Jerusalem thorn	Palo Verde	Parkinsonia aculeata	Retama, Horsebean

English Name	Spanish Name	Botanical Name	Other Names
Jojoba	Jojoba	*Simmondsia chinensis, Simmondsia californica*	Cohobe, Goat Nut, Deer Nut, Quinine Plant
Juliana	Cuachalalate	*Juliana adstringens, Amphyterigum adstringens*	Cuachalate, Cuachalalote
Kidneywood	Palo Azul	*Eysenhardtia polystachya*; also *Caesalpinia bonducella*	Palo Dulce, Palo Cuate, Cualaldulce, Varadulce, Taray
Lavender	Alhucema	*Lavandula spica, Lavandula angustifolia, Lavandula spp.*	
Lemon tree	Limón	*Citrus aurantifolia, Citrus limonium*	
Lemongrass	Té Limón	*Cymbopogon citratus* syn. *Andropogon citratus*	Zacate Limón, Ocozacatl
Lemon-Scented Verbena	Cedrón	*Aloysia triphylla* (formerly *Lippia citriodora*)	Yerba Luisa
Licorice	Orozús	*Glycyrrhiza glabra*	Regaliz, Yerba Dulce, Palo Cuate, Coahtli
Limberbush	Sangre de Drago	*Jatropha dioica, Jatropha macrorhiza, Jatropha spp.*	Sangregado, Palo Sangriento, Sangre de Cristo, Telondilla
Linden	Tila	*Tilia mexicana, Tilia americana, Tilia vulgaris, Tilia spp.*	Flor de Tila, Tilia
Little Trumpet	Anacahuite	*Cordia boissieri*	Trompillo, Camichín, Zalate
Maidenhair Fern	Culantrillo	*Adiantum pedatum, Adiantum spp.*	
Malabar	Malabar	*Solanum verbascifolium*	Berenjena, Berenhenilla, Galantea, Yerba Mora
Mallow	Malva	*Malva rotundifolia, Malva sylvestris, Malva neglecta*	Malva del Campo, Yerba del Negro
Mariola	Mariola	*Parthenium incanum, Parthenium stramonium*; also *Solanum hinsianum*	Ocotillo, Yerba Mora
Mesquite	Mezquite	*Prosopis juliflora, Prosopis glandulosa, Prosopis pubescens*	
Mexican Bird of Paradise	Tabachín	*Caesalpinia pulcherrima* syn. *Poinciana pulcherrima*	Palo Colorado, Brazíl, Noche Buena, Camerón, Barbona, Cabellitos de Angel, Guacamaya, Dwarf Poinciana, Peacock Flower, Barbados Flower
Mexican Dayflower	Yerba del Pollo	*Commelina coelestis, Commelina pallida, Commelina spp.*	Sinvergüenza
Mexican Ground Cherry	Tomate	*Physalis subulata, Physalis angulata, Physalis philadelphia*	Husk Tomato, Tomatillo
Mexican Hawthorn	Tejocote	*Crataegus pubescens, Crataegus mexicanus*	Chisté, Manzanilla, Manzanita

English Name	Spanish Name	Botanical Name	Other Names
Mexican Heather	Cancerina	Cuphea aequipetala, Cuphea jorullensis, Cuphea spp.; also Hemiagium excelsum	Yerba del Cáncer, Alcancér, Calavera, Chanclana, Yerba del Coyote
Mexican Honeysuckle	Muicle	Justicia spicigera syn. Jacobinia spicigera	Muitle, Chuparrosa, Trompetilla, Mayotl, Mozote, Yerba de Añil
Mexican Mock Orange	Jazmín	Philadelphus mexicanus	Mosqueta
Mexican Morning Glory	Jalapa	Ipomoea purga	Raíz de Jalapa, Brionía, Michoacán, Jalap root
Mexican Oregano	Orégano	Lippia berlandieri, Lippia origanoides, Lippia dulcis; also Origanum vulgare	Yerba Dulce, Wild Marjoram, Salvia Real
Mexican Papaya	Papaya	Carica papaya	Melón Zapote, Papaya Real, Papaw, Melon Tree
Mexican Tarragon	Pericón	Tagetes bucida, Tagetes filifolia, Tagetes micrantha	Anís, Yerba de Anís, Anisella, Santa Maria, Periquillo, Curucumín, Flor de Veinte, Yerba del Venado, Cinco Llagas, Mexican Marigold, African Marigold, Sweet Mace
Mexican Thistle	Cardo Santo	Cirsium undulatum, Cirsium mexicanum	Sueldo, Chicalote
Milkweed	Inmortal	Asclepias asperula, Asclepias spp.	Yerba del Indio, Candelilla, Lichens, Candlelit, Yamato, Raíz de Pleurisy, Antelope Horns, Pleurisy Root
Monarda	Orégano del Campo	Monarda menthafolia, Monarda pectinata	Orégano de la Sierra, Monarda
Montezuma Cypress	Ahuehuete	Taxodium mucronatum	Sabino
Mormon Tea	Popotillo	Ephedra torreyana, Ephedra viridis	Cañutillo del Campo, Cañutillo del Llano, Tepopote, Té Mormona, Itamo Real, Retamo Real, Torrey's Ephedra, Desert Tea
Morning Glory	Tumba Vaqueros	Ipomoea stans	Riñona, Espanta Vaqueros
Mountain Mugwort	Altamisa	Artemisia franserioides	
Mugwort	Estafiate	Artemisia mexicana, Artemisia filifolia, Artemisia ludovicana, Artemisia frigida	Istafiate, Ajenjo del País, Romerillo, Wormwood, Silver Sage, Basin Sagebrush, Sand Sagebrush
Nance	Nance	Byrsonima crassifolia	Nanche, Nananche, Nan-Chi
Navajo Tea	Cota	Thelesperma gracile	Té de Cota, Indian Tea, Hopi Tea
Night-Blooming Jessamine	Huele de Noche	Cestrum nocturnum, Cestrum spp.	Yerba del Perro
Nutmeg	Nuez Moscada	Myistica fragans, Myristica officinalis	
Oak	Encino	Quercus gambelii, Quercus spp.	Encino Blanco, Encino Rojo, Roble

English Name	Spanish Name	Botanical Name	Other Names
Orange blossom	*Azahares*	*Citrus sinensis, Citrus aurantium*	*Azahar de Naranjo*
Orange Tree, Bitter orange	*Naranja, Naranja Agria*	*Citrus aurantium, Citrus vulgaris*	
Palo del Muerto	*Palo del Muerto*	*Ipomoea arborescens, Ipomeoa muricoides*	*Palo Santo, Cazahuate Prieto, Arbol del Muerto, Palo Blanco*
Passion Flower	*Passiflora*	*Passiflora edulis, Passiflora mexicana, Passiflora* spp.	*Passionaria, Granadita, Granadilla*
Peach Tree	*Durazno*	*Prumus persica*	*Hojas de Durazno*
Pennyroyal	*Poleo Chino*	*Hedeoma oblongifolia, Hedeoma pulegioides*	*Dwarf Pennyroyal, American Pennyroyal*
Pepper Tree	*Pirú*	*Schinus molle*	*Perú, Pirul, Arbol del Peru*
Peppermint	*Menta*	*Mentha piperita*	
Peruvian Bark	*Quina Roja*	*Cinchona succirubra, Cinchona officinalis*	*Quina Rojo, Chincona*
Pine	*Ocote*	*Pinus teocote, Pinus edulis, Pinus* spp.	*Trementina de Piñon, Aguarrás*
Plumbago	*Alacrán*	*Plumbago pulchella, Plumbago scandens, Plumbago* spp.	*Yerba del Alacrán, Yerba del Pescado, Cola de Iguana, Pañete, Leadwort, Dentallaria*
Poinsettia	*Nochebuena*	*Euphorbia pulcherrima*	*Flor de Pascua del Monte, Catalina, Tabachín*
Pokeweed	*Fitolaca*	*Phytolacca americana*	*Pokeroot, Pokeberry, Inkberry*
Poleo de Monte	*Poleo de Monte*	*Cunila lythrifolia, Cunila longiflora*	*Poleo de Campo*
Pomegranate	*Granada*	*Punica granatum*	
Porter's Loveage	*Oshá*	*Ligusticum porteri, Levisticum porteri*	*Chuchupate, Indian Parsley, Bear Medicine, Colorado Cough Root*
Prickle Poppy	*Chicalote*	*Argemone mexicana, Argemone* spp.	*Cardo Santo, Thistle Poppy, Mexican Poppy*
Pricklenut	*Guázima*	*Guazuma tomentosa, Guazuma ulmifolia*	*Cuaholote, Guasima, Huasima, West Indian mulberry*
Prickly Pear Cactus	*Nopal*	*Opuntia* spp.	*Tuna, Duraznilla*
Puncture Vine	*Abrojo*	*Tribulus cistoides, Tribulus terrestis*	*Abrojo Rojo, Jamaica Feverplant*
Purple Sage	*Cenizo*	*Leucophylbum laevigatum, Leucophyllum texanum, Leucophyllum frutescens*	*Flor de Ceniza, Palo de Ceniza, Chihuahuan, Rain Sage, Texas Range, Silverleaf*
Quassia	*Cuasia*	*Quassia amara*	
Quince	*Membrillo*	*Cydonia oblonga*	

English Name	Spanish Name	Botanical Name	Other Names
Rancher's Tea	Tabaquillo	Hedeoma piperita	Santo Domingo, Té del Monte, Yerba del Borracho
Red Clover	Trébol Morado	Trifolium pratense, Trifolium repens	
Red Dock	Cañaigre	Rumex hymenosepalus	Cañagria, Yerba Colorada, Pie Plant, Wild Rhubarb, American Ginseng
Red Texas Sage	Mirto	Salvia microphylla	Salvia, Chía, Té de Monte
Resurrection Plant	Doradilla	Selaginella lepidophylla, Selaginella cuspidata	Siempreviva, Flor de Piedra, Flor de Rana
Rhatany	Crameria	Krameria lanceolata, Krameria cystisoides, Krameria parviflora	Cramer Plant, Chacate, Cosahui, Mezquitillo
Rocky Mountain Bee Plant	Guaco	Cleome serrulata, Mikanie guaco	Yerba del Indio
Rosemary	Romero	Rosmarinus officinalis	
Rue	Ruda	Ruta graveolens, Ruta chalepensis	Ruta, Lota, Lula, Luta, Lura
Safflower	Azafrán	Carthamus tinctorius	American Saffron, False Saffron
Sage	Chía	Salva hispanica, Salvia cohumbariae	
Sasparilla Root	Zarsaparilla	Smilax medica, Smilax aristolochiaefolia, Smilax mexicana, Smilax spp.	Red China Root, Cocolmeca, Greenbrier
Savory	Té de Monte	Satureja macrostema, Satureja laevigatum	Té de Borracho, Tochil, Tabaquillo Grande, Yerba Buena
Senna	Hojasen	Senna spp., Cassia fistula, Cassia amara, Cassia covesii, Cassi tomentosa (Retama)	Cañafistula, Sen, Té de Sena, Retama, Shower Tree, Monkey Pod Tree
Snake Broom	Escoba de la Víbora	Gutierrezia sarothae, Gutierrezia spp.	Collálle, Yerba de la Víbora, Yerba de San Nicolás
Snakeweed	Yerba de la Víbora	Zornia diphylla	Víborina, Raíz del Víbora
Spearmint	Yerba Buena	Mentha spicata	
Spurge	Golondrina	Euphorbia prostrata, Euphorbia spp.	Yerba de Golondria, Pegahueso, Picachli
Star Anise	Anís de Estrella	Illicium verum	
Stinging Nettle	Ortiga	Urtica dioica, Urtica urens	
Stonecrop	Siempreviva	Sedum dendroideum, Sedum spp.	Cola de Borrego, Doradilla
Storax	Liquidámbar	Liquidambar styraciflua	Ococote, Ococotzl, Styrax
Sunflower	Girasol	Helianthus annus	Mirasol, Flor de Añil

English Name	Spanish Name	Botanical Name	Other Names
Swamp Root	*Yerba Mansa*	*Anemopsis californica*	*Yerba del Manzo, Bavisa, Raíz del Manzo,* Lizard Tail
Sweet Acacia	*Huizache*	*Acacia farnesiana, Mimosa farnesiana*	*Guisache, Palo Huisache, Binorama,* Cassia Flower, Cashaw
Sweet Marjoram	*Mejorana*	*Mejorana hortensis*	*Maté, Yerba Maté*
Tamarind	*Tamarindo*	*Tamarindus indica*	
Tansy	*Tanceto*	*Chrysanthemum vulgare* syn. *Tanacetum vulgare*	*Tanse, Ponso*
Texas Croton	*Barbasco*	*Croton texensis, Croton corymbulosus;* also *Discorea densiflora, Discorea floribunda*	*Pionillo, Palillo,* Dove Weed
Tolu Balsam	*Bálsamo*	*Myroxylon balsamum* var. *Pereirae, Myroxylon* spp.	*Bálsamo de las Indias, Bálsamo Negro del Perú, Bálsamo de Cartagena*
Treadsoftly	*Mala Mujer*	*Croton ciliato-glandulosus*	Scented Croton, *Yerba de la Cruz*
Trumpet Bush	*Tronadora*	*Tecoma stans* syn. *Stenolobium stans*	*Retama, Flor de San Pedro, Flor Amarillo, Palo de Arco,* Yellow Elder
Uva Ursi	*Pingüica*	*Arctostaphylos uva ursi, Arctostaphylos manzanita, Arctostaphylos pungens*	*Manzana, Manzanita, Corallino, Coralillo,* Bearberry
Various chiles	*Chile*	*Capsicum*	*Tlachili, Chiltecpin, Max-ic*
Vegetable Pear	*Chayote*	*Sechium edule*	*Choyotl*
Vervain	*Verbena*	*Verbena canadensis, Verbena carolina, Verbena officinalis, Verbena* spp.	*Dormilón, Moradilla*
Walnut Tree	*Nogal*	*Juglans regia, Juglans mexicana, Juglans major*	
Watercress	*Berro*	*Nasturtium officinale* syn. *Rorippa nasturtium-aquaticum*	
Western Coltsfoot	*Tusilago*	*Petasites palmatus*	
Whistle Tree	*Colorín*	*Erythrina americana, Erythrina flabelliformis*	*Pito, Chilicote, Zompantil,* Coralbean
White Horehound	*Marrubio*	*Marrubium vulgare*	*Manrubio, Mastranso*
White Sapote	*Zapote Blanco*	*Casimiroa edulis*	*Matasano Sapote, Sapotilla, Chapote, Zapote Dormilón*
White Willow	*Sáuz*	*Salix bonplandiana, Salix goodingii, Salix taxifolia, Salix* spp.	*Sáuce, Jarita, Taray, Ahuejote, Negrito*
Wild Cherry	*Capulín*	*Prunus serotina, Prunus capuli, Prunus virginiana*	Black Cherry
Willow Groundsel	*Jarilla*	*Senecio salignus* syn. *Barkleyanthus salicifolius, Senecio flaccidus*	*Yerba del Caballo, Veneno de los Perros, Consueldo, Chilca Atzóyatl*

English Name	Spanish Name	Botanical Name	Other Names
Wormseed	*Epazote del Zorillo*	*Chenopodium graveolens, Chenopodium foetidum* syn. *Teloxys graveolens*	*Yerba del Zorillo, Yerba del Perro*
Wormwood	*Ajenjo*	*Artemisia absinthium*	*Artemisia, Yerba Maestra*
Yarrow	*Plumajillo*	*Achillea lanulosa, Achillea millefolium*	*Plumbajillo, Milenrama, Real de Oro, Alcanfor, Yerba de los Carpinteros*
Yellow Dock	*Lengua de Vaca*	*Rumex crispus, Rumex mexicanus, Rumex pulcher*	*Yerba Colorado, Raíz Colorado,* Curly-leaf Dock
Yellow Oleander	*Ayoyote*	*Thevetia thevetioides*	*Yoyote, Narciso Amarillo,* Bee Still Tree, Giant Oleander
Yucca	*Palmilla*	*Yucca schidigera, Yucca valida, Yucca* sp.	*Amole, Datilla, Lechuguilla,* Spanish Dagger

Page numbers in **boldface** refer to main discussions of traditional treatments.
Page numbers in *italics* refer to illustrations.
For specific plant information, see "The Plants" (pp. 65–203) and "Appendix: Herb List" (pp. 349–58).